FEMINIST EVALUATION AND RESEARCH

D0879322

FEMINIST EVALUATION AND RESEARCH
THEORY AND PRACTICE

Edited by

Sharon Brisolara
Denise Seigart
Saumitra SenGupta

THE GUILFORD PRESS
New York   London

© 2014 The Guilford Press
A Division of Guilford Publications, Inc.
72 Spring Street, New York, NY 10012
www.guilford.com

Printed in the United States of America

This book is printed on acid-free paper.

Last digit is print number: 9   8   7   6   5   4   3   2   1

Library of Congress Cataloging-in-Publication Data is available from
the publisher.

ISBN 978-1-4625-1520-2 (Paperback)
ISBN 978-1-4625-1530-1 (Hardcover)

Preface

As program evaluators, we often operate in the liminal space between research and evaluation; the institutions in (or for) which we work often require both research and evaluation skills from their practitioners. We also self-identify as feminists and have been influenced by feminist theory, women's movements, feminist political action, and the feminists we have known. These identities and experiences have motivated us to practice and contribute to the development of feminist evaluation.

The path leading us to take on the project of promoting and further developing feminist evaluation began in the early 1990s. At that time, the Feminist Issues Topical Interest Group of the American Evaluation Association had just begun promoting the integration of feminist theory and research methods into the practice of evaluation. Early on, progressive evaluators like Donna Mertens, Joanne Farley, and Elizabeth Whitmore were instrumental in advancing the work of practitioners with feminist inclinations and calling attention to the strong need for evaluations that were attentive and responsive to gender and women's issues. We owe a huge debt to these visionary leaders for setting the direction that we now follow. This edited volume is the result of many conversations with these visionaries, among ourselves, and with a growing network of feminist evaluators and researchers who have been looking for ways to incorporate feminist approaches in their evaluation practice. It builds upon our earlier publication "Feminist Evaluation: Explorations and Experiences," a special issue of the journal *New Directions for Evaluation* (Seigart & Brisolara, 2002), which was the first substantive collection of feminist articles to be accepted for publication within the evaluation arena (not that others hadn't tried for several years).

We have strived to present some of the extraordinary work that is being done all over the world by feminist evaluators and researchers, including those in countries and communities that do not respond well to the "f" word ("feminist"). We are indebted to each of the authors whose work appears within this text, and we consider ourselves privileged to present this volume to you, the reader. The following is a brief outline of what each of the chapters holds in store for you. Please be mindful that most chapters include an introduction of concepts along with detailed case examples, but all chapters, whether theoretical or more practical, add rich fodder to the evaluation field for discussion and learning.

Part I

In Part I of this volume, we offer chapters that focus on the theory of feminist evaluation and research, some of the early influences of feminist theory on the evaluation field, the differences between evaluation and research, and the role(s) of the feminist evaluator. In Chapter 1, Sharon Brisolara focuses on the development and application of feminist theory within the evaluation field. She identifies common themes and underlying regularities within many feminist theories that researchers and evaluators can and have applied to their work in order to investigate women's and men's experiences more deeply and from a sometimes unexpected vantage point. Discussion includes a description of the distinct contributions that feminist approaches make to the practices and fields of research and evaluation.

In Chapter 2, Sandra Mathison presents a clear differentiation of research and evaluation. There are key differences between research and evaluation, and understanding these differences is important to situating our understanding of how best to design a feminist approach to our work. This chapter sets the framework for subsequent discussions by defining evaluation and research, describing the similarities and elements common to both, and indicating areas of difference, especially those salient to future and current practitioners interested in integrating feminist principles into their work. The chapter begins by providing basic definitions of research and evaluation elements for the reader's benefit and ends with a brief discussion of the range of evaluator and researcher roles, with their possible overlapping concerns.

In Chapter 3, Elizabeth Whitmore explores in detail the frequently raised challenge to feminist approaches to evaluation and research, as well as to other "nontraditional" approaches, a concern over the role of the practitioner. Within these fields, consideration about the practitioner's relationship with research "subjects," involvement in taking action on findings, intention in integrating theory into design, and self-revelation are salient and often central. What roles are appropriate and possible vary by research and evaluation model. Models that work from the intention of contributing to greater social justice share beliefs about professional roles and responsibilities. As social-justice-focused models, feminist research and evaluation draw from and contribute to this textured conversation. Whitmore extends the discussion on researcher roles begun by Mathison and presents current issues in the debate on what constitutes appropriate professional roles for evaluators and researchers. She discusses the ways in which an interest in social justice has led to the development of models and approaches focused on the promotion of social justice within the fields of research and especially of evaluation. Key social-justice-related models are described in conjunction with the implications of the philosophical underpinnings of these models for project selection, design, method, and researcher/evaluator roles. The discussion raises questions for the reader considering or reconsidering his or her beliefs and values with respect to the role they play as researcher or evaluator. The chapter ends with guidelines for determining, articulating, and monitoring one's role within the context of such structured inquiry.

Chapter 4, by Donna M. Mertens, focuses on the transformative promise of evaluation, particularly for women and other oppressed groups. Addressing the philosophical and theoretical stances that provide frameworks for relevant dimensions of diversity within projects that address the needs of women, the transformative paradigm provides a philosophical umbrella for evaluators who are concerned with issues of discrimination and oppression based on a multitude of dimensions of diversity, including gender, race/ethnicity, disability, deafness, socioeconomic status, refugee or immigrant status, and indigenous status and tribal affiliation. A variety of theoretical frames that provide guidance in working in culturally diverse contexts are discussed in order to derive direction for evaluation methods. Implications for ethical methodological decisions are drawn from the philosophical and theoretical stances.

In the last chapter in this section (Chapter 5), Donna Podems reflects on development programs that aim to change the lives of women, the disempowered, and the "poorest of the poor." Within the international development setting it is generally accepted that if an organization, or government, accepts program funds from a donor, a responsibility to conduct a program evaluation is likely to be attached. While every evaluation approach pursues this knowledge laden with its own, often implicit and often Western, values, few come under as heavy criticism as feminist evaluation when discussed in the international development context. This chapter discusses feminist evaluation and its often more politically, socially, and culturally accepted and incorrectly assumed doppelganger—gender approaches—and suggests that with an in-depth understanding of the history, challenges, and benefits of each, these approaches can bring particular value to various international development evaluations.

Part II

In Part II, the reader will find deeply reflective chapters on the application of feminist theory and methods in a variety of contexts. Authored by evaluators and researchers who have worked and are currently working from a feminist standpoint, these chapters present the challenges, opportunities, and results of applying feminist theory and methods in their work.

In Chapter 6, Kathryn Sielbeck-Mathes and Rebecca Selove address the challenges of involving program staff in a feminist evaluation, particularly with regard to utilization of the results. They examine the problem of substance abuse treatment among traumatized women with co-occurring mental health issues from a feminist perspective. This includes a description of the program, the evaluation design, and outcomes, and a brief overview of frame theory. Strategies to help the feminist evaluator frame the evaluation processes and findings in a language that creates resonance rather than resistance are discussed. Sielbeck-Mathes and Selove remind feminist evaluators to stay closely attuned to their core values and to intentionally strive to understand the core values of those in respective evaluation environments. This awareness, they argue, helps evaluators stay firmly rooted in feminist principles while understanding and considering program stakeholders' values, thus fostering better communication of findings, observations, and recommendations. Frames that foster good communication contribute to better connections and motivate action that can bring about social change to improve the lives of vulnerable women.

In Chapter 7, Tristi Nichols discusses the benefits of utilizing ecological inquiry and feminist approaches in the context of international development. Noting that the crux of feminism is gender equality, Nichols points out that commonly utilized approaches (economist lens, social lens), while useful in elucidating the critical components of progressing toward gender equality, nonetheless present challenges when attempting to apply such constructs in the international development context. Namely, measuring and validating constructs at the community level are challenging processes/endeavors that many stakeholders and field practitioners dare not even initiate. Nichols describes how to design, conduct, and interpret findings of evaluations of international development interventions, ensuring that gender inequality and ecological concerns are fully considered. Pertinent questions to ask throughout the process are examined, and examples of what framing the evaluation with stakeholder values looks like add illumination.

Katherine Hay also addresses the challenges of implementing feminist evaluation in Chapter 8, but in the context of evaluations conducted in India. Noting that the practice of evaluating women's empowerment programs or the "gender" component in development has expanded in recent years, Hay examines (1) the contributions of feminist research (and analysis) to international development theory; (2) the value of feminist evaluation for evaluating development discourse, programs, and projects; and (3) ways to engage in, and use, feminist evaluation in international development. In discussing these issues, Hay makes the case that evaluations informed by feminist analysis lead to opportunities to engender or make equitable development discourse, policies, and programs in the international arena.

Silvia Salinas Mulder and Fabiola Amariles describe their work in Latin America in Chapter 9, reflecting on their practice and contemplating the improvement of evaluation through the utilization of feminist approaches. They share experiences and suggestions on how to make feminist evaluation principles operational in the context of Latin American countries and include examples of and tips about what may or may not work in complex multicultural environments. The chapter, as they describe it, is "reality-based" and "solution-oriented," creatively contributing with effective, new, and inspiring ideas.

Part III

The third part of this volume provides the reader with some very practical examples of feminist research less easily categorized as evaluation. Authored by evaluators and researchers who have worked and are currently working from a feminist standpoint, these chapters present the challenges, opportunities, and results of applying feminist theory and methods in their work.

In Chapter 10, Denise Seigart explores the challenges of incorporating feminist research approaches into the examination of school health programs in the United States, Australia, and Canada. While conducting case studies of school-based health care in these countries, it became apparent to her that inequities in the provision of health care exist and are often related to gender inequities. Racism, sexism, and classism due to religious, economic, and cultural influences were all noted, and these all play a part in the quality and accessibility of health care in these countries. Examples of gender inequities in access to health care are presented, as well as reflections on the challenges of implementing a research project from a feminist perspective. Seigart also highlights the potential for fostering community learning through a feminist research approach, in the context of promoting school-based health care.

In Chapter 11, Alessandra Galiè discusses her work in Syria (prior to the current civil war); her study reflects the findings of an assessment of the empowerment of women farmers from three Syrian villages involved in a Participatory Plant Breeding (PPB) program coordinated at the International Centre for Agricultural Research in the Dry Areas. The assessment adopted four indicators of empowerment (recognition of women farmers, distribution of resources, access to opportunities, and decision making) that were monitored over a period of 4 years (2007–2010). The findings show that PPB has the potential to enhance women's recognition as farmers, facilitate their access to relevant varieties of crop and information, increase their access to opportunities, and support their decision making. Galiè also discusses the difficulties and pitfalls of some of the strategies adopted by the program, and suggests possible adjustments. Finally, the chapter discusses the advantages and shortcomings of the application of the chosen methodology and techniques in the sociopolitical culture and technical context of the research and in the framework of feminist evaluation.

Elaine Dietsch (an Australian midwife) continues the discussion in Chapter 12 as she describes how one research project reflects feminist research values and guidelines. A synopsis of "The Experience of Being a Traditional Midwife" study is provided prior to discussion on how it was informed, influenced, and underpinned by feminist research ideology. The feminist values guiding the conceptualization, design, implementation, data collection, analysis, and dissemination of findings from the study are made explicit. The contributions that feminist research values and guidelines made to the study are also explored. The study is undeniably feminist in spirit, intent, and practical outworking, but was not labeled as such in its proposal, implementation, or dissemination; the reasons for these choices are thoughtfully considered. Lessons learned from working within a feminist research framework are shared with the reader.

Final Reflection

In conclusion, Jennifer C. Greene wraps up this text with her own analysis of all the chapters, as well as her own thoughtful contributions to the field of evaluation. Her thorough and insightful reflections illuminate points made by each author, and add depth and breadth to the ongoing discussion that infuses feminist evaluation and the evaluation field. This book is a foray into the questions we all hold regarding the role of evaluation and research in our societies, the methods we use, the role of the evaluator and/or researcher, the values so many of us hold dear, and the effect we have on programs, policies, and people. We hope that our contribution to the discussions will engage you, and spur you to continue the search for ever better ways to improve our world.

REFERENCE

Seigart, D., & Brisolara, S. (Eds.). (2002). Feminist evaluation: Explorations and experiences. *New Directions for Evaluation, 2002*(96), 1–14.

Acknowledgments

We would like to extend our deeply felt appreciation to everyone who has made this book possible, beginning with the women who initiated the idea of feminist evaluation within the American Evaluation Association. Joanne Farley, Donna Mertens, Bessa Whitmore, and others paved the way for our initial volume on feminist evaluation, struggling for years so that the model would be recognized. Their courage, determination, and insight gave birth to feminist evaluation scholarship and today's community of feminist evaluators.

We are also deeply indebted to the authors represented in this volume and the shoulders upon which they stand. There exists a rich literature of feminist research, methodology, and theory drawing from diverse fields; we owe much to the work of these scholars.

Specifically, we would like to thank C. Deborah Laughton of The Guilford Press for nudging us to follow our dream of bringing the work to fruition when we thought that we couldn't possibly take on one more thing. Jennifer Greene has provided us with inspiration, encouragement, and connection to resources throughout the years; we are very grateful for her generosity. Guilford's reviewers, who were originally anonymous, gave their valuable time to offer cogent comments on the first draft of this work and we benefited from their insight. We would like to thank Wanda S. Pillow, Departments of Gender and of Education, Culture and Society, University of Utah; Lacey Sloan, Department of Sociology, Anthropology, and Social Work, College of Staten Island, The City University of New York; and Wendy L. Hicks, Department of Criminal Justice, Loyola University New Orleans.

Finally, we want to thank our families and loved ones, who have listened to our musings, provided support, occasionally taken up the slack left behind as we worked on chapters, and not excessively asked when we would be done. We feel so fortunate to have so many good, true, loving people in our lives.

Contents

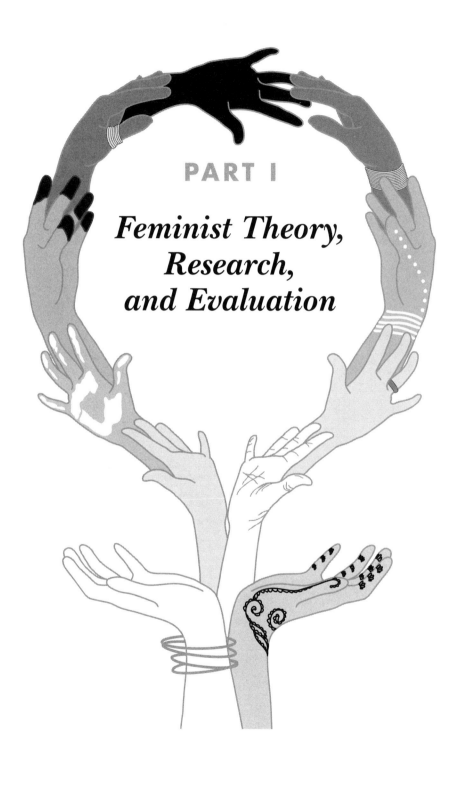

PART I

*Feminist Theory,
Research,
and Evaluation*

CHAPTER 1

Feminist Theory
Its Domains and Applications

Sharon Brisolara

Invitation

If you are new to feminist theory, this book, and this chapter in particular, is an invitation: an invitation to exploring a way of seeing that we believe will shift your worldview in powerful ways. If you have spent years acquainting yourself with the depth and breadth of feminist theory, this chapter may serve as a reorientation to that framework. Regardless of your previous experience, you should know that inquiring about feminist theory is akin to gathering a glass of water from an open fire hydrant, or perhaps a hydroelectric plant spillway. "Feminist theory" is a broad term that describes the application of feminist thought and ideas to a range of disciplines and discourses. Fields as diverse as biology, anthropology, geography, economics, history, literary criticism, sociology, education, theology, and the philosophy of science all have associated feminist theories and have been examined by feminist theorists. In addition, there is a body of work related to feminist research and research methods that has emerged from within particular disciplines but also cuts across disciplinary foci. This introduction presents a brief synopsis of some of the key contributions of diverse feminist theoretical strains. We address some of the primary concerns of feminist research, highlight the key principles on which feminist evaluation is based, and provide an orientation to the work contained within this volume. Think of this chapter, then, as one spoonful of a soup to which many have contributed. If this is your first taste, we hope that you'll drink deeply.

Introduction

As we begin our exploration, let us state from the beginning that there is no one, unifying feminist theory; neither does there exist a consensus on how diverse feminist theoretical contributions should be categorized. There are, however, broad concerns common to a diversity of feminist theories. Most are deeply interested in the nature and consequences of gender inequity. Most forms of feminist theory offer a way of examining and understanding social issues and dynamics that elucidates gender inequities as well as women's interests, concerns, and perspectives. Feminist theories offer critiques of the assumptions, biases, and consequences of androcentric philosophies and practices. Most feminist theories are applied with the intent of contributing to the promotion of greater equity, the establishment of equal rights and opportunities, and the ending of oppression. If you are reading this book, you probably do not have to be convinced of the present need for feminist thought; increasing economic and social disparities within and between nations, the use of rape and sexual violence against women as instruments of war, the continued overrepresentation of women in poverty rates, and persistent legal and political challenges to reproductive rights all speak to the continued need for feminist inquiry and action.

Let us also state that to speak about feminist theory is to allude to a deep and rich literature that has been developed from within and has influenced disciplines as diverse as biology, literary criticism, psychology, journalism, and theology. Even in narrowing our discussion to feminist theory as it informs social science research and program evaluation, we encounter a range of theoretical perspectives and specific contributions to ontology, epistemology, and methodology. Neither this book nor this chapter pretends to offer a comprehensive review of the theoretical underpinnings upon which feminist social science research and feminist evaluation are built. Rather, the reader will find summaries of theories and issues associated with selected key theoretical perspectives and ideas about how feminist theory contributions can be integrated into and strengthen research and evaluation more broadly.[1] The intention of this chapter, together with the remaining chapters in Part I of this volume, is to provide a framework from which feminist research and evaluation practice can be better understood and implemented.

The histories of feminist theory and feminism as an activist social movement are rich, dating at least to the late 18th century in Western nations if measured by the published word. Initially focused on voting rights, Western forms of feminism have developed from an inquiry into patriarchy and the consequences of sexism to a focus on the multiple interconnected structures of oppression that constrain human potential. Feminist thought has drawn from a broad range of studies and discourses, many of which will be discussed briefly in the following sections. In recent years, feminist theory has significantly contributed to the idea that sex and gender are inextricably linked to race, ethnicity, class, sexual identity, age and ability, and that the work of the feminist researcher/evaluator is to understand the dynamics in play at the nexus of these identities from a feminist perspective. Each of the most prominent feminist theories has contributed significantly to what it means to use a feminist perspective within social research and program evaluation.[2]

Prominent Feminist Theories

Any discussion of feminist theory limited to the length of a chapter is, perforce, partial. Moreover, how to best categorize groups of theories and which groups of theories should be included are a matter of debate; that is, experts in feminist theory, like experts in other fields, will differ in their categorization of theories and in terms of which theoretical perspectives they believe to be most salient to a volume like this one. Theories and philosophies, for example, have been categorized by nation of origin (as in German-inspired, French-oriented, Latin American-developed), by philosophical traditions (such as Marxist or postmodern), as related to stages in the Western feminist movement (first wave, second wave, etc.), and by the key issues or concerns addressed by particular theories. Indeed, some have suggested that how to categorize diverse feminist theories and philosophies is a philosophical issue in itself (Braidotti, 2003).

We begin our discussion of feminist theories with an overview of feminist empiricism, followed by broad categories of theoretical traditions commonly cited as being influential within social science research and evaluation. These include standpoint, critical, postmodern/poststructural, global/postcolonial, queer and lesbian, and black feminist, Chicana, indigenous, and race-focused theories. Each of these theories draws from a rich literature, each has had significant influence in multiple fields, and each also has its critics. Summaries of these categories are presented as a point of departure from which the reader can deepen her or his knowledge about feminist research and evaluation and engage in critical dialogues about these issues.

Feminist Social Research Theories

Feminist Empiricism

While not a theory per se, feminist empiricism is a useful point of departure from which to understand other feminist theoretical traditions. By "empiricism," we mean the idea that the only source of knowledge humans can access is that which we experience (and measure) through our senses. As such, feminist empiricism is firmly grounded in positivist ideals and practices such as a striving for objectivity and truth, a belief that the social and natural worlds are knowable and accessible, and a reliance on methodologies established within and sanctioned by mainstream scientific communities. While many other feminist theoretical traditions eschew the core values of positivism, feminist empiricists integrate positivist practices and feminist perspectives in ways that critique the practices and products of the traditional scientific establishment. For feminist empiricists, this effort involves attending to social and political context, including women and their experiences in scientific questioning in order to account for androcentric biases, and paying attention to perspectives and experiences typically ignored or obscured (Leckenby, 2007, pp. 28–34).

Critics of feminist empiricism have claimed that adherents of this framework have adopted an uncritical view of experience. They also charge that feminist empiricists assume that knowledge exists outside or apart from social forces and wrongly believe that science will correct its androcentric biases on its own without feminist theoretical insights (*Stanford Encyclopedia of Philosophy*, 2013). However, feminist empiricists describe more complex positions than those cited by skeptics. In fact, feminist empiricism, as it has developed, has blended political goals and empiricist practices, has critiqued and suggested expansion of positivism in order to allow for a wider embrace of women's experiences, and has promoted the idea that knowledge can best be understood by exploring the role of communities as agents and producers of knowledge (Hundley, 2007; Leckenby, 2007; Longino, 1990).

Standpoint Theories

At the center of standpoint theory is the idea that where we are socially situated (i.e., where we stand) matters and has important implications for social and political power and the creation of knowledge. Put another way, standpoint feminist theory is "an attempt to combine the politics of location with a more specific scientific methodology" (Braidotti, 2003, p. 200). To be sure, there are multiple feminist standpoint theories with somewhat different methodological approaches and varying interests in understanding the nature and scope of knowledge. However, standpoint theory as a body of literature has had a profound influence on the development of feminist theory and methods and is still among the theories in use by feminist researchers and evaluators.

Influenced by the women's political movements of the 1960s and 1970s and the anti-positivist thought that followed, feminist standpoint theory was developed in the late 1970s through the 1980s by philosophers such as Allison Jaggar (1989), sociologist of science Hilary Rose (1987), science historian Donna Haraway (1991), sociologists Dorothy Smith (1974) and Patricia Hill Collins (1990), political philosopher Nancy Hartsock (1983), and philosopher of science Sandra Harding (1983) (also see Harding, 2012; MacKinnon, 1999). Standpoint theories, like many feminist theories, are also deeply indebted to post-Marxist and critical theories particularly regarding their focus on the effects of power on the production and validation of knowledge. Standpoint theorists critiqued not only male-centered and biased theories and approaches but also the objectifying, positivist epistemologies on which they were based. The sociologists noted above recognized the diversity of women's experiences (shaped as they are by culture, race, and class) but focused on the unique gender standpoints that result in differences in how men and women think, and what they think about, and what they regard as important. Given the fact that elements of research (e.g., its methods, categories, assumptions, ways of knowing, writing style) were created and regularly shaped by male discourse, resulting in the silencing of women's experiences and perspectives, these theorists advocated for immersing oneself in the "lived experiences" of women, beginning where they were (Chafetz, 1998).

Feminist standpoint theory can be thought of as having three main claims: that knowledge is socially situated; that the ways in which marginalized groups are socially situated allows people in these groups to be aware of dynamics and ask questions unavailable to others; and that research should begin with the lives of those marginalized for this reason in order to better understand power dynamics (*Internet Encyclopedia of Philosophy*, 2012).

As a result, theorists proposed approaches that would unearth the differences in standpoints by questioning categories and assumptions; gathering claims to knowledge from people through relationships, cooperative interactions, and/or connectedness; seeing through the eyes of women experiencing oppression; and integrating political struggle or action with scientific methods. They not only advocated beginning with women's lived experiences, but also critiqued the possibility of scientific objectivity and the dynamics of power and domination that exist within scientific practice (Braidotti, 2003; Brooks, 2007; *Stanford Encyclopedia of Philosophy*, 2013).

At various stages in the development of standpoint theory, critics have charged that women and women's experiences were being represented as if there was an essential element or condition that constituted "women"; they also charged that some theorists had abandoned traditional standards of objectivity and had embraced relativism, and that they privileged women's experiences. Sandra Harding, in her extensive writings on standpoint theory, has documented the transformation of standpoint theory over the past 30 years, and the persistence of such opposition. She also notes the diversity of standpoint theories and these theories' contributions to the scientific enterprise, particularly in its focus on subjugated understandings that can lead to insights, challenges, and tendencies otherwise difficult to identify (Brooks, 2007; Harding, 1990, 1992, 2012).

Critical Theories, Poststructural Theories, and Postmodern Theories

Another, albeit not cohesive, set of feminist theories are often considered together as critical, poststructural, or postmodern. Gannon and Davies (2012) describe *postmodernism* as having "targeted for demolition the centrality of the individualized human subject, the dominance of rationality as a mode of knowing, and the realist claim that language can describe the real world" (p. 65). In describing this field for feminist researchers and theorists, Gannon and Davies lay out five principles of feminist approaches to postmodernist, poststructuralist, and critical theories. The first is that, given that all perspectives are situated, we must be wary of and must rethink the concept of objectivity. Similarly, attention must be paid to writing/discursive practices through which "versions of the world" are created; reflexive attention to language used, and the implications of this language, are very important from a feminist perspective. A related principle is the need for awareness of how/when/that one adopts binary categories that limit perception, understanding, and imagination and result in exclusions, particularly when categories become tightly associated with one another (such as "male" with "rationality"). Although these theoretical perspectives assume different positions on issues of power and agency, all three hold that power relations are established and maintained through discourse and positions assumed within these discourses and that agency and emancipation are contingent and limited. A final principle summarized by these writers is the importance of being skeptical, of deeply questioning what is assumed to be true or accepted knowledge for all of the reasons stated above (Gannon & Davies, 2012).

Critical Theory

Feminist critical theory draws more directly from neo- and post-Marxist thought than poststructural or postmodern theories. Most often, critical theory within the sociological tradition refers to the Frankfurt school, the Institute for Social Research led by Theodor W. Adorno, Max Horkheimer, Herbert Marcuse, and others. The original project of the Frankfurt school was to explore why Marx's predictions regarding a socialist revolution did not evolve as expected and to understand how Marxism could be relevant given emerging 20th-century capitalism (Agger, 1991; see also York & Mancus, 2009). Moving away from the positivist materialism of Marxist theory, critical theory focused social researchers' attention on the assumptions underlying their understanding of reality and how reality can be known. As such, there was a shift from materialism to idealism, from a focus on labor to a focus on ideology (York & Mancus, 2009).

Critical theorists joined others in a critique of positivism, with its emphasis on prediction and control and cause and effect, as limiting not only the ability to see and understand current social dynamics and social facts, but also to comprehend the possibility of new social configurations or realities. Positivism, then, was seen as another contributor to false consciousness (particularly within capitalist societies) and to the sense that the existing social order was inevitable and rational, not historically contingent or changeable. Critical theorists, particularly in the early stages of critical theory work, focused on issues of domination and exploitation (external as well as internal limitations) (Aggers, 1991; Bronner, 2002; York & Mancus, 2009). Feminist critical theorists such as Benhabib (1986) further examined the existence of domination and exploitation within social structures such as the family and promoted feminist perspectives and approaches as methods for envisioning possibilities for social transformation. Other commonalities among various feminist critical theories is a political commitment to gender equality, a commitment to making gender a focus of analysis, and a methodological commitment to describing the world in ways that have a greater correspondence with women's lived experiences (Rhode, 1990). Critics of feminist critical theory have charged that, despite a focus on social change, no widely accepted method for achieving such change is proposed (Martin, 2002).

Postmodern and Poststructural Theories

Postmodern theories, broadly speaking, are epistemological, philosophical paradigms that also critique positivist research for its claims to be able to predict or understand and for its attempt to present the researcher as separate from the individual or object being "studied." These theories are not exclusively feminist, not easily bounded or categorized, and have had significant influence in a wide swath of fields such as anthropology, literary criticism, sociology, psychology, quantum physics, and theology. The ideas of postmodern and poststructuralism were greatly shaped by Foucault's critique of modernity and humanism in which he made problematic modern forms of social institutions, knowledge, rationality, and subjectivity. These modern forms were then offered as sites and constructs of power and domination (Best & Kellner, 1991). Francois

Lyotard, Jacques Derrida, and others further critiqued the ability of social theory to explain modern existence (modernity) and to contribute to progressive social change (Antonio & Kellner, 1994). Feminist writers such as Judith Butler (1993), Patti Lather (1991), and Nancy Fraser (see Fraser & Nicholson, 1990) integrated a feminist perspective and understanding to postmodern and poststructural theories. Key feminist postmodern theorists noted that postmodernism and feminism were "natural allies." Postmodern thought offered and reinforced new methodological ideas including a skepticism about generalizations, particularly those based on white, Western perspectives (Nicholson, 1990).

Early critics of postmodern feminism warned of a potential slide into relativism; they were concerned about the deconstruction of the category of gender and abandonment of theory. Feminist postmodern advocates responded to this concern by pointing to new opportunities, made possible through this alliance, of more clearly situating concepts and categories within particular historical and cultural contexts and the ability to embrace multiple, rich, and sometimes contradictory aspects of our individual and collective identities (Fraser & Nicholson, 1990; Haraway, 1990).

Global and Postcolonial Theories

Postcolonial theories, which received much attention in the 1990s, are an offshoot of postmodern theories. After writers like Pierre Bourdieu examined colonialism as "a racialized system of domination rooted in coercion" (Go, 2013, p. 56), postcolonial theorists moved from a more Marxist, materialist, economic interpretation to an examination rooted in race and power and a distinction between "Northern" and "Southern" theories, the latter focusing on concerns of those oppressed through colonization. The influence of postcolonial work was felt across disciplines and was sharpened through the work of literary theorists Gayatri Spivak and Edward Said (Said, 1994; Spivak, 1990). While similarly concerned with the role of discourse in shaping reality and constraining possibilities, postcolonial theories offer important insight into the Western bias and assumptions that permeate social theory and social institutions, thereby constraining perceived solutions. Such theories also often focus on the effects of cultural diversity (between as well as within groups) and are interested in sites and strategies of resistance.

There exist a diversity of postcolonial theories and feminist postcolonial theories and there have also been significant challenges to these theories. And yet, "postcolonialism remains a useful conceptual framework for the practice of (radical) critique: its emphasis on resistance, and its historically grounded analysis of continuing social inequalities, make it well equipped to explore and interrogate contemporary myths of unitary nationhood, as well as to examine and combat the legacy of the colonial past" (Huggan, 1993, pp. 62–63). Feminist postcolonial theorists have also contributed to furthering the examination of Western biases within some forms of feminism and/or feminist movements. Feminist postcolonialism has also emphasized how women, women's bodies, and women's spheres of influence can be simultaneously sites of oppression and sites of resistance, and can both inform and be informed by existing social systems (DeCaires, 2010).

In recent years, there has been more scholarship devoted to the dynamics and effects of globalization on feminist theory. Feminist social movements such as ecofeminism illustrate the global nature of not only social action, but attention to the global *situatedness* of policy, political economies and capital, and social institutions. Women from "non-Western" nations have participated in and written about solidarity, resistance, and how to decolonize theory and research practice (Mohanty, 2003; Mohanty, Russo, & Torres, 1991, among others). Feminist scholars have focused on the absence or near absence of women's concerns or feminism in treatments of globalization as well as the assumptions focused on dominant narratives such as of the internationalization of capital and economic restructuring. In *Globalization and Feminist Activism*, M. E. Hawkesworth (2006) describes globalization as an engendered phenomenon pointing to "new modes of gender power and disadvantage" related to the globalization or outsourcing of reproduction (international adoptions), intimacy and companionship (mail-order brides, sex trafficking), and care and concern (e.g., the growth of occupations filled primarily by women including paraprofessionals who move from lower income to wealthier nations to assume child and elder care responsibilities).

Postcolonial feminism, then, arose as the result of the challenges of postcolonial critiques in an attempt to widen the scope of those critiques, examine how gender interacts with other systems of oppression and domination, and attend to the ways in which Western feminist scholarship could homogenize the experience of "third-world women." The contributions of feminist postcolonial approaches have led to a deeper, clearer understanding of the nature of globalization and the multiple ways in which colonization and imperialism have deeply affected the material, psychological, and social experiences of women. Critics of feminist postcolonial thought have charged that such a focus on differences divides the feminist movement, negatively affecting the potential and power of all women. The counterargument to this criticism has been that such differences of experience and perspective cannot be ignored and that such awareness can move feminist theorists and activists to new ways of working *across* differences.

Black Feminist, Chicana, Indigenous, and Race-Based Feminist Theories

Often considered in concert with postcolonial and cultural theorists, and sometimes integrated into discussions of standpoint theory, feminist theories that focus on race, or race and culture, have offered unique contributions to the feminist theoretical literature. Chicana as well as Latin American feminists, black feminists and womanists, and indigenous feminists have played significant roles in refiguring feminist theory's conceptualization of race and racialization (see Anzaldúa, 1987; Chilisa, 2012; Collins, 1990; Garcia, 1997; hooks, 1984). Encounters between more mainstream feminist theory and theories focusing on race and ethnicity have not always been easy. Black and Chicana feminists sought to educate theorists, practitioners, and others to the exclusion of groups of women and the authority that had been ceded to white, Western, middle-class feminist discourse. Together with postcolonial theories, these literatures had an important role in highlighting issues of race, the existence of multiple feminisms, and the deconstruction of the notion of a category ("woman") that could represent a cohesive or coherent whole (Ang, 1995; Bhavani & Coulson, 2003). The work of Patricia Hill Collins (1990) was seminal in promoting the discussion of race within sociology and in focusing attention on the intersections of race, class, sexuality and sex, and nation. Other claims of her work include the role of the experience of oppression in providing new and important insights into reality and the existence of multiple, overlapping systems of oppression. An expanding literature from Latin American writers and the work of Chicana feminists have illuminated the connection between identity, power, and difference and how a lack of attention to these intersections remarginalizes women (Anzaldúa, 1987; Garcia, 1997; Moraga & Anzaldúa, 1981). In addition to these critiques, indigenous feminists have written about the importance of celebrating women's power as expressed through the celebration of motherhood and women's relationships with each other and the utilization of the experience of marginalization as a source of insight (Chilisa, 2012; Fennell, 2009).

Similarly to critics of postcolonial feminist thought, some have expressed concern that too great an emphasis on difference has the potential to further divide and to hinder workers' ability to perceive common goals and characteristics. Proponents of these perspectives have responded that such theories offer critical ways of understanding realities and that it is incumbent upon feminists to learn and implement new ways of fostering solidarity in the new global and diverse contexts in which we find ourselves.

Sex, Sexuality, Queer, and Lesbian Theories

Although various feminist theories took on issues of identity and difference and increasingly embraced methods of recognizing the ways in which race, class, and sex as well as gender are inextricably interlocked, it took the work of lesbian, gay, bisexual, transgender, transsexual, and intersex (LGBTI) scholars and queer theory to illuminate and problematize the uncritical use of sex and gender in many inquiry traditions. Queer theory, in particular, has contributed to the growing awareness of heteronormative language, assumptions, and practices, the artificial categorization of two sexes (Delphy, 2001; Fausto-Sterling, 1993; Hood & Cassaro, 2002), gender as socially constructed (Butler, 1993; Scott, 1986), and the multiple faces of gender oppression and gender-sex identities (see Johnson, 2012). Queer theory within sociology emerged at the end of the 1980s during which time lesbian and gay studies were becoming institutionalized in academic halls; queer theory integrated and expanded on the work of Michel Foucault and feminist poststructuralists in attempting to disrupt this institutionalization and the social control and domination it implied (Green, 2007). Queer theory has since developed in variety and richness with many theoretical stances and contributions subsumed within the larger heading of queer theory.

Like many feminist theories, queer theories see sexual identities and gender as socially constructed and historically situated. Both feminist theories and queer theories work to illuminate the institutionalized and systematic nature of gender discrimination and oppression. Feminist theories had focused on female sexuality and society's focus on reproduction; later, both feminist theorists and queer theorists drew on Foucault's work on sexuality and the idea of bodies and pleasure as sites of "resistance to the apparatus of sexuality" (Chow, 2003; Foucault, 1980; Halperin, 1998, pp. 94–95). Queer theory has pushed feminist theory beyond a focus on the inclusion of female heterosexual and lesbian sexuality and sexual identity to an awareness of the multiple gender, sex, and sexuality exclusions reproduced even within some feminist work. What constitute the key contributions of queer theory to social science research will be viewed differently by different proponents; for our purposes we note a few key elements. The first is an acknowledgment of the critical role of interpretation, in particular of disrupting past events and theories and challenging what is assumed to be "normal." Within this disruption or adjacent to it is an explicit rejection of subjugation in its many forms. Queer theory has also stood for the "primacy of politics over identity" and the importance of engaged, assertive political action in service of social change (Green, 2007; Rudy, 2010). In embracing such politics, queer theorists have taken perhaps the strongest stand on the role of action within research and evaluation.

Critics of queer theory have questioned the usefulness of "queer" as a theoretical perspective, particularly given its integration or cooptation by mainstream forces. Others have been troubled by the loss of a specific focus on lesbian or transgender or transsexual identities. As is true of other action-focused epistemologies, queer theory-informed social science research is also sometimes criticized for being more political than scientific. Advocates of queer theory, however, maintain that one of the "points" of queer theory is to not only resist the confines of particular identifications, not only to "trouble" them, but to show that they are fictitious. Another is to show that what is queer theory, indeed, what is anything, is in a perpetual state of formation, reconstitution, and becoming (Butler, 1993; Jagose, 1996; Johnson, 2012). Jagose, the author of Queer Theory, claims, "The extent to which different theorists have emphasized the unknown potential of queer suggests that its most enabling characteristic may well be its potential for looking forward without anticipating the future. Instead of theorizing queer in terms of its opposition to identity politics, it is more accurate to represent it as ceaselessly interrogating both the preconditions of identity and its effects" (Jagose, 1996).

Feminist Research Challenges

As Table 1.1 makes clear, feminist theories related to research have presented multiple challenges to research practice. While other research approaches have had to respond to these challenges, feminist evaluation and research have made significant contributions to the literature on understanding and engaging in inquiry. These challenges and contributions can be broadly categorized as being epistemological, ontological, and methodological. In the following section, we review a summary of the challenges posed by feminist theorists for research, and how feminist researchers have approached these challenges in their work.

Challenges to Epistemology (the Nature and Scope of Knowledge)

Within each evaluation and research approach is an implicit, if not explicit, understanding of what constitutes social reality and how it can best be "known." Feminist researchers and evaluators claim that our understandings, even when aggregated with those of others, are partial. Knowledge

TABLE 1.1. Key Concepts, Claims, and Theorists

Theories	Key concepts and claims	Selected theorists
Feminist empiricism	• Holds that social and natural worlds are knowable and measureable. • Integrates positivist practices and feminist perspectives. • Critiques scientific practice as insiders. • Argues that androcentric views bias results; value judgments are important in rigorous inquiry.	Sandra Harding Sharyn Clough Helen E. Longino Lynn H. Nelson Richmond Campbell
Standpoint	• Emphasizes the importance of social positioning, situatedness. • Critiques positivism and role of male discourse in shaping research practices and institutions. • Suggests that different standpoints provide unique insights. • Advocates political action with research.	Patricia Hill Collins Donna Haraway Sandra Harding Nancy Hartsock Allison Jaggar Hilary Rose Dorothy Smith
Critical	• Critiques positivism. • Focuses on the existence of power, domination, and exploitation. • Works toward social transformation. • Makes methodological choices that connect descriptions of the world with women's lived experiences.	Seyla Benhabib Judith Butler Patti Lather Catherine MacKinnon Deborah L. Rhode
Postmodern, poststructural	• Presents a critique of positivist research and the separation of researcher from subject/object of study and urges reconsideration of "objectivity." • Requires reflexive attention to language and skepticism. • Critiques the ability of social theory to contribute to social change. • Recommends the deconstruction of modernity, social institutions, and knowledge.	Hélène Cixous Nancy Fraser Donna Haraway Luce Irigaray Linda Nicholson Gayatri C. Spivak
Global and postcolonial	• Examines the role of dominant discourse in shaping reality. • Examines interaction between gender and other systems of oppression. • Investigates Western biases/assumptions and the effects of the colonial past. • Urges awareness of how sites of oppression can also be sites of resistance. • Discusses changing modes of gender power and advantage/disadvantage.	Kum Kum Bhavani M. E. Hawkesworth Maria Mies Chandra Mohanty

(continued)

TABLE 1.1. *(continued)*

Theories	Key concepts and claims	Selected theorists
Race-based, black feminist, Chicana, and indigenous feminist	• Highlights race and issues associated with race; racializes "whiteness." • Understands and celebrates women's power from culturally rooted identities. • Examines the connections among identity, power, race, class, sexuality, and sex. • Offers new way to engage in solidarity.	Ien Ang Gloria E. Anzaldúa Kum Kum Bhavani Bagele Chilisa Patricia Hill Collins Alma M. Garcia bell hooks
Sex, sexuality, lesbian, and queer	• Examines the multifaceted nature of gender and gender oppression. • Raises awareness of hetero-normative assumptions and the artificial nature of binary sex categories. • Advocates the role of assertive/aggressive action and politics in the name of disrupting accepted understandings of what is considered "normal."	Judith Butler Rey Chow Christine Delphy David M. Halperin Annemarie Jagose Jacqueline Scott

is situated; it exists relationally and must be considered within its context. What constitutes knowledge depends on the culture, social milieu, and time in which it is created or shared. Feminist researchers use knowledge to refer to facts as well as shared understandings, both of which have been influenced and shaped by patriarchal paradigms. Recognizing that knowledge shared through and produced by the inquiry is contingent reinforces the feminist researcher's interest in attending to those voices typically silenced or ignored and in accounting for androcentric biases.

Another related critique of masculine epistemology is the privileging of logic and rationality as dominant, authoritative, or exclusive ways of knowing while other forms are largely devalued. Feminist researchers, drawing on work from a range of fields including the philosophy of science, have worked for the validation of multiple sources of knowledge and ways of knowing. Hawkesworth (1989), for example, claimed that "perception, intuition, conceptualization, inference, representation, reflection, imagination, remembrance" are also ways of knowing (p. 551); recent developments in the field of neuroscience have increased scientific understanding of how decisions are made and how situations are understood through these mechanisms. Writers like Hawkesworth advocated for an acknowledgment of these forms of knowing within research and the importance of drawing more specifically from them in structured and unstructured ways. From this perspective, emotions, intuition, and relationships (whether interaction with other human beings, the natural world, or one's own subject matter) serve as legitimate sources of knowledge. Researchers Stanley and Wise stated this point strongly, urging feminist researchers to explicitly utilize the self as data source and instrument much as ethnographers or anthropologists might do (Stanley & Wise, 1989). Their now classic study of their own experience of harassment proved to be a powerful illustration of the possibilities of this approach.

Feminist evaluators have written previously about how Jane Goodall, who worked with chimpanzees, and Barbara McClintock, who worked with grains of maize, both acknowledged the importance of empathy, love, and affection in deepening their understanding of their subject matter and their ability to reach new insights (in Keller, 1985). Feminists have also written about emotions as important sources of knowledge. Rather than viewing emotions as being separate from rationality, Jaggar (1989) has described emotions as "ways in which we engage actively, even construct the world" (pp. 152–153).

In addition to focusing on who is generating the defining questions of science and of scientific studies, what can be considered knowledge, and how knowledge is generated, feminists also raised awareness that science and society have limited who is considered a legitimate source or producer of knowledge. An important aspect of attending to silences was the recognition that the very individuals who were not granted authority to speak or claim or guide discourses were the very ones possessing insight unavailable to others in more privileged positions. Ordinary people, nonscientists, and scientists from different racial, cultural, and socioeconomic backgrounds who possessed ideas shaped by their very different experiences in the world were not "sanctioned" by science as individuals capable of generating knowledge: more typically, they were the ones to be studied so that knowledge could be derived through analysis by researchers who were educated in certain ways and have certain credentials. Some feminist social scientists rejected the idea that anyone, including scientists, could become experts in the lives of others (Stanley & Wise, 1989); some focused specifically on what is lost in such attempts, and others emphasized the importance of individuals' participation in the construction of meaning surrounding issues of significance to them. Feminist sociologists and others have further criticized the tendency to usurp the knowledge of others on ethical grounds and urged a greater emphasis on the needs, interests, concerns, and involvement of the people who are the foci of the studies conducted (Harding, 1992), as well as greater transparency and accountability by researchers.

Challenges to Ontology (the Nature of Being, Reality, or Existence)

Most postpositivists hold that there is no coherent "reality" that can be discovered or predicted; no research methods, no matter how faithfully implemented, will unearth "the truth". Feminist social scientists were among the loudest voices during the 1980s and 1990s, describing science as "a social construct, its inquiries and methods shaped by relations of power, specific historical contexts, dominant ideologies, and the standpoint of the scientist" (Spalter-Roth & Hartman, 1999, p. 336). The theoretical perspectives outlined have been active in critiquing positivism and strict adherence to the scientific method and randomized controlled experiments. And yet feminist researchers have assumed a range of positions on this topic including the use of positivist traditions by some feminist empiricists. As Hesse-Biber (2012) notes, "positivism per se is not the enemy of all feminist inquiry, rather the adversary is how positivist principles of practice are deployed in some mainstream research projects" (2012, pp. 8–9).

Feminist researchers most concerned about positivism have presented cogent critiques of objectivity and offered alternative constructions. As an initial stage of this critique, feminist empiricists attempted to work within traditional social science research paradigms while critiquing misogynist bias as an important obstacle to obtaining objective knowledge (Harding, 1983; Hawkesworth, 1989). As previously noted, some feminist empiricists continue to value the use of more traditionally accepted research methods. For feminist empiricists, objectivity was possible but required removing some key systemic biases. These included promoting more women to important positions within scientific institutions, encouraging a greater number of women to choose careers in science, and ensuring that there were a greater number of studies that focused on women and women's experiences. Later, feminist writers working within the field of international development were quick to point out the inefficacy of what became a simplistic "add women and stir" approach. Such a response, they argued, merely extended the authority of the existing paradigm (Smith, 1972).

Although feminist theorists contend that there is no one "truth" or "reality," it is possible to have conditions or experiences that are similar and somewhat constant within particular contexts. Bringing multiple and diverse perspectives to a social situation in order to raise awareness of these underlying regularities (Harding, 1990) is one of the tasks of feminist inquiry. According to feminist researchers involved with such issues, feminist objectivity criteria include accountability (to those being researched and to feminist values), positioning (acknowledging one's social positions and identities), and a consciousness of the partiality of the limits of research. Truman draws from Harding and others in positing that a feminist objectivity is not neutral, and that it can be achieved through the use of reflexive processes that elucidate some of the assumptions and perspectives partially hidden even to their authors (Bhavani, 1993; Harding, 1992; Truman, 2002). Such a position invites greater participation in research or evaluation dynamics and promotes democratic principles. Illuminating these underlying tendencies and the forces that constrain or promote them is one of the gifts of feminist inquiry and feminist evaluation. Hawkesworth has noted, "In the absence of claims of universal validity, feminist accounts derive their justificatory force from their capacity to illuminate existing social relations, to demonstrate the deficiencies of alternate interpretations, and to debunk opposing views" (1989, p. 557).

Challenges to Methodology

Initial feminist challenges to methodology focused on methods and the strict and seemingly arbitrary division between quantitative methods that were thought to lead to "objective" knowledge and qualitative (as well as other) ways of understanding reality deemed invalid in uncovering reality. Feminist researchers noted that all methods and instruments are inherently fallible, yielding partial answers to our partial, fallible questions. The human instrument is fallible as well and even quantitative instrumentation thought to be objective is, as social scientist Donald Campbell (1978) later said, based on qualitative knowing. Beyond the creation of instruments, the selection of even quantitative measures, data collection, and data analysis are all influenced by human frailties. Indeed, they may be even more profoundly influenced if they are considered to be immune from such biases. With respect to methods, feminist social scientists have often (but not exclusively) advocated for the use of qualitative methods as an important means of unearthing unexamined perspectives, complex dynamics, and silenced voices. They have further advocated the use of mixed methods, using a variety of both quantitative and qualitative methods, within research and evaluation designs. There has similarly been a focus on integrating a multiplicity of methods, values, and even paradigms within other evaluation and research models that have challenged traditional scientific practice (Brisolara, 1998; Green, 2007).

However, there are no methods, even ones implemented with the intention of understanding complexity or based on the development of some form of relationship, that in themselves conform to feminist principles. Even within qualitative interviewing, for example, unequal power relationships between researcher and interviewee exist and it can be difficult to negotiate the waters of representation. Negotiating representation, for example, suggests attending to the inherent dangers and contradictions in deciding how representation occurs, how the narrative and discourses produced are negotiated, and how decisions regarding what is analyzed and published and where findings are published are made (DeVault & Gross, 2012). Such a line of questioning makes clear the need for conscious attention to methodology.

The development of feminist methodology owes much to feminists working within the philosophy of science. A central aim of the philosophy of science is the question of whether or not social sciences or social inquiry can or should mirror the natural sciences in its methodology, a question that necessarily strikes at the core of what is the scientific enterprise (*Internet Encyclopedia of Philosophy*, 2012). Fonow and Cook, pioneers in writing on feminist methodology (see Fonow & Cook, 1991; Harding, 1987), recently described feminist methodology as involving "the description, explanation, and justification of techniques used in feminist research and scholarship" and as being "an abstract classification that refers to a variety of methodological stances, conceptual approaches, and research strategies" (Chakravarty, Cook, & Fonow, 2012, p. 693). These authors further describe feminist methodologies as including perspectives on how to understand social reality, assessments of particular techniques and methods, and the creation of feminist-informed research designs and questions on the multidimensionality of women's lives and gender relationships. As such, feminist methodologies pay close attention to the ethical, policy, and political consequences of the practice of inquiry and strategize research dissemination accordingly.

Volumes have been (or could be) written on any of these topics, including ethical issues and responsibilities to the needs of the stakeholders of feminist research projects given real and implied relationships. In this section, given the emphasis on methodology, we will address one more critical concept: that of multidimensionality or intersectionality of identities and perspectives. Intersectionality has been used to embrace history, encompass and refer to the space where gender relations, physical/personal/sexual characteristics, socioeconomic indications, and cultural/national/transnational identities intersect and overlap. Of particular interest has been an inquiry into the nexus of sex, race, ethnicity, and class (see Bhavani, 1997). Within feminist literature broadly writ, this is sometimes approached as an effort to understand "difference." A more textured understanding of intersectionality involves apprehending not only the intersections where identities cross one another, but the interconnections that are configured with one another (Bhavani & Talcott, 2012). Such a perspective demands active engagement in order to understand an individual holistically, and yet allows for the possibility of further inquiry into additional differences. The concept of intersectionality also helps to illuminate how race, class, and gender are intimately integrated and continually construct each other (Davis, 2008). Because there are no strict guidelines for using intersectionality as a theory or framework, the concept, despite the limitations of its use, "encourages each feminist scholar to engage critically with her own assumptions in the interests of reflexive, critical, and accountable feminist inquiry" (Davis, 2008, p. 79).

In this section we have referred to feminist research in the broadest of terms as research that occurs within a range of disciplines. In the discussion that follows, our focus will be on feminist evaluation, a particular model of evaluation that is used to guide the assessments of and inquiry into programs and projects.

Feminist Evaluation: Concepts, Responses, and Inquiries

Although evaluators have been engaged in work that they considered to be feminist evaluation for some time, it was not until 2002 that a special journal issue was published outlining the basic tenets of this approach to evaluation (Seigart & Brisolara, 2002). A similar proposal for such a volume was made earlier by Elizabeth Whitmore, Donna Mertens, and others; however, reviewer comments made clear that mainstream journals were not yet ready for what was considered a radical approach to evaluation. Seigart and Brisolara built upon that original proposal. The shaping or gathering of the proposed feminist evaluation principles drew strongly from feminist research, imbued as it was with feminist theory. Feminist evaluation, however, was also shaped by and helped to shape emerging evaluation models and approaches seeking to more fully engage and include stakeholders, to give space to underrepresented voices, and to work for social justice. The controversy that these aims sparked was not unanticipated; these approaches did not merely suggest new ways of conducting evaluations. They raised questions about the meaning of utility, the role and responsibilities of the evaluator, and what relationship can or should exist between evaluation and social justice objectives. More broadly, such models challenged historically accepted notions about what can be known, including what constitutes reality and truth, and what are the most ethical and effective ways of understanding a program, its outcomes, and dynamics (Brisolara & Seigart, 2012).

Feminist Evaluation and Other Evaluation Models

As the evaluation field has grown and the need for and use of evaluation has diversified, so too has the array of evaluation models developed. An evaluation model lays out an approach to evaluation typically based on a particular theory of evaluation, often favoring some methodologies over others. Models provide an explicit or implicit perspective on the relationship of the evaluator to stakeholders, the evaluator's role in the project (see Whitmore, Chapter 3, this volume), and use of evaluation findings. Models are born from practice and experience as well as from theoretical developments and are often a response to perceived social and economic needs or dynamics. Evaluation practitioners often become skilled in a range of models and select models based on the social, political, and organizational context of the program they are evaluating and their assessment of which approach would best serve the programs or stakeholders' needs. (In this sense, the term *practitioner* refers to evaluators working primarily in the field rather than as academicians with the resources and particular needs of universities.) As Podems (Chapter 5, this volume) notes, practitioners often draw from more than one model when engaging in their work.

Feminist evaluation shares an affinity with a range of evaluation models and has learned from these models as well. Stakeholder-based evaluation models, for example, urged practitioners to include key stakeholder groups within the evaluation and address key stakeholder values within the evaluation design. Democratic evaluation valued pluralism and a studied recognition of power relationships and accountability to stakeholders (MacDonald & Kushner, 2005). Fourth-generation evaluation, while more of a paradigm than a model, was a groundbreaking work that helped shape the debate about what constitutes reality, validity, and objectivity while proposing alternative concepts and processes for these traditional terms (Guba & Lincoln, 1989). Within the past decade, other more explicitly collaborative models have emerged and gained prominence. One of the most influential has been participatory evaluation (e.g., Weiss & Greene, 1992; Whitmore, 1998), which calls for the involvement of key stakeholders, including those historically considered the "subjects" of the evaluation, in all (or most) elements of the evaluation: design, data collection, analysis, and reporting. Empowerment evaluation (Fetterman, 2000) contributes a focus on participant empowerment through the evaluation process. Emancipatory and critical action research (McTaggert, 1991; Noffke & Somekh, 2005), and the use of multiple theoretical lenses from marginalized communities/perspectives, were among other precursors to transformative evaluation (Mertens, 2009). Transformative evaluation provides guidance in designing and implementing evaluation (and research) that promote social justice aims. (See Mertens, Chapter 4, this volume, for a discussion on applying a transformative feminist stance.) Recently, Michael Quinn Patton's (2010) developmental evaluation has contributed new understandings about how to work with social innovators by applying complexity concepts (such as nonlinearity, emergence, and dynamic adaptations) to improve innovation and evaluation use.

While practitioners are able to combine models and perspectives and some other models focus on social justice aims, feminist evaluation makes a unique contribution to the evaluation field. First, it offers an approach that begins with an acknowledgment and examination of the structural nature of inequities beginning with gender as a point of departure. Second, it offers guidance in examining multiple identities that cannot be abstracted or reduced to only sex, race, class, or ability. Feminist evaluation advocates active engagement in social action, although how one defines "active engagement" varies by practitioner and feminist perspective. It draws from rich and engaged philosophical, methodological, and epistemological literature. Furthermore, feminist evaluation responds to a significant need in this particular historical period. One need look no farther than the use of rape as an instrument of war in the Congo, India, Bosnia, and Sudan; continued female genital mutilation; and the divisive discourse around reproductive health care in contemporary U.S. political discussions to gain a sense of how using a feminist lens might contribute to our understanding of and approach to solving these issues.

Key Feminist Evaluation Principles

In our 2002 volume, we proposed six principles of evaluation. These principles constitute the frame on which the feminist evaluation canvas is stretched. They are drawn from the feminist theories described in this chapter as well as from previously conducted feminist research. Each principle is related to a vision of the nature of knowledge, the nature of social reality and inquiry, and the nature of social justice and knowledge creation. To conduct a feminist evaluation means to integrate a response to these concepts within one's work.

In this chapter, eight feminist evaluation principles are described; these principles serve as a guide to methodological decisions and approaches. Other chapters in this volume provide insight into implementing a feminist evaluation in particular contexts with particular challenges. In this section, the principles and perspectives that guide decisions are briefly discussed along with some of the related questions the feminist evaluator may bring to bear on her or his work.

Concepts Related to the Nature of Knowledge

The first feminist evaluation concept related to knowledge and knowledge creation is:

1. Knowledge is culturally, socially, and temporally contingent.

Knowledge is deeply connected to a particular time, place, and social context and it is incumbent upon feminist evaluators to recognize the "situatedness" of this knowledge. This concept limits the evaluator's claims to generalizability and increases the evaluator's attendance to the specific social context in order to better understand the factors shaping actors, relationships, and situations. Contextualizing the program requires investigating and describing relevant social, cultural, economic, power, and identity issues and asking questions from these points of departure, recognizing that such questions may bring to light previously unseen conditions or dynamics that affect the program's (or participants') outcomes or possibilities.

Feminist evaluation holds that everyone engaging in the evaluation context possesses contingent and partial knowledge and all such knowledge is filtered through the knower. One's historical realities, identities, and experiences shape what one sees and doesn't see. To put it another way, stakeholders, participants, and evaluators all possess contingent knowledge, and therefore it is critical that these diverse perspectives contribute to the design of the evaluation (the questions guiding the evaluation, selection of appropriate methods, and interpretation of results) in meaningful ways. More will be said about this participation later.

Similarly, because knowledge is filtered through the knower, it is important that the identities and commitments of the feminist evaluator be made known to others involved in the evaluation and be evident in written accounts. As Harding (2012) suggests, the practitioner should not consider such attempts at transparency (or "confessions") to be sufficient information for a reader seeking indications of bias or for a researcher interested in making balances of power more equitable; neither should it constitute the end of reflexive efforts. And yet, it is an important step toward these ends and so feminist evaluation encourages active engagement in honest self-reflection and disclosure.

The second feminist principle related to knowledge states that:

2. Knowledge is a powerful resource that serves an explicit or implicit purpose.

Feminist evaluators hold that, within an evaluation project, evaluators interact with knowledge that is owned and created by stakeholders and participants. Further, the evaluator role is to help facilitate the articulation of knowledge that emerges from the evaluation. Those in control of gathering and disseminating knowledge usually decide whether or not knowledge is recognized as a resource of and for the people who create, hold, and share that knowledge. Evaluators also largely determine how that knowledge is utilized. A feminist evaluation perspective acknowledges that those collecting data are in a position of power with the ability of sharing (or not sharing) what is learned, for giving credit (or not) to those who have shared information or knowledge, and for guiding what is to be done with knowledge unearthed. With that power comes responsibilities that feminist evaluators believe should be rooted in relationships.

Knowledge is considered a resource in part because it will serve those who acknowledge its presence. It will serve a purpose, whether that be personal edification and clarity, policy development, program improvement, or political action. Typically, knowledge serves both implicit and explicit purposes. An ethical stance attempts to make initial intended purposes and possible uses that emerge through inquiry known to all who might be affected by the evaluation. Feminist evaluation principles also suggest that evaluators engage with participants to discover and articulate the important uses to which evaluation findings should be dedicated (see Table 1.2).

Concepts Related to the Nature of Inquiry

Program evaluation usually involves an investigation into the nature and dynamics of a program, and evaluation models provide guidance into how one engages in inquiry within the program setting, the methods one uses, and what are legitimate subjects of inquiry. Feminist evaluation begins with the following understanding:

> 3. Evaluation is a political activity; evaluators' personal experiences, perspectives, and characteristics come from and lead to a particular political stance.

No one is value-free; the human beings involved in some capacity within evaluations have political perspectives, positions, interests, and commitments that shape their actions. The contexts in which evaluations operate (programs, organizations, communities interactions) are politicized and imbued with asymmetrical power relationships. Relationships of power influence which programs are acceptable and funded; who has authority to make decisions within organizations (or other contexts) are constrained not only by bureaucratic structures, but also by political realities. Evaluation, as an enterprise, is also a political activity; the types of evaluation sanctioned, partnerships developed through evaluation, what is learned, how it is learned, what is shared, and the interaction between governance and evaluation are all political in nature (Chelimnsky, 1987; see also Taylor & Balloch, 2005; Weiss, 1987).

Not only are human beings political, but so too are methods of inquiry themselves imbued with biases, reflecting the dominant ideologies within which they were created. As feminist theory critiqued positivist and mainstream theories for its sex-, class-, gender-, and race-biased assumptions, feminist evaluation reminds us that methods of inquiry are

TABLE 1.2. Feminist Evaluation Positions on Feminist Concepts Related to the Nature of Knowledge and Associated Questions

Concepts	Positions	Questions
Knowledge is culturally, socially, and temporally contingent.	• Feminist evaluation contextualizes programs and findings in their social, cultural, economic, and historical contexts and asks questions that reflect these understandings. • Feminist principles encourage evaluators to make their own identities and interests in the program clear and known. • Involvement and participation by a range of stakeholders in the evaluation, including program participants, is important to widening understanding of program realities.	• What are the prevalent social issues and cultural values of various stakeholders? • How do current understandings differ from understandings from the recent past? • Considering various stakeholders, what is needed in order to recognize and elicit meaningful and credible results in this context? • What forms of communicating findings would participants find most credible or appropriate?
Knowledge is a powerful resource that serves an explicit or implicit purpose.	Feminist evaluators make initial intended purposes and possible uses that emerge through inquiry known to all who might be affected by the evaluation and engage with participants to discover and articulate the other important uses of findings.	• Who/what gatekeepers to sources of knowledge exist? • In what ways are the types of knowledge of interest already utilized by stakeholders? • What are the consequences of sharing/not sharing what is learned? • For whom are we producing "knowledge" and for what purposes?

not sacrosanct social facts to which we must adjust. Put another way, feminist evaluation proposes the following guideline:

> 4. Research methods, institutions, and practices are social constructs.

As social constructs, research and evaluation methods, institutions, and practices have been influenced by dominant ideologies, including patriarchy. They are a product of their culture and time as well as the theories, academic traditions, and perspectives of those responsible for creation of particular methods. Even the most quantitative of psychometric scales rely on theories and assumptions about which indicators to use and what constitutes a condition—depression, for example. An often-used example of the affect of changing norms on diagnosis of mental illness is the "mad woman in the attic," the practice of isolating or institutionalizing women exhibiting what might now be described as hysteria or depression.

Evaluation models also take a position on how one comes to know what is learned through inquiry. Beyond methods, inquiry is concerned with what constitutes legitimate forms, such as rationality, of acquiring knowledge. Our fifth principle states that:

5. There are multiple ways of knowing.

Feminist theory suggests that particular ways of knowing, such as logic, are privileged over others by those with the power to sanction or privilege certain ways of knowing. This privileging is so engrained within Western culture that the initial questioning of why and if this should be the case was a radical idea indeed. Feminist evaluation urges evaluators to employ a variety of ways of knowing, using intuition, emotions, and love as legitimate sources of insight into problems or program dynamics (see Table 1.3). Such a position does not excuse an evaluator from rigorous implementation of methods or faithful following of the research design. It does, however, acknowledge that there are sources of insight that are not rationally obtained. Recent developments in the field of neuroscience have vindicated this principle by demonstrating that "split-second" decision making often occurs as the result of a rapid review of previous experiences and knowledge processed in such a way that subjects report not knowing how they decided or how they knew what they knew.

Concepts Related to Social Justice

One might assume that feminist evaluation would concentrate exclusively on women. Many feminist evaluators do orient their work toward women's lived experiences and the disparity in outcomes that women face related to their sex; for many others, however, a recognition of the multiple identities inherent in any individual and the deconstruction of binary (male–female) sexual categories has resulted in a more appropriate focus on gender inequities. In recent years, women's studies programs located within Western universities have reflected this concern, including courses on sexual identity and on multiple forms of oppression. So, too, feminist evaluation acknowledges that inequity based on gender and sexual identity is ubiquitous, a powerful manifestation of oppression, but not the only and sometimes not the most salient source of oppression. As a result, an important principle of feminist evaluation states that:

TABLE 1.3. Feminist Evaluation Positions on Feminist Concepts Related to the Nature of Inquiry and Associated Questions

Concept	Positions	Questions
Evaluation is a political activity; evaluators' personal experiences, perspectives, and characteristics come from and lead to a particular political stance.	Feminist evaluation approaches a project seeking to understand the political nature of the context from the very beginning of the project through reflexive processes, engagement with stakeholders, open-ended inquiry, and establishing trust among research participants.	• Whose voices are ostracized or limited in this context? • What power issues exist among stakeholders? • To what extent do power differences need to be addressed in order to allow for fuller participation? • To what extent can power imbalances safely and ethically be acknowledged? • To what extent is a feminist evaluation possible? • What personal political stances might interfere with an ability to see or represent project politics and what steps can be taken to mitigate this effect?
Research methods, institutions, and practices are social constructs.	• Methods are not value-neutral. • Through mixing methods, thinking critically about how to give space to silences, and using inclusive approaches, evaluators can work to counteract the influence of limiting ideologies.	• What procedures and stances do we introduce to ensure that we are making the best effort to understand program context and dynamics? • Who is asking the questions and from what position? • Whose voices or what perspectives are potentially excluded or diminished using the methods proposed?
There are multiple ways of knowing.	Feminist evaluation honors and searches for multiple ways of knowing, in part through deep and real engagement of a range of stakeholders.	• What ways of knowing are valued in this (cultural, social) context (e.g., stories, emotions, artistic representations)? • Do these ways of knowing vary by stakeholder/participant group? • Which forms of knowledge have the highest credibility (and does this depend on the source of information)?

6. Gender inequities are one manifestation of social injustice. Discrimination cuts across race, class, and culture and is inextricably linked to all three.

The spirit of this principle suggests that an awareness of and attention to gender inequities is a point of departure for more deeply understanding the multiple effects of discrimination and existing power dynamics. Gender, of course, is not a synonym for biological sex; to avoid disciplinary privileging, let us use the World Health Organization's (2013) definition of gender: "the socially constructed roles behavior, activities and attributes that a particular society considers appropriate for men and women." Beginning with examination of gender inequities offers the potential for new perspectives and insights as well as additional possibilities for engagement given that inequities based on sex or sexual identity are still frequently overlooked or underestimated. However, sex is not a facet of personhood that can be abstracted from other important identities including race, ethnicity, class, culture, sexual identity, age, and physical ability. Viewing a program or context using a feminist evaluation lens in the spirit of this principle is to examine gender as interacting with and being mutually constitutive of other key identities.

As a result, men can be the subjects of feminist evaluation as well as being feminist evaluators themselves; Truman's feminist evaluation of a sexual health needs assessment conducted with men is one illustration of how a feminist evaluation lens can be effectively used in powerful ways. In this case, Truman (2002) used such a perspective to expose new insights into the multiple sexual health needs of gay men who were the target population for a community-based organization.

Just as gender is socially constructed, so too is discrimination based on gender. Discrimination, the prejudiced treatment of individuals based on personal characteristics, is not enacted solely by individuals. Discrimination permeates social systems and is embedded within the policies and practices of social institutions. Our seventh principle proposes the following:

7. Discrimination based on gender is systemic and structural.

In other words, discrimination based on gender (like other forms of discrimination) is perpetuated through social norms that shape and restrict possibilities for women through the policies, practices, and structures of social institutions such as educational institutions, the government, the military, the media, the family, religious institutions, and within organizations. Discriminatory practices are so embedded within structures and systems that they are not easily recognized and are often assumed to be part of the "way things are" within a given structure. Using a feminist perspective disrupts these assumptions and seeks a deeper understanding of how power and oppression interact and play out within the unexamined facets of the context at hand.

Issues of action and social justice are often addressed at the end of discussions about a particular model. It is true: evaluation models have become increasingly aware of the importance of ensuring that evaluations are useful and actually utilized. Even more than much applied research, evaluation is commissioned for a particular use, and yet that fact in and of itself does not guarantee use. Patton's (1978) utilization-focused evaluation highlighted this issue for the field and provided support and guidance to those committed to better serving those in need of evaluation as well as simply doing good work with the potential for making a difference. The salience of this issue to the profession is evident in the continued success of Patton's volume, now in its fourth edition. Those interested in utilization often point to the resources of time, money, and energy invested in evaluations, resources otherwise available to program activities, as reasons for making utilization an ethical imperative.

Feminist evaluators take this imperative even further, proposing that:

8. Action and advocacy are considered to be morally and ethically appropriate responses of an engaged feminist evaluator.

Controversies about the appropriate role of an evaluator abound, to be sure, an issue discussed further by Whitmore (Chapter 3, this volume). Taking action to promote social justice while keeping in mind the interests and needs of those whose lives are being studied is the ethical standard for feminist evaluation. To see, and especially to unearth, injustice invokes responsibilities; we see a reflection of this belief in Western law (e.g., mandated reporting laws, sanctions for withholding information). While practitioners of some evaluation models find action and advocacy roles anathema to the evaluation enterprise, feminist evaluators are not alone in embracing, when appropriate, an engaged advocacy position, as previously noted. Indeed, Mertens's contribution to this volume (Chapter 4) contains a detailed description of the transformative evaluation model used in conjunction with a feminist lens. The trust developed within relationships, the interests of stakeholders, and the recognition of power and oppression are all factors leading to a principle of action and advocacy for feminist evaluation.

Action can take many forms, from assuring adequate and strategic dissemination of findings, to taking extra steps to ensure that evaluation findings are reviewed and acknowledged by those with power to make decisions, to engaging in activities aimed at altering the balance of power through political pressure. It is critical, however, that the type and degree of action be appropriate to the individual evaluation context. Just as feminist evaluators perceive an ethical imperative to act on their findings, the consequences of such action will be shouldered by the evaluation's most vulnerable participants. It is important, therefore, that feminist evaluators deeply consider the potential cultural, social, and political consequences of the forms of action or advocacy they choose.

Evaluators, like most researchers, are typically external to the communities or programs that they study. Advocacy, even on behalf of beneficiaries reportedly disenfranchised, can have multiple and not wholly predictable consequences. Consider rural women microenterprise owners who are beneficiaries of a nongovernmental organization that provides them with loans and training. They may be correct in their assessment that the interest rates they are receiving are higher than necessary or that women of color are poorly treated and provided inferior services. And yet the same women may resist advocacy given the limited other opportunities that exist for women in their isolated communities and legitimate fears of being shut out of the program or other community services given the political structure and the fact that a few people make decisions about many services. Feminist evaluation urges evaluators to engage participants in conversations about knowledge that emerges through the evaluation and about their fears and concerns related to advocacy, respecting participants' wishes regarding potential action on findings (see Table 1.4). It can sometimes be difficult to discern where advocacy is most appropriate. For example, women from certain cultures obtain circumcisions for their daughters, regardless of health promotion or other efforts, fearing that they will otherwise be unworthy for marriage. In such cases, should a feminist evaluator explore advocating for the young girls, for those women seeking to change social norms, or for some other related cause? Discerning answers to such questions can be difficult, and should not be approached in isolation or without the deep involvement of participants.

Engaging in Feminist Evaluation and Research: Using a Feminist Lens

The discussions of feminist research and evaluation in this chapter are intended to provide guidance in understanding the theoretical underpinnings of both as well as guidance in beginning to apply feminist principles within social science research practice. This volume contains several detailed examples of feminist evaluation and research projects conducted in a variety of settings and drawing from diverse disciplines. Within each chapter, authors discuss the practical matters they needed to address in

TABLE 1.4. Feminist Evaluation Positions on Feminist Concepts Related to Social Justice and Associated Questions

Concept	Position	Questions
Gender inequities are one manifestation of social injustice. Discrimination cuts across race, class, and culture and is inextricably linked to all three.	Feminist evaluation begins its investigation by examining sex and sexual identity and expands its inquiry to understand how gender interacts with, shapes, and is shaped by other critical identities.	• In what ways are women (men, bisexual, transgendered people, etc.) treated differently within the program and how do their experiences and outcomes differ? • How does viewing participants/stakeholders from the perspective of class illuminate program dynamics? • In what ways do class, race, and gender combine to expand or contract possibilities for participants?
Discrimination based on gender is systemic and structural.	Efforts must be made to uncover policies and practices that lead to discrimination if programs and outcomes are to be more accurately understood. Care must be taken, however, to investigate what the possible repercussions of bringing these dynamics to light might be.	• What structural and gender inequities exist within this context? • What are the personal, social, and political consequences of these inequities? • What are the consequences of bringing systemic and structural inequities to light?
The purpose of knowledge is action.	Advocacy with or for people central to the evaluation, such as facilitating action on evaluation findings, is one of the most important intended outcomes of the evaluation. In order for advocacy to be ethical, the evaluator must discuss possible actions with participants most likely to be affected by advocacy and respect their experiences and concerns.	• What is the appropriate role of the evaluator given the circumstances and potential consequences of advocacy? • What are evaluation participants' most pressing needs for action, according to them? • What is gained and lost by acting? By not acting?

order to successfully complete their project as well as an examination of how to implement a project in keeping with feminist research or evaluation. As we conclude our discussion of feminist theory, I'd like to frame these case studies with some thoughts on approaching our work using a feminist lens.

Feminist theorists and practitioners alike advise adoption of a feminist lens in apprehending the context of inquiry, one's role, and the data gathered; in selecting analytical strategies and articulating interpretations; and in crafting and acting upon findings. But what does that mean? How to develop a feminist lens may be as personal as the way that one builds trust within a research relationship. In part, strategies must be compatible with one's learning style and perhaps even personality to be successful. In this volume alone, the reader will find a variety of examples and suggestions for how to develop and apply a feminist lens in conducting one's work.

However, to use a feminist lens implies several steps that are helpful to consider. Before one is able to cultivate a feminist perspective, one must develop an awareness and recognition of the perspective through which one is currently viewing the world. This is no small matter; it is not necessary to be grounded in psychological literature to know that human beings often live and work without critically examining the internal assumptions, values, norms, and beliefs that shape their actions and interactions. And yet we know what can be gained through attention to hidden and overt dynamics of power and internalized oppression such as Foucault described (1975) and the consequences of unrecognized absorption of racism, sexism, and other forms of discrimination described so eloquently by bell hooks (1984, 1995).

Feminist evaluation and research offer suggestions for becoming aware of one's perspectives, biases, and stances. Reflexivity, for example, is a useful tool. *Reflexivity* can be thought of as actively seeking to be conscious of and to understand the cultural, political, and ideological situatedness of the subjects we study, of those who are audiences for our studies, and of ourselves (Hertz, 1997). It involves a recognition that we assume and bring multiple identities into the evaluation or research context with us as do the people we study and that there are larger forces (e.g., geopolitical conflicts, power inequities, and differences) that affect what we know, have access to understanding, and how we understand. Reflexive processes urge us to deconstruct and understand what shapes who we are and our interactions in the evaluation and research field and to communicate these understandings and struggles through our work. Within feminist research practice, reflexivity has come to mean "analyses of how the production of ethnographic knowledge is shaped by the shifting, contextual, and relational contours of the researcher's social *identity* and her social situatedness or *positionality* (in terms of gender, race, class, sexuality and other axes of social difference), with respect to her subjects" (Nagar & Geiger, 2007, p. 269).

Claims about the usefulness and possibility of the reflexivity have been vigorously contested. And yet, at a fundamental level, the notion of reflexivity combines an invitation to become aware of one's perspective and potential blind sides, as well as to thoughtfully document one's developing perspective. Such an enterprise involves transparency, is sometimes described as a truth-telling that allows others to see possible biases or interests, and assumes that much can be discerned through such processes. Another facet of reflexivity mentioned earlier is the intentional deconstruction or disturbance of written representation of research contexts and people's lives in an effort to reveal biases, challenge assumptions, and highlight what remains unknown. Both transparency and deconstruction, we should note, involve relationship and dialogue. They do not happen in isolation.

There are limits to our ability to know ourselves, certainly, and to perceive the biases in the discourses and forms of representation that we create; furthermore, engaging in reflexive practices does not alter power relationships in the field. Certainly, the idea that the use of standard reflexive practices protects against the most egregious forms of essentialization has received a fair amount of deserved criticism (Stacey, 1991; Wasserfall, 1997). However, feminist researchers and evaluators still often invoke reflective practices that are based in interaction or engagement with (or sometimes relationship with) those conducting research and those who are the subject of inquiry, aware of its limitations. We enter into conversation and listening deeply to each other as well as examining, through interaction and investigation, the processes and structures at play within particular contexts (DeVault, 1999b; Nagar & Geiger, 2007). The practice and intention of reflexivity can contribute both to an understanding of one's own positionality and perspectives as well as a way of problematizing the research context.

Using a feminist lens also implies a knowledge of feminist principles or perhaps of feminist theory. Such knowledge does not require an advanced degree in women's studies; rather, a feminist perspective is informed through the written word (including theory and carefully conducted studies), examined experiences, relationships, and engagement in feminist ideas. There are no particular orthodox feminist treatises to which to ascribe or feminist positions to adopt. In fact, some even contend that one does not have to consider oneself a feminist to use a feminist lens (see Podems, Chapter 5, this volume). And yet adopting a feminist lens requires knowledge of feminist thought and a recognition of the feminist principles one believes to be operating in the world.

With a conscious awareness of this feminist perspective and keeping key principles in mind, applying a feminist lens is facilitated by asking questions informed by that perspective. Some suggest that their feminist perspective informs the way they see the world to such an extent that application of the perspective is a natural, perhaps inevitable, occurrence. However, asking particular types of questions as well as exploring new and unexpected questions are all hallmarks of applying a feminist lens. The tables included in the discussion of feminist evaluation principles pose many classic and useful questions. Broader questions (e.g., Whose voices are not being heard? Which perspectives are being silenced and why?) can be used to orient oneself to the context at hand. More specific questions such as those about knowledge or power (e.g., For whom are we producing "knowledge" and for what purposes? What is the appropriate role of the evaluator given the circumstances and potential consequences of advocacy?) can lead to powerful insights not easily accessible through many other modes of inquiry. Questions informed by a feminist perspective permeate the process of inquiry; they are present in the research or evaluation design; they are reflected in the choice and structure of data collection methods; they shape how accountability and validity are addressed; and they guide interpretation, analysis, writing, and dissemination of results.

At its broadest, using or applying a feminist lens implies a cultivated consciousness of one's perspectives and intention; it also involves examining the research context from the angles suggested by this view. Developing an awareness of one's perspective, of course, is an iterative and continual process formed by experiences and new ideas. It requires, in addition to a degree of vulnerability and honesty, an engagement in the world of ideas, in relationships, and situations. Many researchers and evaluators do not have the luxury of in-depth, sustained engagement sometimes available through an ethnographic or anthropological study; for many researchers and evaluators, engagement implies a presence and degree of commitment to the evaluation or study and the cultivation of authentic relationships. It requires returning again and again to the context of inquiry with the intention of examining key issues and dynamics from multiple angles in an attempt to understand dynamics not readily visible. The involvement of participants in the evaluation/research design, sharing emerging findings with participants and critical, honest outsiders/ colleagues, and ongoing structured self-reflection (including reflection on written accounts) have all been proposed as important strategies for deeper engagement in the evaluation/research setting.

Looking Forward

And so we end this chapter as we began, by offering this volume as an invitation to explore feminist theory and the power and possibility of feminist research and evaluation. We are excited about the ideas that the work within this volume will generate and the potential for expanding the field of feminist ideas.

NOTES

1. Notable among these resources is a recent overview of traditions and current issues related to feminist research, the *Handbook of Feminist Research: Theory and Praxis* (Hesse-Biber, 2012); the most significant work on feminist evaluation prior to this volume is "Feminist Evaluation: Explorations and Experiences" (Seigart & Brisolara, 2002).
2. The differences between research and program evaluation will be discussed in depth in Chapter 2 of this volume. For now, let us distinguish evaluation from research by describing *evaluation* as the application of research methods to a social program or intervention in order to make decisions about its merit or worth and to contribute to its improvement or quality.

REFERENCES

Agger, B. (1991). Critical theory, poststructuralism, postmodernism: Their sociological relevance. *Annual Review of Sociology, 17,* 105–131.

Ang, I. (1995). Other women and post-national feminism. In B. Caine & R. Pringle (Eds.) *Transitions: New Australian feminisms* (pp. 57–73). London: Allen & Unwin.

Antonio, R. J., & Kellner, D. (1994). Postmodern social theory: Contributions and limitations. In D. Dickens & A. Fontana (Eds.), *Postmodernism and social inquiry* (pp. 127–152). New York: Guilford Press.

Anzaldúa, G. (1987). *Borderlands/la frontera: The new mestiza.* San Francisco: Aunt Lute Press.

Best, S., & Kellner, D. (1991). *Postmodern theory: Critical interrogations.* New York: Guilford Press.

Benhabib, S. (1986). *Critique, norm, and utopia: A study of the foundations of critical theory.* New York: Columbia University Press.

Bhavani, K. K. (1993). Tracing the contours: Feminist research and feminist objectivity. *Women's Studies International Forum, 16*(2), 95–104.

Bhavani, K. K. (1997). Women's studies and its intersections with "race," ethnicity and sexuality. In D. Richardson & V. Robinson (Eds.), *Thinking feminist* (pp. 27–48). New York: New York University Press.

Bhavani, K. K., & Coulson, M. (2003). Race. In M. Eagleton (Ed.), *A concise companion to feminist theory* (pp. 73–92). Malden, MA: Blackwell.

Bhavani, K. K., & Talcott, M. (2012). Interconnections and configurations: Toward a global feminist ethnography. In S. N. Hesse-Biber (Ed.), *Handbook of feminist research: Theory and praxis* (2nd ed., pp. 135–153). Los Angeles: Sage.

Braidotti, R. (2003). Feminist philosophies. In M. Eagleton (Ed.), *A concise companion to feminist theory* (pp. 195–214). Malden, MA: Blackwell.

Brisolara, S. (1998). The history of participatory evaluation and current debates in the field. In E. Whitmore (Ed.), Understanding and practicing participatory evaluation. *New Directions for Evaluation, 80*, 25–42.

Brisolara, S., & Seigart, D. (2012). Feminist evaluation research. In S. N. Hesse-Biber (Ed.), *Handbook of feminist research: Theory and praxis* (2nd ed., pp. 135–153). Los Angeles: Sage.

Bronner, S. E. (2002). *Of critical theory and its theorists.* New York: Routledge.

Brooks, A. (2007). Feminist standpoint epistemology: Building knowledge and empowerment through women's lived experience. In *Feminist research practice, a primer* (pp. 53–82). Thousand Oaks, CA: Sage.

Butler, J. (1993). *Bodies that matter: On the discursive limits of "sex."* New York: Routledge.

Campbell, D. T. (1978). Qualitative knowing in action research. In M. Brenner, P. Marsh, & M. Brenner (Eds.), *The social contexts of method* (pp. 184–209). London: Croom Helm.

Chafetz, J. S. (1998). Feminist theory and sociology: Underutilized contributions for mainstream theory. *Annual Review of Sociology, 23*, 97–120.

Chakravarty, D., Cook, J. A., & Fonow, M. M. (2012). Teaching, techniques, and technologies of feminist methodology: Online and on the ground. In S. N. Hesse-Biber (Ed.), *Handbook of feminist research: Theory and praxis* (2nd ed., pp. 693–709). Los Angeles: Sage.

Chelimnsky, E. (1987). The politics of program evaluation. *Society, 25*(1), 24–32.

Chilisa, B. (2012). *Indigenous research methodologies.* Thousand Oaks, CA: Sage.

Chow, R. (2003). Sexuality. In M. Eagleton (Ed.), *A concise companion to feminist theory* (pp. 93–110). Malden, MA: Blackwell.

Collins, P. H. (1990). *Black feminist thought: Knowledge, consciousness and the politics of empowerment.* New York: Routledge.

Davis, K. (2008). Intersectionality as buzzword: A sociology of science perspective on what makes a feminist theory successful. *Feminist Theory, 9*(1), 67–85.

DeCaires, D. N. (2010). Mapping a return to feminist solidarity (or "diving into the wreck" again). *Feminist Theory, 11*(1), 95–104.

Delphy, C. (2001). Rethinking sex and gender. In M. Evans (Ed.), *Feminism: Critical concepts in literary and cultural studies.* New York: Routledge & Kegan Paul.

DeVault, M. L. (1999a). *Liberating method: Feminism and social research.* Philadelphia: Temple University Press.

DeVault, M. L. (1999b). Talking and listening from women's standpoint: Feminist strategies for interviewing and analysis. In *Liberating method: Feminism and social research* (pp. 59–83). Philadelphia: Temple University Press.

DeVault, M. L., & Gross, G. (2012). Feminist qualitative interviewing: Experience, talk and knowing. In S. N. Hesse-Biber (Ed.), *Handbook of feminist research: Theory and praxis* (2nd ed., pp. 206–236). Los Angeles: Sage.

Fausto-Sterling, A. (1993). The five-sexes: Why male and female are not enough. *Life Sciences, 33*(2), 20–25.

Fennell, S. (2009). *Decentralizing hegemonic gender theory: The implications for educational research* (RECOUP Working Paper No. 21). Cambridge, UK: Cambridge University, Development Studies and Faculty of Education.

Fetterman, D. (2000). *Foundations of empowerment evaluation: Step by step.* Thousand Oaks, CA: Sage.

Fonow, M. M., & Cook, J. (1991). *Beyond methodology: Feminist scholarship as lived research.* Bloomington: Indiana University Press.

Foucault, M. (1975). *Discipline and punish: The birth of the prison.* Paris: Gallimard.

Foucault, M. (1980). *The history of sexuality: Vol. I. An introduction* (R. Hurley, Trans.). New York: Vintage.

Fraser, N., & Nicholson, L. J. (1990). Social criticism without philosophy: An encounter between feminism and postmodernism. In L. J. Nicholson (Ed.), *Feminism/postmodernism* (pp. 19–38). New York: Routledge.

Gannon, S., & Davies, B. (2012). Postmodern, post-structural, and critical theories. In S. N. Hesse-Biber (Ed.), *Handbook of feminist research: Theory and praxis* (2nd ed., pp. 65–91). Los Angeles: Sage.

Garcia, A. M. (1997). *Chicana feminist thought: The basic historical writings* (Vol. 1). New York: Routledge.

Go, J. (2013). Colonial and postcolonial theory in Pierre Bourdieu's early work. *Sociological Theory, 31*(1), 49–74.

Green, A. (2007). Queer theory and sociology: Locating the subject and self in sexuality studies. *Sociological Theory, 25*(1), 26–45.

Guba, E. G., & Lincoln, Y. S. (1989). *Fourth-generation evaluation.* Newbury Park, CA: Sage.

Halperin, D. (1998). Forgetting Foucault: Acts, identities, and the history of sexuality. *Representations, 63*, 93–120.

Haraway, D. (1990). A manifesto for cyborgs: Science, technology, and socialist feminism in the 1980s. In L. J. Nicholson (Ed.), *Feminism/postmodernism* (pp. 190–233). New York: Routledge.

Haraway, D. (1991). Situated knowledges. In *Simians, cyborgs, and women* (pp. 183–201). New York: Routledge.

Harding, S. (1983). Why has the sex/gender system become visible only now? In S. Harding & M. Hintikka (Eds.), *Discovering reality: Feminist perspectives on epistemology, metaphysics, methodology, and philosophy of science* (pp. 311–325). Dordrecht, The Netherlands: Reidel.

Harding, S. (1987). *Feminism and methodology: Social science issues.* Bloomington: Indiana University Press.

Harding, S. (1990). Feminism, science and the anti-Enlightenment critiques. In L. J. Nicholson (Ed.), *Feminism/postmodernism.* New York: Routledge.

Harding, S. (1992). Re-thinking standpoint epistemology: What is "strong objectivity." *Centennial Review, 36*(3), 437–470.

Harding, S. (2012). Feminist standpoint. In S. N. Hesse-Biber (Ed.), *Handbook of feminist research: Theory and praxis* (2nd ed., pp. 46–64). Los Angeles: Sage.

Hartsock, N. (1983). The feminist standpoint: Developing a ground for a specifically feminist historical materialism. In S. Harding & M. Hintikka (Eds.),

Discovering reality: Feminist perspectives on epistemology, metaphysics, methodology, and philosophy of science (pp. 283–310). Dordrecht, The Netherlands: Reidel.

Hawkesworth, M. E. (1989). Knowers, knowing, known: Feminist theory and the claims of truth. *Signs: Journal of Women in Culture and Society, 14*(31), 533–559.

Hawkesworth, M. E. (2006). *Globalization and feminist activism.* Lanham, MD: Rowman & Littlefield.

Hertz, R. (1997). Introduction: Reflexivity and voice. In R. Hertz (Ed.), *Reflexivity and voice* (pp. vii–xvii). Thousand Oaks, CA: Sage.

Hesse-Biber, S. N. (Ed.). (2012). *Handbook of feminist research: Theory and praxis* (2nd ed.). Los Angeles: Sage.

Hood, D. W., & Cassaro, D. A. (2002, Winter). Feminist evaluation and the inclusion of difference. In D. Seigart & S. Brisolara (Eds.), Feminist evaluation: Explorations and experiences. *New Directions for Evaluation, 2002*(96), 27–40.

hooks, b. (1984). *Feminist theory: From margin to center.* Boston: South End Press.

hooks, b. (1995). *Killing rage: Ending racism.* New York: Holt.

Huggan, G. (1993). *The post-colonial exotic: Marketing the margins.* New York: Routledge.

Hundley, C. (2007). Feminist empiricism. In S. N. Hesse-Biber (Ed.), *Handbook of feminist research: Theory and praxis* (2nd ed., pp. 28–45). Thousand Oaks, CA: Sage.

Internet encyclopedia of philosophy: A peer reviewed academic resource. (2012). Feminist standpoint theory.

Jaggar, A. (1989). Love and knowledge: Emotion in feminist epistemology. In A. Jaggar & S. Bordo (Eds.), *Gender, body, knowledge* (pp. 145–169). New Brunswick, NJ: Rutgers University Press.

Jagose, A. (1996). Excerpt from queer theory. *Australian Humanities Review.* Retrieved July 24, 2013, from *www.australianhumanitiesreview.org/archive/Issue-Dec-1996/jagose.html.*

Johnson, K. (2012). Transgender, transsexualism, and the queering of gender identities. In S. N. Hesse-Biber (Ed.), *Handbook of feminist research: Theory and praxis* (2nd ed., pp. 606–626). Thousand Oaks, CA: Sage.

Keller, E. F. (1985). *Reflections on gender and science.* New Haven, CT: Yale University Press.

Lather, P. (1991). *Getting smart: Feminist research and pedagogy with/in the postmodern.* New York: Routledge.

Leckenby, D. (2007). Feminist empiricism: Challenging gender bias and "Setting the record straight." In S. Hesse-Biber & P. L. Leavy (Eds.), *Feminist research practice, a primer* (pp. 27–52). Thousand Oaks, CA: Sage.

Longino, H. E. (1990). *Science as social knowledge.* Princeton, NJ: Princeton University Press.

MacDonald, B., & Kushner, S. (2005). Democratic evaluation. In S. Mathison (Ed.), *Encyclopedia of evaluation* (pp. 109–113). Thousand Oaks, CA: Sage.

MacKinnon, C. (1999). *Toward a feminist theory of state.* Cambridge, MA: Harvard University Press.

Martin, J. (2002). *Feminist theory and critical theories: Unexplored synergies* (Research Paper No. 1758). Stanford, CA: Stanford Graduate School of Business.

McTaggert, R. (1991). *Action research: A short modern history.* Geelong, Victoria, Australia: Deakin University Press.

Mertens, D. (2009). *Transformative research and evaluation.* New York: Guilford Press.

Mohanty, C. T. (2003). *Feminism without borders: Decolonizing theory, practicing solidarity.* Durham, NC: Duke University Press.

Mohanty, C. T., Russo, A., & Torres, L. (1991). *Third-world women and the politics of feminism.* Bloomington: Indiana University Press.

Moraga, C., & Anzaldúa, G. (Eds.). (1981). *This bridge called my back: Writings by radical women of color.* Watertown, MA: Persephone Press.

Nagar, R., & Geiger, S. (2007). Reflexivity and positionality in feminist fieldwork revisited. Revised final draft of the published chapter. In A. Tickell, E. Sheppard, J. Peck, & T. Barnes (Eds.), *Politics and practice in economic geography* (pp. 267–278). London: Sage.

Nelson, L. H. (1990). *Who knows: From Quine to a feminist empiricism.* Philadelphia: Temple University Press.

Nicholson, L. J. (1990). Introduction. In L. Nicholson (Ed.), *Feminism/postmodernism* (pp. 1–18). New York: Routledge.

Noffke, S. E., & Somekh, B. (2005). Action research. In B. Somekh & C. Lewin (Eds.), *Research methods in the social sciences* (pp. 89–96). London: Sage.

Patton, M. Q. (1978). *Utilization-focused evaluation.* St. Paul, MN: Sage.

Patton, M. Q. (2010). *Developmental evaluation: Applying complexity concepts to enhance innovation and use.* New York: Guilford Press.

Rhode, D. L. (1990). Feminist critical theories. *Stanford Law Review, 42*(3), 617–638.

Rose, H. (1987). Hand, basin, and heart: A feminist epistemology for the natural sciences. In S. Harding & J. E. O'Barr (Eds.), *Sex and scientific inquiry.* Chicago: University of Chicago Press.

Rudy, K. (2010). Queer theory and feminism. *Women's studies: An Inter-disciplinary Journal, 16*(32), 195–216.

Said, E. (1994). *Culture and imperialism.* New York: Routledge.

Scott, J. (1986). Gender: A useful category of historical analysis. *American Historical Review, 91*(5), 1053–1075.

Seigart, D., & Brisolara, S. (Eds.). (2002). Feminist evaluation: Explorations and experiences. *New Directions for Evaluation, 2002*(96), 1–114.

Smith, D. E. (1972, June). Presentation for the meeting of the American Academy for the Advancement of Science (Pacific Division), Eugene, OR, June 1972, p. 93.

Smith, D. E. (1974). Women's perspective as a radical critique of sociology. *Sociological Inquiry, 44,* 7–13.

Spalter-Roth, R., & Hartman, H. (1999). Small happiness: The feminist struggle to integrate social research with social activism. In S. Hesse-Biber et al. (Eds.), *Feminist approaches to theory and methodology: An interdisciplinary reader* (pp. 333–347). New York: Oxford University Press.

Spivak, G. (1990). *The post-colonial critic: Interviews, strategies, dialogues* (S. Harasym, Ed.). New York: Routledge.

Stacey, J. (1991). Can there be a feminist ethnography? In S. Berger Gluck & D. Patai (Eds.), *Women's words: The feminist practice of oral history* (pp. 111–120). New York: Routledge.

Stanford Encyclopedia of Philosophy. Retrieved July 25, 2013, from *plato.stanford.edu/entries/feminism-epistemology/#empiricism*.

Stanley, L., & Wise, S. (1989). "Back into the personal" or: Our attempt to construct "feminist research." In S. Bowles & R. D. Klein (Eds.), *Theories of women's studies* (pp. 192–220). London: Routledge & Kegan Paul.

Taylor, D., & Balloch, S. (Eds.). (2005). *The politics of evaluation: Participation and policy implementation*. Chicago: University of Chicago Press.

Truman, C. (2002). Doing feminist evaluation with men: Achieving objectivity in a sexual health needs assessment. In D. Seigart & S. Brisolara (Eds.), Feminist evaluation: Explorations and experiences. *New Directions for Evaluation, 2002*(96), 71–82.

Wasserfall, R. R. (1997). Reflexivity, feminism, and difference. In R. Hertz (Ed.), *Reflexivity and voice* (pp. 150–168). Newbury Park, CA: Sage.

Weiss, H. B. (1987). Family support and education in early childhood programs. In S. Kagan, D. Powell, B. Weissbourd, & E. Zigler (Eds.), *America's family support programs* (pp. 133–160). New Haven, CT: Yale University Press.

Weiss, H. B., & Greene, J. (1992). An empowerment partnership for family support and education programs and evaluation. *Family and Science Review, 5,* 131–149.

Whitmore, E. (Ed.). (1998). Understanding and practicing participatory evaluation. *New Directions for Evaluation, 1998*(80), 1–99.

World Health Organization. (2013). Retrieved from *who.int*.

York, R., & Mancus, P. (2009). Critical human ecology: Historical materialism and natural laws. *Sociological Theory, 27*(2), 122–149.

CHAPTER 2

Research and Evaluation
Intersections and Divergence

Sandra Mathison

Introduction

Within the discipline and practice of evaluation there is confusion about how precisely research and evaluation are different. Add the adjective "feminist" to both and the confusion may be amplified. This chapter discusses the similarities and differences between research and evaluation generally, and concludes by introducing the core ideas of feminist research and evaluation; the full articulation of feminist evaluation is left to other authors in this book.

Contrasting Research and Evaluation

Offering a definition of *evaluation* as the process and product of making judgments about the value, merit, or worth of an evaluand does little to answer the perennial question: What is the difference between evaluation and research? This question about differences between evaluation and research is fueled by the fact that evaluation as a discipline draws on other disciplines for its foundations, and especially the social sciences for its methods. As evaluation has matured as a discipline and profession this question is sometimes posed to clarify what is distinct about evaluation. This delineation of a profession of evaluation is also tied to a discussion of who is and can be an evaluator. What knowledge and skills does evaluation require, and how does this differ from the knowledge and skills of social science researchers? Scriven suggests evaluators must know how to search for unintended and side effects; how to determine values within different points of view; how to deal with controversial issues and values; and how to synthesize facts and values (Coffman, 2003–2004).

Although there are arguments that evaluation and research, especially applied social science research, are no different, in general, evaluators do claim there is a difference, but that the two are interconnected. Because evaluation requires the investigation of what is, doing evaluation requires doing research. In other words, determining the value, merit, or worth of an evaluand requires some factual, descriptive knowledge about the evaluand and perhaps similar evaluands. But, of course, evaluation requires more than "brute" facts about evaluands (Coffman, 2003–2004). Evaluation also entails the explicit synthesis of facts and values in the determination of merit, worth, or value. *Research*, on the other hand, investigates factual knowledge but may not necessarily involve valuing and therefore need not (although may) include evaluation.

Attempting to provide a clear, unambiguous description of the difference between research and evaluation can too easily rely on dualistic arguments, when indeed most dualisms constrain rather than enable understanding. Making this distinction can be further obfuscated by explaining evaluation–research differences by using other dualisms, such as the all important fact–value dichotomy. One long-standing view on the fact–value distinction, inherited from Humean skepticism, is that values cannot be deduced from facts, that is, we cannot decide what ought to be the case just because we know what is the case. In this version, research is more about establishing the facts and valuing is more about deciding what ought to be the case. Another perspective eschews the notion that value judgments are statements of personal preference and treats both facts and values as interconnected and constitutive of one another, that is, facts don't exist separate from values and vice versa (Putnam, 2002). This view that facts and values are constitutive still does not necessarily imply that knowing the value of an evaluand is the same as knowing what to do about the evaluand. In other words, knowing the value of something (a program or product) doesn't seamlessly entail what we need to do in the future (dis/continue funding the program or buy a product), and so the knowledge about an evaluand differs logically from prescriptions. (See Taylor, 1961, for a thorough discussion of this perspective.) Doing research requires values and value judgments, but it isn't always the case that the primary objective of research is valuing, whereas this is the sine qua non of evaluation.

The similarities and differences between evaluation and research relate often to the purpose of each (that is, the anticipated outcome of doing research or evaluation), the methods of inquiry used, the roles of inquirers, and how one judges the quality of evaluation and research. More often, evaluation is focused on the particular, whether that is a program, policy, or intervention, and research is focused on the general, whether that is a theory, construct, or policy area. Both evaluation and research may lead to decisions and action, although evaluation often does so at a microlevel while research more often has an impact at a macrolevel. Evaluation borrows data collection and analysis strategies from many disciplines including the social sciences, but increasingly the evaluators are developing data collection strategies that emphasize the centrality of stakeholders' values and perspectives. Research, on the other hand, is bound by the methodological traditions within a particular social science discipline (such as anthropology, psychology, or sociology). In both evaluation and research, the inquirer's role ranges from objective outsider to knowledgeable insider and from the detached to the fully engaged. The inquirers' role in both evaluation and research is dependent on epistemological assumptions and the particular skills most central to a particular paradigm. Evaluation is judged by its usefulness, particularly its contribution to improvement, learning, and change, and decision making, while research is judged by its generation of theoretical knowledge.

These attributes of both research and evaluation are further elaborated in the following sections.

Defining Social Science Research

Social science research theory and practice is complex and reflects foundational differences in ontology and epistemology, and so any characterization of research must acknowledge this diversity. Recognizing the differences in epistemology is a good place to start. Research methodologies are connected to three primary theories of knowledge: objectivism, social constructivism, and subjectivism. Crotty (1998) argues that perspectives and research methodologies are aligned with these theories of knowledge (an objectivist theory of knowledge is associated with neopositivism, which favors experimental designs, and a social constructivist theory of knowledge is associated with interpretivism, which favors methodologies like symbolic interactionism). The following sections acknowledge and illustrate these differences, albeit in a sometimes oversimplified way.

Purpose

Research can serve a number of purposes, but most fall into one of three categories: exploration, description, or explanation. Exploratory research may be done for a number of reasons including satisfying one's curiosity, testing the feasibility of a more extensive or intensive study, or testing and developing techniques to be used in subsequent research studies. Exploratory studies are not confined to any particular epistemological paradigm and exploration is useful for neopositivist and interpretive research. Within a neopositivist framework, exploratory research often paves the way for testing the feasibility of scaling up a study or determining a clear research focus. Within an interpretivist paradigm, exploratory research may well be concomitant with the methodology; such is the case, for example, with grounded theory methodology.

Much research is done to describe the current state of some social domain. A good example of descriptive research is population census studies, the purpose of which is to accurately describe characteristics of a population including race, ethnicity, age, gender, household size, and income. Other examples include actuarial studies, most research done by demographers, product use research, and surveillance studies that describe the incidence patterns of human behaviors and conditions (like smoking, obesity, or homelessness). Some interpretive research methodologies are primarily descriptive, including, for example, ethnography and symbolic interactionist research studies. Descriptive studies address the questions of who, what, when, and where.

The third purpose of research is to provide explanations, the why question. Often explanatory research builds on exploratory and descriptive research studies, thus making sense of data by examining relationships and building more abstract constructs and theories to account for the nature of the social world. For example, crime statistics are descriptive, but when we begin to explore why there are differences (like why crime rates are higher in some cities than in others) then the purpose of the research is explanatory. Again, all paradigms of research include explanation, although the forms of explanation differ—neopositivist researchers look for causal relationships while interpretivist researchers look for coherent middle-range theoretical frameworks.

While these are commonly understood purposes of research, there are research perspectives that focus on change. The most practical of these is action research, which is meant to solve an immediate problem. Action research is a process wherein individuals share a felt need for change and work collectively to define and remedy the problem through an action research spiral of planning (including data collection), acting, reflecting, and revising the plan (Carr & Kemmis, 1986; Schön, 1983). Action research may look very much like participatory evaluation, especially when participatory evaluation has a transformative intent and emphasizes the creation of democratic processes and empowering opportunities for everyone involved in the program or organization (Cousins & Whitmore, 1998). Other critical social science research approaches may envision change more theoretically, such as is the case with Marxist analysis, dialectics, and critical ethnography.

A distinction between theoretical and applied research can also be made, a difference in expectation about whether the research provides immediate, tangible, and useful results or more general knowledge. The goal of theoretical, or what is sometimes called "basic research," is to explore the social or physical world without any necessary expectation that a useful, tangible result will be found. For example, theoretical research might ask questions such as "How does social class reproduce itself?" or "What is the biological basis of emotions?" Basic research is often done to test theories and make broad generalizations, and may be seen as the foundation upon which applied research is built.

Applied research may build on basic, theoretical research but its purpose is to solve practical problems. Applied research might ask questions like "What is the best way to teach children to read?" or "How can this disease be cured?" The currently used term "evidence-based practice" is an example of the connection between research and the development of knowledge for specific areas of practice, such as health care, counseling, teaching, and so on. Some applied research looks very much like evaluation, especially if the research is oriented to improvement of the human condition, but differs because of the expectation that the results of applied research will be useful in solving a problem across many sites and contexts. Action research is a kind of applied research that is specifically about seeking solutions within a particular context and resembles some forms of participatory evaluation.

Methods

Research methods are the ways in which researchers collect and analyze evidence, and these vary considerably. While methods are not inherently connected to particular research paradigms, it is the case that neopositivist-oriented research is more likely to use experimental, quasi-experimental, and survey designs, and to employ statistical analysis. Interpretivist research, on the other hand, is more likely to employ observation and interviewing, and to employ thematic approaches to data analysis.

The methods used in research are often tied to disciplinary traditions, and while there is always variation within a specific discipline, patterns do emerge. For example, one is likely to find that those educated as psychologists favor quasi-experimental and experimental methodologies and statistical analysis of data, in contrast with those educated as anthropologists who favor field work, observation, open-ended interviewing, and thematic analysis of data.

Researcher Roles

When researchers adopt an objectivist epistemology, their role is one of distant, dispassionate, and neutral inquirer. A key aim for the researcher is to avoid influencing the research context or participants, actions that are presumed to introduce bias in answering research questions.

Researchers who adopt a social constructivist or subjectivist epistemology may also adopt dispassionate and objective roles, but are more likely to see themselves as part of the research context. Depending on the relationship of the researcher to the research context, they may be seen as insiders (i.e., members of a social context that grants privileged access to knowledge) or outsiders (i.e., outsiders who are granted access to knowledge as an other) (Merton, 1972). Adler and Adler (1987) provide more detail in describing three interpretivist researcher roles: (1) peripheral member, who observes but does not participate in the core activities of the social context; (2) active member, who participates in activities of the group without committing to the values within the social context; and (3) complete member, who is already a member of the group or who becomes integrated into the social context during the course of the research (this is also referred to as "going native").

Additionally, within this research paradigm, the researcher is often seen as the "instrument," the primary data collection strategy, and therefore there is significant emphasis placed on the importance of the researcher's reflexivity, a systematic approach to reflection within the research context. This reflection on personal experience and attributes and their intersection with the research context is seen as key to developing a warranted and clear description or explanation of a social context. For example, Peshkin (1988) describes his "research I's" while studying a fundamentalist Christian school, which are key to an ongoing process of understanding how his subjectivity is related to his interpretations of school–community relations.

Judging Quality

Research is generally expected to make a contribution to knowledge, and at the core this is the key criterion for judging its quality. In addition, the appropriate use of methods and the transparency of the research design contribute to confidence in the contribution the research makes. The indicators of quality differ depending on the research paradigm: in neopositivist research validity, reliability, replicability, and generalizability are key, while in interpretivist research credibility, transferability, dependability, and confirmability are key. In general, researchers are expected to acknowledge and contextualize their work within bodies of related theory and research, make convincing arguments with evidence, and contribute generalized knowledge.

While it is generally assumed that research is about creating generalizable knowledge that is clearly an overstatement and does not represent the diverse contributions research may make. For example, "an historical analysis of the causes of the French revolution, an ethnography of the Minangkabau, or an ecological study of the Galapagos may not be conducted in order to generalize to all revolutions, all matriarchal cultures, or all self-contained eco-systems" (Mathison, 2007, p. 190).

Defining Evaluation

Evaluation, like research, is not a singular or coherent theory or practice. Indeed some considerable effort has been made in attempting to describe the various assumptions underlying evaluation approaches that account for differences in evaluation practice (see Alkin, 2004; Shadish, Cook, & Leviton, 1991). Alkin and Christie (2004) assert the root of all evaluation is accountability and systematic social inquiry, but they distinguish among evaluation approaches and theories based on the primacy given to the use of the evaluation process and findings, the methods employed, or the valuing aspect. Each of these three emphases becomes a branch on their "evaluation theory tree."

Differences in evaluation approaches also, to a large extent, mirror the epistemological differences in research described previously. Some approaches to evaluation adopt a neopositivist framework and see the discernment of value, merit, and worth in a discovery of what works and how change happens. A good example of this approach is realist evaluation (Pawson & Tilley, 1997), which "focuses on developing explanations of the consequences of social actions that contribute to a better understanding of why, where and for whom programs work or fail to work" (Henry, 2005, p. 359). Realist evaluation does this by identifying and testing mechanisms that produce programmatic outcomes. These sit on Alkin and Christie's "methods" tree branch.

Other approaches to evaluation adopt a social constructivist epistemology, such as participatory evaluation, which involves program stakeholders in decisions about planning, doing, and reporting an evaluation. Participatory evaluation has been further divided into practical participatory evaluation or transformative participatory evaluation (Cousins & Whitmore, 1998). The former values participation in the evaluation to increase ownership in and usefulness of evaluation studies. The latter more explicitly incorporates the idea that evaluation should promote social justice and change through the inclusion of and attention to oppressed and disenfranchised stakeholders. These approaches sit on Alkin and Christie's "valuing" tree branch.

Other approaches are more aligned with a pragmatism, a focus on doing evaluation that is useful for decision making, improvement, and empowerment. Perhaps the most widely cited example is Michael Patton's utilization-focused evaluation and more recently developmental evaluation (Patton, 1997, 2010). While Patton's Utilization Focused Evaluation provided a framework for identifying why and how evaluation practice could be more useful at a programmatic level, developmental evaluation extends those concerns in light of what Patton perceives as inevitable complexity in social problems, contexts, and the examination of innovative solutions that must be incorporated into evaluation practice. These approaches sit on Alkin and Christie's "use" tree branch.

Purpose

In part the definition of evaluation defines its purpose: *evaluation* is both the process and product of determining the value, merit, or worth of an evaluand. While some research may be evaluative, most research is not, but the judgment component is essential to evaluation. Determining the value of an evaluand can be done for a number of reasons: to determine if goals are met; to determine outcomes, both anticipated and unanticipated and intended and unintended; to improve the evaluand; to make decisions about an evaluand (including decisions about adopting, funding, or dismantling the evaluand); to inform public discourse and policy about an evaluand; and to demonstrate accountability.

Evaluation is usually seen as relevant to understanding and judging a particular evaluand, although that evaluand may be small and local (like a single program to support local food production) to large and global (like a global policy on environmentally sustainable agriculture). Unlike research, evaluation is always about looking for solutions to problems that are tangible and meaningful in the immediate future.

Methods

Like research, the methods for collecting and analyzing evidence in evaluation often reflect the disciplinary tradition within which evaluators are educated. For example, Lum and Yang (2005) investigated the methods choices of criminal justice evaluators and found that these evaluators (whose primary academic discipline was generally criminology) favored nonexperimental methods, such as forensics.

Evaluation has by and large drawn on the social sciences for its methods and so the ways evidence are collected and analyzed are similar to those used by researchers. In part, because many evaluators were educated within social science traditions, especially psychology and sociology, and to a much lesser extent anthropology, ways of establishing empirical evidence have been informed by these traditions. Thus, evaluators use experiments, survey methods, observations, interviews, and so on. Because evaluation necessarily addresses issues like needs, costs, ethicality, feasibility, and justifiability, evaluators have also turned to other disciplines, such as jurisprudence, journalism, arts, philosophy, accounting, and ethics, for ideas on methods.

In addition, as the discipline of evaluation matures there are methods that have been developed specifically for evaluation, for determining value, merit, or worth. For example, Davies and Dart (2005) have developed the "most significant change" method. This method

> involves the collection of significant change (SC) stories emanating from the field, and the systematic selection of the most significant of these stories by panels of designated stakeholders or staff. The designated staff and stakeholders are initially involved by "searching" for project impact. Once changes have been captured, various people sit together, read the stories aloud and have regular and often in-depth discussions about the value of these reported changes. When the technique is implemented successfully, whole teams of people begin to focus their attention on program impact. (p. 8)

Another example is Brinkerhoff's "success case method," which is a relatively simple two-step storytelling-based procedure for identifying potential and likely successful job performance (Brinkerhoff, 2005). The success case method borrows various methods (surveys, key informants, in-depth interviewing) from various disciplines (e.g., sociology, journalism) and packages them in a distinct way that informs the key feature of evaluation, that is, to determine the value, merit, or worth of an evaluand.

While collecting evidence in an evaluation context often looks quite similar to research, the context in which the methods are used or the ways they are packaged sometimes reveals the explicit judgment component of evaluation by the search for success (such as in the success case method), or the positive (such as in appreciative inquiry), or change (such as in the most significant change method).

Evaluator Roles

Because evaluation theory and practice is not unified into one perspective, there are many roles evaluators occupy (Mathison, 2005).

Evaluators variously see themselves as objective inquirers, technicians, values-committed inquirers, change agents, facilitators, collaborators, and educators. These different role conceptions place differing emphasis on the importance of creating a focus for the evaluation, data collection and analysis, reporting, and stakeholder engagement. King and Stevahn (2002) identify three components to all evaluator roles: the relationships between the evaluator and evaluation participants, the relationship between the evaluator and the organization, and the evaluator's conflict management and resolution strategies.

Stakeholder engagement as a component of the evaluator's relationship to evaluation participants is unique to evaluation and indeed cuts across all perspectives on how evaluation should be conducted. Over time, evaluation practice has come to be defined by sensitivity to and engagement of stakeholder perspectives, albeit in different ways. Realist evaluators, for example, may especially pay attention to collecting value positions of stakeholders to interpret the meaning of data, while participatory evaluators may partner with evaluation participants in conceptualizing, doing, and/or reporting the evaluation. What is notable is that this commitment to stakeholder engagement is a critical distinction between research and evaluation.

Evaluators are either internal or external, that is, they work within the organization or program they are evaluating or they do evaluation for hire. While there are certainly organizational research units and therefore internal researchers, the commonplaceness of internal evaluation practice makes this distinction more salient in determining an evaluator's role (Mathison, 2011). The practice of an internal or external evaluator may look similar, but the different roles create unique tensions and demands including the need to juggle high standards for evaluation with organizational commitments and loyalties (Mathison, 1991).

Judging Quality

The quality of evaluation builds on notions similar to the quality of research and there is an expectation that the descriptions and explanations about evaluands are accurate, but in addition evaluation is judged by its utility, feasibility, and propriety. These dimensions for judging the quality of evaluation are clear in the Metaevaluation Checklist, which is based on the Program Evaluation Standards (Stufflebeam, 1999).

While evaluations can make contributions to more general knowledge, the typical expectation is that evaluation is useful within a clearly defined context within which the evaluation occurred. This context may be extensive (even national or international in scope) or quite local.

What Does the "Feminist" Adjective Add to Contrasting Research and Evaluation?

Defining Feminism

Feminism is defined in many ways, but common to most definitions is the idea of challenging gender inequality. "Feminism is: (a) a belief that women universally face some form of oppression or exploitation; (b) a commitment to uncover and understand what causes and sustains oppression, in all its forms and (c) a commitment to work individually and collectively in everyday life to end all forms of oppression" (Maguire, 1987, p. 79). While feminism begins with the assumption that all human beings, women and men, are of equal worth, a feminist perspective also adopts the assumption that culturally men are typically more valued than women. As a consequence of this cultural valuing of men, women face myriad forms of oppression that must be named to be overcome.

Putting women first sometimes means a feminist perspective is useful for understanding issues of gender more broadly, including masculinity, which is a component of feminine identity and experience. Men's liberation, whether conceived of as a liberation from patriarchy or matriarchy, confronts gender inequality by challenging men's privileged institutionalized and lived experiences (Messner, 2000).

Feminist Research

If feminism is about uncovering and redressing oppression and unequal treatment of women, then the purpose of feminist research can be understood as the process by which this occurs. Like research in general, feminist research explores, describes, and explains the conditions of women's lives. "By documenting women's lives, experiences and concerns, illuminating gender-based stereotypes and biases, and unearthing women's subjugated knowledge, feminist research challenges the basic structures and ideologies that oppress women" (Brooks & Hesse-Biber, 2007, p. 4). Brooks and Hesse-Biber (2007) continue by emphasizing feminist research's action orientation, a feature that distinguishes feminist research: "Feminist research goals foster empowerment and emancipation for women and other marginalized groups, and feminist researchers often apply their findings in the service of promoting social change and social justice for women" (p. 4). These goals therefore emphasize both the "invisibility and distortion of female experience" (Lather, 1988, p. 571).

Feminist Research Methodology

Feminist research generally steps outside the boundaries of the debates about quantitative and qualitative research, and indeed historically feminist research has been and can be done within any paradigm. In other words, any research methodology can be pressed into service to document gender inequalities and to provide direction for emancipation from those oppressive inequalities. Three perspectives dominate the discussions about feminist research methodology: feminist empiricism, standpoint feminism, and feminist postmodernism.

Feminist empiricism adopts a realist ontology, an objectivist epistemology, and employs traditional social science research methods. Unlike empiricism, though, feminist empiricism is critical of the practice of science, if not its foundations, and looks to both study women's issues and to obviate gender bias in research techniques including biased instrumentation, male-dominated sampling, and asking research questions that emphasize women's experiences. There is much criticism of the conservatism of feminist empiricism including the constraints that empiricism has on new and alternate ways of reasoning and that scientific standards are themselves a product of patriarchy (Hundleby, 2012).

Feminist standpoint research aligns closely with the definitions of feminism and women's political movements. Standpoint approaches put women's experiences at the center of the research and declare that women are best positioned to understand those experiences. This methodological approach favors a social constructivist epistemology, blurs the roles of researcher and researched, and emphasizes the importance of researcher reflexivity. This approach places greatest emphasis on what women do, and the concrete experiences of their lives; for example, Jaggar (1997) connects women's everyday nurturing activities with their skill in expressing and reading emotions. But feminist standpoint research also emphasizes the oppressiveness of women's experiences and the unique perspective this gives women in understanding the social world, which, in turn, provides a means for understanding desirable social change. A challenge for feminist standpoint research is that there are multiple and diverse feminine standpoints, standpoints that derive from the intersection of gender with race and/or class, for example. Nonetheless, feminist standpoint research methodologies remain a dominant feminist research approach.

Related more to critical theory and a rejection of foundationalism, feminist postmodernist research is focused more on contrasts than universal understandings and critiques unitary notions of woman and gender (Fraser & Nicholson, 1990). In part, postmodern feminist research attempts to deal with the differences among women, rejecting the universalist idea or grand narrative of woman's experience.

Although there are clear and important differences among feminist research methodologies, there are several common elements. Stanley and Wise (1990) include the relationship between researcher and researched; the importance of the researcher's autobiography; the critical role of reflexivity; experience as the focus of the research; and complex questions of power. One would obviously add an attention to gender as a central construct. Feminist research can be thought of as a normative framework for inquiry.

Feminist Research Methods

Discussions of feminist research often eschew a claim that there are feminist research methods and claim that any and all research methods may be used in service of the gender-focused and problem-focused nature of feminist research. And indeed, feminist researchers adapt research methods, often through collaboration with research participants, to include gender issues, to acknowledge and explore subjective experiences, and to empower research participants. Interviewing, ethnographic field work, surveys, and action research, for example, are adapted to meet the goals of feminist research (Hesse-Biber, 2012). For many feminist researchers, the adoption of methods that have the potential for engaging and empowering women are appealing. One example of such methods are visual- and image-based approaches as exemplified, for example, in the Academy Award-winning documentary film *Born into Brothels: Calcutta's Red Light Kids* and the visual storytelling of PhotoVoice (Wang, 1999; Wang & Burris, 1994).

The feminist researcher's adaptation of research methods is similar to the evaluator's adaption of research methods, molding them to a particular interest in lived gendered experiences in the former instance or making value judgments in the latter instance.

Feminist Evaluation

Like all evaluation approaches, feminist evaluation is fundamentally about ascertaining the value, merit, or worth of an evaluand, but with particular attention "to gender issues, the needs of women, and the promotion of change" (Seigart, 2005, p. 155). Feminist evaluation is not the evaluation of women's programs, but rather, as Seigart (2005) explains, it is a perspective that casts a critical and gender-focused eye on all programs. This perspective reflects the foundational feminist framework that informs all feminist evaluations. While addressing and redressing women's oppression, some feminist evaluation attends also to other social conditions of oppression, such as race, class, ethnicity, sexual orientation, and ableness—what Mertens (2005) calls "a transformative feminist approach."

Most often the core elements of feminist evaluation are those summarized in Sielbeck-Bowen, Brisolara, Seigart, Tischler, and Whitmore (2002, pp. 3–4):

- Feminist evaluation has as a central focus the gender inequities that lead to social injustice.
- Discrimination or inequality based on gender is systemic and structural.
- Evaluation is a political activity; the contexts in which evaluation operates are politicized; and the personal experiences, perspectives, and characteristics evaluators bring to evaluations (and with which we interact) lead to a particular political stance.
- Knowledge is a powerful resource that serves an explicit or implicit purpose.
- Knowledge should be a resource of and for the people who create, hold, and share it. Consequently, the evaluation or research process can lead to significant negative or positive effects on the people involved in the evaluation/research. Knowledge and values are culturally, socially, and temporally contingent. Knowledge is also filtered through the knower.
- There are multiple ways of knowing; some ways are privileged over others.

Feminist evaluation shares many of the attributes of participatory, empowerment, and democratic evaluation approaches, those evaluation approaches that rest on the "valuing" and "use" limbs of Alkin and Christie's (2004) evaluation theory tree. Indeed transformative evaluation (Mertens, 2009), empowerment evaluation (Fetterman, 2001), critical theory evaluation (Freeman, 2010), transformative participatory evaluation (Cousins & Whitmore, 1998), and deliberative democratic evaluation (House & Howe, 1999) are all approaches that provide a foundation for feminist evaluation. Coupled with a feminist perspective, including concerns about women's oppression and emancipation, any of these evaluation approaches becomes feminist evaluation.

The Practical Importance of Distinguishing Evaluation from Research

I have argued that there is a distinction between evaluation and research, but have also tried to illustrate that drawing a line between the two is neither easy nor straightforward. Because of the diversity of both evaluation and research perspectives, it is easy to find evaluation and research that are difficult to distinguish, and to find evaluation and research that look dramatically different. This is no less the case when one is describing feminist evaluation or feminist research.

A key similarity is that both evaluation and research use many of the same strategies for collecting and analyzing evidence, that is, they share a common ancestry with regard to methods. While some methods are now being developed within the discipline of evaluation, especially methods that focus on perceived change or success, nonetheless what counts as evidence remains quite similar for evaluation and research.

A key difference is in the purpose or expected outcome. By definition, evaluation is about valuing. Research, which is the pursuit of theoretical descriptions or explanations, necessarily involves values (because facts and values are inextricable) but need not and often does not involve valuing. Another key difference is that evaluation is about the particular, whether that is a program, policy, or intervention, and research is about the general, whether that is a theory, construct, or policy area. Evaluation is judged by its usefulness, particularly its contribution to improvement, learning and change, and decision making, while research is judged by its generation of theoretical knowledge.

Evaluators and researchers alike want their work to matter, whether within a particular context or in a more abstract theoretical way. Evaluators, however, shoulder a necessary burden of ensuring that evaluation as a practice is relevant, useful, and responsive to clients, particular contexts, and social problems. It is this burden that most especially behooves us to be clear about when we are doing evaluation and when we are doing research.

REFERENCES

Adler, P., & Adler, P. (1987). *Membership roles in field research*. Newbury Park, CA: Sage.

Alkin, M. (2004). *Evaluation roots: Tracing theorists' views and influences*. Thousand Oaks, CA: Sage.

Alkin, M., & Christie, C. A. (2004). An evaluation theory tree. In M. Alkin (Ed.), *Evaluation roots: Tracing theorists' views and influences* (pp. 12–66). Thousand Oaks, CA: Sage.

Brinkerhoff, R. O. (2005). The success case method: A strategic evaluation approach to increasing the value and effect of training. *Advances in Developing Human Resources, 7*(1), 86–101.

Brooks, A., & Hesse-Biber, S. N. (2007). An invitation to feminist research. In S. N. Hesse-Biber & P. Leavy (Eds.), *Feminist research practice: A primer*. Thousand Oaks, CA: Sage.

Carr, W., & Kemmis, S. (1986). *Becoming critical: Education, knowledge and action research*. Lewes, UK: Falmer.

Coffman, J. (2003–2004, Winter). Michael Scriven on the differences between evaluation and social science research. *The Evaluation Exchange, 9*(4).

Retrieved July 30, 2012, from *www.gse.harvard.edu/hfrp/eval/issue24/expert.html*.

Cousins, J. B., & Whitmore, E. (1998). Framing participatory evaluation. In E. Whitmore (Ed.), Understanding and practicing participatory evaluation. *New Directions for Evaluation, 1998*(80), 5–23.

Crotty, M. (1998). *The foundations of social research*. Newbury Park, CA: Sage.

Davies, R., & Dart, J. (2005). *The most significant change technique: A guide to its use*. Retrieved July 30, 2012, from *www.mande.co.uk/docs/MSCGuide.pdf*.

Fetterman, D. (2001). *Foundations of empowerment evaluation*. Thousand Oaks, CA: Sage.

Fraser, N., & Nicholson, L. J. (1990). Social criticism without philosophy: An encounter between feminism and postmodernism. In L. J. Nicholson (Ed.), *Feminism/postmodernism* (pp. 19–38). New York: Routledge.

Freeman, M. (Ed.). (2010). Critical social theory and evaluation practice. *New Directions for Evaluation, 2010*(127), 1–98.

Henry, G. (2005). Realist evaluation. In S. Mathison (Ed.), *Encyclopedia of evaluation* (pp. 359–367). Thousand Oaks, CA: Sage.

Hesse-Biber, S. N. (Ed.). (2012). *Handbook of feminist research: Theory and praxis*. Thousand Oaks, CA: Sage.

House, E. R., & Howe, K. (1999). *Values in evaluation and social research*. Thousand Oaks, CA: Sage.

Hundleby, C. B. (2012). Feminist empiricism. In S. N. Hesse-Biber (Ed.), *Handbook of feminist research: Theory and praxis* (pp. 28–45). Thousand Oaks, CA: Sage.

Jaggar, A. M. (1997). Love and knowledge: Emotion in feminist epistemology. In S. Kemp & J. Squires (Eds.), *Feminisms* (pp. 188–193). Oxford, UK: Oxford University Press.

King, J. A., & Stevahn, L. (2002). Three frameworks for considering evaluator role. In K. E. Ryan & T. A. Schwandt (Eds.), *Exploring evaluator role and identity* (pp. 1–16). Charlotte, NC: Information Age Publishers.

Lather, P. (1988). Feminist perspective on empowering research methodologies. *Women's Studies International Forum, 11*(6), 569–581.

Lum, C., & Yang, S. (2005). Why do evaluation researchers in crime and justice choose non-experimental methods? *Journal of Experimental Criminology, 1*, 191–213.

Maguire, P. (1987). *Doing participatory research: A feminist approach*. Amherst: University of Massachusetts Press.

Mathison, S. (1991). Role conflicts for internal evaluators. In S. Mathison (Ed.), Authority in internal evaluation. *Evaluation and Program Planning, 14*(2), 173–179.

Mathison, S. (2005). Evaluator roles. In S. Mathison (Ed.), *Encyclopedia of evaluation* (pp. 146–147). Thousand Oaks, CA: Sage.

Mathison, S. (2007). What is the difference between evaluation and research? And why do we care? In N. L. Smith & P. Brandon (Eds.), *Fundamental issues in evaluation* (pp. 183–196). New York: Guilford Press.

Mathison, S. (2011). Internal evaluation: Historically speaking. In B. Volkov &

M. Baron (Eds.), Internal evaluation in the 21st century. *New Directions for Evaluation, 2011*(132), 13–24.

Mertens, D. M. (2005). Feminism. In S. Mathison (Ed.), *Encyclopedia of evaluation* (p. 154). Thousand Oaks, CA: Sage.

Mertens, D. M. (2009). *Transformative research and evaluation.* New York: Guilford Press.

Merton, R. K. (1972). Insiders and outsiders. *American Journal of Sociology, 78*(1), 9–47.

Messner, M. (2000). *Politics of masculinities: Men in movements.* Oxford, UK: AltaMira Press.

Patton, M. Q. (1997). *Utilization-focused evaluation: The new century text* (3rd ed.). Thousand Oaks, CA: Sage.

Patton, M. Q. (2010). *Developmental evaluation: Applying complexity concepts to enhance innovation and use.* New York: Guilford Press.

Pawson, R., & Tilley, N. (1997). *Realistic evaluation.* London: Sage.

Peshkin, A. (1988). In search of subjectivity: One's own. *Educational Researcher, 17*(7), 17–21.

Putnam, H. (2002). *The collapse of the fact/value dichotomy and other essays.* Cambridge, MA: Harvard University Press.

Schön, D. A. (1983). *The reflective practitioner: How professionals think in action.* New York: Basic Books.

Seigart, D. (2005). Feminist evaluation. In S. Mathison (Ed.), *Encyclopedia of evaluation* (pp. 154–157). Thousand Oaks, CA: Sage.

Shadish, W. R., Cook, T. D., & Leviton, L. C. (1991). *Foundations of program evaluation: Theories of practice.* Thousand Oaks, CA: Sage.

Sielbeck-Bowen, K., Brisolara, S., Seigart, D., Tischler, C., & Whitmore, E. (2002). Exploring feminist evaluation: The ground from which we rise. *New Directions for Evaluation, 2002*(96), 3–8.

Stanley, L., & Wise, S. (1990). Method, methodology and epistemology in feminist research processes. In L. Stanley (Ed.), *Feminist praxis* (pp. 20–60). London: Routledge.

Stufflebeam, D. (1999). *Metaevaluation checklist.* Retrieved July 30, 2012, from *www.wmich.edu/evalctr/archive_checklists/program_metaeval_10point.pdf.*

Taylor, P. (1961). *Normative discourse.* Englewood Cliffs, NJ: Prentice-Hall.

Wang, C. C. (1999). PhotoVoice: A participatory action research strategy applied to women's health. *Journal of Women's Health, 8*(2), 185–192.

Wang, C., & Burris, M. A. (1994). Empowerment through photo novella: Portraits of participation. *Health Education and Behavior, 21*(2), 171–186.

CHAPTER 3

Researcher/Evaluator Roles and Social Justice

Elizabeth Whitmore

Introduction: What Does It Mean When We Talk about Role?

Volkov (2011) defines a role as "an explicitly and implicitly expected function performed and behavior associated with a particular position in an organization" (p. 27). Further, "roles are also a translation of professional values, priorities and principles into behaviors and courses of action to deliver desired results." Thus, evaluators are expected to perform their function—conducting an evaluation or leading the process—in a particular way; they bring a certain status and thus expected behavior to the role. Expanding the traditional role beyond that of technical expert is well supported in the literature (Volkov, 2011).

What makes the role of the feminist different or unique? The task of this chapter is to respond to that question.

We can draw guidance from feminist researchers[1] who have explored more deeply what "role" means. Hesse-Biber and Leavy (2007), for example, see the researcher's role as bringing together/incorporating "interpretation, subjectivity, emotion and embodiment into the knowledge building process, elements historically associated with women and excluded from mainstream positivist research. Indeed, many feminist researchers have begun to illuminate potential new sources of knowledge and understanding precisely within the lived experiences, interpretations, subjectivities and emotions of women" (p. 13). These become "tools for knowledge building and rich understanding" (p. 13). The researcher's role is certainly not static, however. It can vary from detached observer to complete participant, depending on the situation, what is desired, and what may be possible in a given circumstance (p. 202). It is also critical to recognize that what role the researcher plays and how is intimately tied to her or his own worldview, history, and biography. There is no objectivity; we need to be aware that we are deeply grounded in our own location and life experience. All this is applicable to evaluation. Though evaluation and research may look quite similar, evaluation is more typically associated with producing information for decision making, while research more often generates knowledge that can be transferred to other settings (Mertens, 2009). (Mathison, Chapter 2, this volume, elaborates on this topic.)

To start, here are some general thoughts about the feminist evaluator role.

■ Feminist evaluation is an "engaged praxis" that is "imbued with theory but pragmatic in implementation" (Brisolara & Seigart, 2007, p. 292). This describes the evaluator role, in that the practice is based firmly in feminist principles, outlined in earlier chapters. "What is critical is that an evaluator is well versed in the tenets of feminist theories and familiar with a particular feminist framework" (Brisolara & Seigart, 2007, p. 291). There is an extensive and rich theoretical literature on feminism and feminist research. There is much less on feminist evaluation and little on the role—what the evaluator does and how to put the theory into practice.

■ There are many feminisms and thus many roles. How these play out will depend on the purpose of the evaluation, its consequent set of potential designs, and above all the principles and values that undergird the practice. Being up-front and communicative about one's stance is an essential and ongoing process. Even when a feminist evaluator is clear at the beginning of an evaluation process, differing perspectives are likely to occur along the way and thus meanings and expectations may need to be revisited throughout the process.

■ It is methodology, rather than method, that is of interest in how a feminist evaluator plays out the role. Methods (or techniques) are of less importance here; rather it is methodology that counts. Methods in feminist evaluation (how we collect data) are limited (there are only so many ways we can collect information), but it does matter which methodologies (lenses through which we do our evaluation) and epistemologies (our knowledge bases) we use (Pillow, 2002, p. 15). Feminist researchers and evaluators may use conventional and unconventional methods, depending on the situation. "Emergent methods as a process include assorted combinations of methods and feminist methodologies" (Moss, 2007, p. 374).

▪ The evaluator's role depends on the context, and on her or his personal characteristics, experiences, and preferences (Brisolara & Seigart, 2007, p. 297). What may work in one situation or with one group of stakeholders may not work with another. This notion is hardly new, but the evaluator enters the situation with a set of experiences and tools and will naturally draw on them in new situations. And every evaluator is, above all, an individual; we bring ourselves to this process, quirks and all. Self-awareness and reflexivity are thus essential skills in adapting one's role to a given set of circumstances. Reflexivity is more fully discussed in the section (below) on capacity building.

▪ It is important to emphasize that both women and men can be feminist evaluators. While it is often assumed that feminist evaluators will be women, that is not necessarily the case. Feminism is a state of mind, a framework, an understanding of the world, and necessitates a deep commitment to gender equity. Men can be (and some are) feminists; not all women are. At the same time, in many cultures, women may be more comfortable with female evaluators or researchers, while men may respond better to male investigators, no matter how skilled and committed one may be (Ahmed, Lewando-Hundt, & Blackburn, 2011).

One starting point for this chapter is the 2002 *New Directions for Evaluation* special issue (No. 96) on feminist evaluation. In one article, Beardsley and Miller (2002) outline a set of broad expectations for the feminist evaluator, including being sensitive to power dynamics among stakeholders, conducting a gender analysis of stakeholder interactions, and validating the personal and collective experiences (p. 69). Beardsley and Miller do not tell us how to do this in any detail, however. This current chapter expands on these expectations by offering a more detailed discussion of what a feminist evaluation means in terms of what the evaluator actually says and does.

My Own "Awakening" to Feminism

It wasn't until the 1970s that I really "woke up" to the feminist message. A divorce (after 19 years of marriage) opened up a whole new world of possibilities for me, including graduate school. A colleague began sharing some articles that certainly resonated with my experience. I saw incidents, in both my work and personal life, that I had previously misinterpreted, ignored, or explained away, in a wholly different light. For example, when I expressed an interest in getting involved in politics, my husband's response was "I'll divorce you if you do that." Having been brought up in the 1950s, in a white, middle-class American, suburban household, my role as a woman (read: wife and mother) was to serve my husband. Whatever needs, interests, or ambitions I might have would have to come second. This was a deeply written script for me. What I had so readily understood, and accepted, as simply not possible, or my fault, I now recognized as something quite different. While that doesn't or shouldn't eliminate some serious self-examination, the articles put my experience in a context I had not fully appreciated. I've never looked back and thus feminist evaluation was an "of course" for me when I eventually got into the field of evaluation. Though the general feminist lens is now quite mainstream—few (overtly at least) oppose equal rights for women—it is the more subtle resistance (structural barriers, attitudes, processes) that require our ongoing attention.

The feminist evaluator thus has her or his hands full, needing to be constantly adept both at planting seeds and at "hearing" the cues. These are not easy "skills" and certainly not ones addressed in evaluator training.

This chapter is built around two major sections. First, I offer a detailed discussion of the roles played by a feminist evaluator and links to underlying feminist assumptions and principles. A second section looks at some contrasting models, including the level of stakeholder involvement, general evaluator roles, and what a feminist lens would add. This is intended to give the reader an overview of differing evaluation purposes and models, and how these play out in terms of the evaluator role. Finally, I look at some key issues emerging from the discussion.

Feminist Evaluator Roles

Table 3.1 summarizes key feminist evaluator roles and what these imply specifically in terms of practice (what the evaluator says and does). At the same time, it draws their connection to underlying assumptions and feminist principles, clarifying the continuity between theory and practice. In the discussion (below), I use examples from my own and others' experience to illustrate exactly what this could mean in practice.

Four issues cut across all roles: First is the importance of clarifying what these roles mean, which one(s) are to be emphasized in any particular circumstance, and formally negotiating expectations with an evaluand. Second, the personal characteristics, experiences, and preferences of the evaluator will dictate which role(s) she or he best plays. Not everyone can do everything equally well, so self-knowledge and confidence in

TABLE 3.1. Roles of a Feminist Evaluator and Implications for Practice

Role	Practice (what the evaluator does)	Skills and attitudes needed	Element (or underlying assumption)	Principle
Facilitator	• Start with lived experience. • Build trust. • Explore/embrace differences. • Use inclusive language. • Share own experience. • Balance power/authority, control.	• Listening (verbal and nonverbal) • Posing relevant questions. • Conflict management • Promoting dialogue, mediating • Giving and receiving feedback • Organizational skills • Openness, patience	• Participants as experts in their own lives; participants' lived experience as primary source of knowledge • Making space for voice • Dealing with difference (cultural competence)	Multiple ways of knowing
Educator	• Build capacity. • Raise consciousness (illuminating existing social relations, etc.). • Encourage reflexivity (own and others).	• Asking provocative questions • Naming • Challenging androcentric bias	• Personal is political • Importance of reflexivity	Knowledge is situated
Collaborator	• Make space for all voices. • Share power/control. • Strive for consensus.	• Share own stories • Assuming a partnership role	• Valuing cooperation (vs. competition); participation	Democratic values/principles
Technical advisor/ methodologist	• Share various possibilities for design, etc. • Help integrate feminist evaluation theory into design.	• Using nonjargon language • Translating complex concepts into easy-to-understand steps and processes	• Evaluator training/expertise to be openly shared with participants	Sharing knowledge and power
Activist/ advocate	• Stimulate cognitive dissonance. • Push participants to take action.	• Asking hard/provocative questions	• Importance of follow-through when inequality detected	Gender/ sex equity; social justice

63

one's strengths (and limitations) is essential. Third, implicit in all roles is cultural competence; it is essential that all evaluators, regardless of their approach, understand and practice principles of cultural competence, such as those outlined in the American Evaluation Association's (AEA) public statement on Cultural Competence in Evaluation (*www.aea.org*). All roles, however implemented, require this. And finally, building trust with and among the stakeholders is integral to all roles. Without this base, very little of any validity will happen.

Facilitator

A facilitator practicing from a feminist perspective starts with the lived experience of the stakeholders, giving voice, making space for all voices (Seigart & Brisolara, 2002). "The focus is on analyzing gender in context . . . on the 'dailiness'—the daily lived experiences previously seen as mundane—of women's lives" (Pillow, 2002, p. 16). This begins the process of building trust—among stakeholders and with the evaluator—so essential to effective interaction. There are a wide variety of team-building exercises and techniques, needed especially when internal (or external) tensions block effective interaction and decision making.[2]

> The evaluator explores and embraces differences and knows how to effectively balance power and control with a group. "The challenge for an evaluator is to construct or stitch together the various parts of the narrative, to make connections and lay open for discussion and reflection competing interpretations and points of conflict. . . . [She or he] strives to bring in as many voices as possible in order to make these partial connections, to reveal limited truths. (VanderPlatt, 1995, p. 92)

This process enhances mutual awareness, and captures complexity.

There is a range of skills a facilitator brings to the table. She or he is good at posing relevant questions, promoting dialogue, mediating, managing conflict, knowing when to take charge (or not), noticing and "reading" nonverbal communication, giving and receiving feedback (both positive and negative), organizing skills, keeping the discussion "on track" but recognizing and encouraging "creative" sidetracks when they occur. An understanding of group dynamics is essential knowledge for facilitators. An openness to ideas and contrasting perspectives, and patience, are fundamental attitudes as well. Doing all of these well is a tall order; they involve not only skills (that can be learned and refined through practice), but attitudes, which require self-awareness, flexibility, openness, and humility.

Language

A good facilitator ensures that language is inclusive, avoids jargon, and is sensitive to differing forms of expression, experiences, and perspectives. She or he encourages participant interaction, supports others' ideas, and validates the entire process. Language also reflects cultural competence and a skilled evaluator understands the many subtleties when working across cultures. For example, in the African tradition, circumlocution rather than an exact definition is considered appropriate. A direct statement is seen as crude and unimaginative. In addition, in the African tradition, the team must have people who are perceived to be the right people for the job (Mathison, 2005, pp. 96–101).

Then there is communication without words, nonverbal communication. "One of the primary tools of oppression of women is the maintenance of silence about their experiences and perspectives" (Ward, 2002, p. 54, citing Tolman & Szalacha, 1999). Silence is communication and can have many meanings. Breaking silence is one thing, working with it quite another. Interpreting the silence requires respect, that is, attentiveness to what one is "hearing." Silence involves both vigilance and compassion, as sometimes language is inadequate to express feelings that have no words (DeVault & Gross, 2007). Similarly,

> as women, we are often aware of how much language doesn't adequately express what we mean. We're forever up against how words we want to use that have developed a pejorative meaning. So awkward language and different uses of words is something else I'd say as feminists we listen for. And when we hear intimations of this, we stop, and try to open up and look into the gap. At the same time, as feminists, we're particularly aware of silencing and all its subtle power and of the ongoing need to honor that, and to take measures to encourage and support that silence being broken. (Heather Menzies, personal communication)[3]

The facilitator takes her or his time, works with small groups, individual work sheets, whatever helps a person to speak. Some of this depends on a person's predisposition and attitudes—openness and respect for others, her or his sense of personal security, comfort with emotions, not needing to be "center stage." Some are skills that can be learned, such as active listening, sensitivity to nonverbal communication, and cultural awareness.

"Soft" (People) Skills

The facilitator role involves a set of "soft" (people) skills, not often taught in evaluation training programs. The process aims to engage the stakeholders in dialogue about a range of issues related to the evaluation of a given program and/or organization. These skills include listening (really listening), which DeVault and Gross (2007) call radical, active listening. This involves a fully engaged relationship whereby the researcher listens for gaps and silences and considers what meanings might lie beyond the explicit speech. Being an active listener is being attentive to the complexity of human talk—the pauses and patterns of speech and emotion and placing these in context. Radical, active listening helps create knowledge that challenges rather than supports ruling regimes (Hesse-Biber & Piatelli, 2007, pp. 149–150). Good facilitators are comfortable in sharing personal experiences appropriately, are flexible, patient, always able to "work on their feet." They know how to keep people motivated, project positive body language and energy, and are comfortable with feelings.

Though some have assumed that women may do a better job when interviewing other women, that may not be enough when crossing class and cultural boundaries. Kohler-Riessman (1987) contrasts an interview with a middle-class Anglo woman and a working-class Puerto Rican woman and concludes that the narratives were so differently constructed that major misunderstandings resulted. While the Anglo told her story chronologically, the Puerto Rican organized her narrative episodically. The (Anglo) interviewer found the episodic way of describing an experience confusing and scattered, and kept trying to force the interviewee's story into a chronological format. The author urges greater attention to awareness of one's own way of telling a story and how this may differ from the way others tell theirs.

The ability to recognize and interpret nonverbal behaviors is highly culturally specific. In some cultures, eye contact with a woman is considered provocative, for example. One also has to retain a sense of humor. In a (social work) training workshop I conducted with a group of northern Cree, in Quebec, the participants responded positively to my suggestion of a role play. Within a few minutes, however, most had quietly slipped out of the room. Oops. Time out. What's going on here? I went outside to find them all feeling some consternation, not knowing how to tell me that my understanding of a role play, involving a spontaneous dialogue, was clearly different from their understanding. They were more comfortable with a structured process. We all had a good laugh at the "miscommunication" and we used it as a moment to talk about the challenges of working across cultures.

The practices and skills described above reflect a set of underlying assumptions essential to good feminist practice. Participants are assumed to be experts in their own lives and it is also assumed that their lived experience is a primary source of knowledge. Feminist practice presupposes that all voices should be heard (though perhaps not equally valued), that culture underlies and shapes our thinking (both the stakeholders' and the evaluators'), and thus that cultural competence is essential for all evaluations, including feminist evaluations. These practices, skills, and assumptions all draw from the principle of multiple ways of knowing, an essential theoretical principle in feminist thought (Belenky, Clinchy, Goldberger, & Tarule, 1986).

Brisolara and Seigart (2007) suggest some key questions that a feminist evaluator might ask: "In what ways are women (men, bisexual and transgender people, etc.) treated differently within the program, and how do their experiences and outcomes differ? In what ways do class, race, and gender combine to expand or contract possibilities for participants" (p. 280)?

I offer an example from my own experience.

In the early 1990s, I was the outside evaluator for a "goat cooperative" project in the southern United States. The cooperative was located on the Rio Grande River, just a short "wade" (in the dry season) across to Mexico. The U.S. Department of Agriculture had funded this project in part to offer a source of alternative income for poor goat farmers in the region in order to counteract the temptation of money offered by drug smugglers. The co-op needed a midproject evaluator and they were looking for someone who could do a participatory evaluation and who spoke Spanish. I, a middle-aged white lady from urban Canada who certainly knew nothing about goats, arrived on the scene and immediately encountered two problems. One was major hostility between two older (white male) Anglo co-op members, who were in leadership positions. And two: I was promptly pulled aside by one of the women and told that as a woman, "You can't talk to the men." How to proceed? Fortuitously, at the time, there was a (male) consultant there who agreed to team up with me, at least initially. This allowed me/us to conduct initial interviews to get a sense of the situation. Together we also attempted to mediate the conflict between the two Anglo men, ultimately to no avail. But we did set up a series of workshops including all co-op members (half of whom were Mexican and spoke no English; the other half unilingual "Anglos"). Good facilitation skills were essential in this situation, and with all communication translated (with the help of the daughter of a Mexican co-op member), I worked through an evaluation that started with their experience in the co-op, and moved through an assessment of their goals and objectives, plans for the future, and yes, the role of women in the co-op (for details, see Whitmore, 1998).

Educator

Another feminist evaluator role is that of educator. Two key aspects of this role are highlighted here in terms of practice: capacity building and reflexivity.

Capacity Building

There is an extensive literature on capacity building in many fields (Simmons, Reynolds, & Swinburn, 2011). In thinking about capacity building in evaluation, the questions arise: Why would feminist evaluators engage in capacity building? For what purposes? What capacities are we talking about? Who is assumed to need them? What are evaluators assuming about what stakeholders already know or don't know?

When we talk about "capacity building," it is implicit (and sometimes explicit) that stakeholders lack certain knowledge or skills and that part of our role is to "teach" them, or build their capacity to perform evaluation tasks. While it is reasonable to assume that many stakeholders do not possess sophisticated technical evaluation skills, it is surely presumptuous, and even arrogant, to assume that they bring no knowledge or skills to the process. Evaluators need to approach this issue with care and respect, as the term can carry with it a certain patronizing undertone. Stakeholders' understandings and language may be different but they bring valuable experience, knowledge, and skills to the process, and evaluators need to recognize, value, and invite their contributions. At the same time, evaluators need to build our own capacity, for our knowledge and skills are also incomplete. Capacity building is thus a mutual process.

In addition to particular skills and knowledge exchange, capacity building involves consciousness raising, illuminating existing social relations between women and men, how these have developed over time, cultural norms, and the power dynamics implicit in them. This links people's current life situations with the wider social, political, and economic context. The process is shared—both the stakeholders and the evaluator pose provocative questions and challenge hidden assumptions that reveal underlying androcentric biases. Many women (and some men) are well aware of the multiple forms of oppression of women and how they are deeply embedded in the institutions of society. Naming these oppressions brings them out into the open where they can be discussed and strategies developed to address them.

Reflexivity

Reflexivity is also essential to the role of educator in feminist evaluation, starting with her or his own subjectivity (Brisolara & Seigart, 2007; Patton, 2002). It "requires a more complex understanding of the many ways in which one's own presence and perspectives influence the knowledge and actions that are created" (Stuart & Whitmore, 2006, p. 157). The identity and social location of all participants, including the evaluator, cannot be ignored, as these profoundly influence our worldview, our understanding of any given situation, and how we interact with others. "If the evaluation practitioner is uninformed regarding her/his own identities (collective and individual) or social location, or those of the participants, then relevant issues may remain unexamined" (Hood & Cassaro, 2002, p. 33). Ultimately, evaluation is "socially situated," and thus interpretations are rooted in the biases and taken-for-granted assumptions of those involved, including both the evaluator and the stakeholders (Beardsley & Miller, 2002, p. 59). The question, posed by Brisolara and Seigart (2007, p. 280), is thus: "How is the role of the evaluator shaped and bounded by her/his personal experiences and characteristics?" Educator skills are similar to those of a facilitator, but emphasis is put on asking provocative questions, naming what is happening (or has happened), and challenging the implicit androcentric bias in the status quo and taken-for-granted "truths." "Facts are not given but constructed by the questions we ask of events" (Lather, 1991, as quoted in VanderPlatt, 1995, p. 90). The evaluator might ask, for example: "What is the nature of the structural and gender inequities within this context? Hesse-Biber and Leavy (2007, p. 144) emphasize the importance of reflecting on difference in feminist research:

> Reflexivity also reminds us of the important role difference plays in our research. Difference enters every facet of our research process. It guides the projects we select, informs the questions we ask and directs how we collect, analyze, write and interpret our data. Differences should be explored and embraced, for ignoring and disavowing them could have negative effects on your data and overall project.

Underlying these practices and skills is the feminist assumption that the personal is political. Both capacity building and reflexivity also abide by the feminist principle that knowledge is not detached from its environment, but rather is fully situated within a context. Here is an example from my own experience: In the late 1990s, I conducted a participatory evaluation of the Besserer Street Drop in Centre for street-involved youth located in downtown Ottawa. To do this, I hired six youth who used the centre and trained them to conduct an evaluation. While I brought the technical knowledge and skills to this process, they brought knowledge and lived experience of the centre and the world of street-involved youth. In teaching them the basics of evaluation, I had to put often complex concepts into plain language. So instead of design, I asked "What do we want to know?" Instead of instruments, I asked "How can we find out (what we need to know)?" Instead of sample, I asked "Who should we talk to?" The youth taught me the language of the streets, much to their amusement, as lifestyles and opinions differed between such subgroups as "skaters," "goths," "punks," and "twinkies." Trust building among them (they were from different subgroupings) and with me was an ongoing challenge, especially when I noted gender biases among them. They were less defensive when such biases and practices were raised about the centre as a whole and in the broader context. All through this evaluation, I was not only in an educator role, but also served as a facilitator, a collaborator, a technical expert, an advocate, and sometimes a referee. (For further details, see Whitmore & McKee, 2001.)

Collaborator

"Feminist evaluations must strive to collaboratively incorporate the participant stakeholders' and the evaluators' voices into the evaluation design and implementation, circumventing the hierarchical organizations context" (Beardsley & Miller, 2002, p. 57). The evaluator as collaborator assumes an equal relationship with stakeholders, as much as is realistically possible. Once this kind of relationship has been established, the evaluator/collaborator strives to make space for all voices, shares power and control, and whenever possible reaches out for consensus in terms of decision making. She or he shares her or his own experience and perspectives and welcomes those of stakeholders. The role of being a partner means a commitment to equality of power and authority in decision making. One option is to build a collaborative evaluation team, consisting of stakeholders committed to the process. This will involve attending to the relationships among team members and consciously working to build trust and confidence with one another.[4] This role reflects the valuing of cooperation rather than competition, and democratic participation. A deep commitment to democratic values and principles underlie this role.

Sielbeck-Bowen, Brisolara, Seigart, Tischler, and Whitmore (2002, p. 6) emphasize the point that collaboration does not guarantee fairness. It can mask the real power of the evaluator, who normally has greater control over the evaluation process and product, though this can depend on the partner organization, its characteristics, and its knowledge of evaluation. The balance of power and control is an ongoing process, and will need to be negotiated explicitly.

Hesse-Biber and Leavy (2007) discuss collaborative interviewing styles in feminist research (p. 15).

> What is feminist about each interview style, however, are the *types of questions* feminists ask. Research that gets at an *understanding of women's lives and those of other oppressed groups*, research that promotes *social justice and social change*, and research that is mindful of the

> *researcher–researched relationship* and the *power and authority* imbued in the researcher's role are some of the issues that engage the feminist researcher. Feminist researchers practice reflexivity throughout the process. This practice keeps the researcher mindful of his/her personal positionality and that of the respondent (Hesse-Biber & Leavy, 2007, p. 117; emphasis in original)

Attention is paid to the interview as the co-construction of meaning (p. 128).

Beardsley and Miller (2002) offer an example of a collaborative evaluation, using a feminist framework. The evaluation was of a women's substance abuse education program that provided educational and relapse prevention services, primarily to lower-income women. They created a nonhierarchical evaluation team, consisting of core staff members (the program coordinator, supervisor, and executive director) and their specific roles, based on their expertise, were negotiated in initial face-to-face meetings. Clients were not included because of confidentiality issues, but, as their voices were considered of equal value to their own and those of other stakeholders, the team found various other ways to incorporate everyone's voices. For example, the team developed cooperative imagery, using herstory[5] as a way to collaboratively engage in the process. Feminist ideals provided the framework for negotiating the team's processes, such as consensus decision making, recognition of power differentials, and team building. "In short, the process of the evaluation took on a role equal to the product or outcome of the evaluation" (p. 62). The team concluded that "group processes developed in the initial meetings allowed us [the team] to collaboratively work through our disagreements" (p. 67).

The methodology consisted of three phases, designed collaboratively by the team, to evaluate professional training services ("Are we changing the system?"), identify educational needs of high-risk women ("Are we doing what we should be doing?"), and determine program effectiveness ("Have we made a difference?"). The feminist framework shaped survey questions, for example, to test professionals' beliefs about substance-abusing women, they were asked to agree/disagree with the statement: "I would feel more uncomfortable working with an alcoholic female than an alcoholic male" (p. 65).

Though this example is used here to illustrate a collaborative evaluator role, the authors recognize the overlap with that of facilitator. They list a number of expectations, including encouraging a feminist model of leadership, balancing power dynamics, facilitating trust building in participants' interactions, and promoting ongoing gender and sociopolitical analysis (p. 68).

Technical Advisor/Methodologist

All evaluators, by definition, bring technical expertise and experience to an evaluation. In a feminist evaluation, the methodologist role focuses on sharing various possibilities for designing and implementing the evaluation, rather than imposing a preassumed design. She or he integrates feminist theoretical principles and theory into the design. So, for example, Humble (n.d.) poses a set of questions to ask when planning and implementing a (development) project. Here is a brief selection:

Project Design and Appraisal
- How might the project affect women's and men's workloads and their access to and control over resources? Does the project have the potential to put extra work on women, and will women be compensated for their contribution to the project if their workloads are increased? Are women's interests and needs as mothers and as nonmothers both being taken into consideration?
- Is there a process for consultation with organizations and communities about the objectives and activities of the project? Are both women and men being consulted? Which women, and which men? What are the mechanisms for consultation (meetings, interviews, surveys, etc.)? Are there barriers that might affect women's ability to participate in consultations on a basis of equality with men, such as heavy domestic responsibilities, lack of access to information, lack of mobility, deference to men in mixed-sex settings, difficulty in talking to outsiders, fear of retribution? How might barriers be overcome?

In Project Implementation and Monitoring
- Has an appropriate gender balance among field staff and project workers (including management) been established in order that both male and female target-group members are able to access project services and participate in activities, and in order that both men's and women's needs and perspectives are incorporated into the project decision-making structures?
- Has the potential for community resistance to women's empowerment activities or organizational resistance to female managers been assessed? Is there potential for backlash against women participants or staff? How can resistance be addressed? What mechanisms for ongoing consultation with project participants are in place for quality checks and results monitoring? Do these mechanisms ensure that both women's and men's views are being heard? Which women and which men?

In Project Evaluation and Renewal

- Were there any negative effects of the project on women and men, their workloads, their access to control over resources, or their social status? Were such effects anticipated at the planning stage? Were the negative effects on women or men adequately compensated for by other benefits from the project?
- Did the project have any positive social and gender equity outcomes that were unexpected at the planning stage? How should these results be understood? Is it possible to anticipate these kinds of outcomes in the next project phase or in other projects?

The feminist evaluator willingly shares her or his technical knowledge and expertise with participants so that they can fully understand what is happening, what certain terms mean, how to implement a particular technique, and how to interpret data and the pros and cons of various reporting possibilities. In this way, the evaluator shares her or his knowledge while guiding the inquiry process.

An example from my own experience illustrates this role. In the late 1980s, I conducted an evaluation of a single expectant mothers prenatal program. These mothers were reluctant to attend mainstream prenatal classes for several reasons. One, the classes were held in hospitals or other downtown facilities, considered "alien territory" to the single mothers, in addition to being a long bus ride away. In addition, the women attending such classes were usually accompanied by their husbands, which made the single mothers feel out of place. The single expectant mothers' program was held in a nearby neighborhood center, familiar to them, and the program had been designed specifically with their needs in mind.

I hired a team of the program participants to be co-evaluators and together we designed the evaluation, collected and analyzed the data, and wrote a report. We integrated questions about gender into the participant questionnaire, such as "Did the classes help you understand your rights as a mother in the hospital?" In crafting the report, we would first discuss it, I would draft the section, and together we would go over it. They flagged the jargon ("them big professor words"), which we discussed and agreed to either include or eliminate. This was also an opportunity for them to learn the vocabulary and be able to use it accurately. After the study was completed, for example, the team presented the results to a broader audience (at a university conference) which resulted in increased confidence and self-esteem, as these women rarely felt "heard" by those they considered more powerful: "I can do this! They were really interested in what we had to say!" They also recognized the value of their own experience and expertise. Later, we discussed why they felt they could obtain better information than I, a university-trained evaluator.

You're dealing with a lot of people on social assistance and welfare.

You're dealing with real hard to reach, low self-esteem people. And when they see anybody coming in that they think is high class or has anything to do with welfare and you working with them, they are scared to death that you're going to squeal on them. . . . They [the respondents] are just scared you work with those people [social work-ers], you deal with them, you're high up there so that they can't trust you 'cuz you're right in with them. But we're not in with them [social workers] and we're not in there to tear them apart. And I think they really know that. (in Whitmore, 1994, p. 82)

Activist/Advocate

Activism and/or advocacy are explicit elements in feminist evaluation (Patton, 2002, p. 104). If, as House (1993) asserts, "evaluation research was invented to solve social problems," our task goes beyond the evalua-tion itself (p. 11). "In our advocacy for a more just world, it is our conten-tion that feminist evaluation can contribute far more than any evalua-tion that does not consider feminist issues or utilize feminist approaches" (Sielbeck-Bowen et al., 2002, p. 110). Ward (2002) explicitly includes col-laboration with advocates and activists in her guidelines for feminist eval-uation. Advocacy and activism thus become an integral part of what we do. At the same time, Patton (2010, p. 163) warns us about maintaining professional boundaries, staying focused on the evaluative tasks, and not getting involved in the actual program work.

Activism takes many forms—from conducting solid research to col-laborating with others to achieve a mutual goal, to lobbying and demon-strating (Whitmore, Wilson, & Calhoun, 2011). It can take the form of advocating for the inclusion of marginalized groups in a sample (Mertens, 2009). It can mean involving feminist advocates in the evaluation process (e.g., on a collaborative panel or advisory committee) (Beardsley & Miller, 2002). Feminist evaluators frequently work with activist organizations (Truman, 2002). This certainly means the evaluator must be explicit about the feminist principles that guide the work. It also may mean following up once a report has been completed. When issues of gender equity (or other inequities) have been revealed, the feminist evaluator would be remiss in not becoming engaged, in some way, in addressing those injustices.

However, it is critical that the evaluator not take the lead in this, but rather "accompany" the stakeholders in their efforts. The notion of accompaniment is consistent with feminist processes (Wilson & Whit-more, 2000, p. 116). Accompaniment (or *acompañamiento*) is a term used by Latin Americans to describe an approach that embodies "a process of sharing and mutual support . . . based on mutual knowledge, a com-mon commitment and solidarity" (Wilson & Whitmore, 2000, p. 103). It is grounded in deep respect for the experience and wisdom of those with whom we work. Ultimately, we accompany our partners' process for it is they who will make the final decisions, especially about what to do with findings and how to proceed.

Considerable work has been done around evaluating advocacy efforts. A relatively new Topical Interest Group (TIG) in the AEA focuses on advocacy and public policy. Though driven primarily by funders' interest in evaluating advocacy efforts, rather than by activists themselves, the challenge is "how best to align evaluation practice with real-world advocacy work" (Riessman, Gienapp, & Stachowiak, 2007, p. 2). Substantially absent from advocacy evaluation is the voice of the advocates themselves (Innovation Network, 2008). Most advocacy/activism evaluation currently focuses on policy change, which Guthrie, Justin, Tom, and Foster (2005) describe as "too narrow" because it overlooks "the work building up to policy change and the implementation of policy once passed." Other authors share the belief expressed by Guthrie et al. (2005) that effectiveness has been too restrictively defined in the advocacy field (Coffman, 2007; Miller, 1994; Miller, 2004). The activist role, then, has an important contribution to make, especially as it is manifested through a feminist lens.

The evaluation profession itself has been an advocate for certain policies. For example, internally, it has actively promoted diversity in the field (Christie & Vo, 2011; Collins & Hopson, 2007; Mertens, 2009; see also the Building Diversity Initiative of the AEA, *www.aea.org*). Likewise with cultural competence (Hood, Hopson, & Frierson, 2005; Thompson-Robinson, Hopson, & SenGupta, 2004; see also the Statement on Cultural Competence in Evaluation (2011), *www.aea.org*). At the same time, AEA has vigorously advocated for certain public policy positions, such as the statement on high-stakes testing (2002) and on the U.S. federal government's proposal on scientifically based evaluation methods (2003) (*www.aea.org*).

Table 3.2 contrasts several evaluation focus areas and their relevant models and evaluator roles. (This is by no means an exhaustive list, but is a selection of models for illustrative purposes.)

Depending on the situation, of course, these models can and do overlap, but for purposes of this discussion, I have separated them. The intent here is in no way to imply a judgment of any model, but rather to elaborate upon them, using a feminist lens. Brisolara and Seigart (2007) pose a critical question here: "Are the feminist aims of the project or evaluation better served by bringing a feminist perspective to a different evaluation model and sacrificing other elements?" All are valid, depending on the context, but could be sharpened in their attention to gender equity. Adding a feminist lens would certainly enhance the quality of the data and increase the validity of the findings. A conscious choice needs to be made, however. Introducing a feminist model in a context that could

TABLE 3.2. Contrasting Models and Evaluator Roles

Purpose	Model/design	Context	Stakeholder involvement	Evaluator role	Feminist lens
Precision; measurement objectivity	Experimental & quasi-experimental evaluation designs	Simple (using Snowdon & Boone, 2007)	None; only as "subjects"	Detached, technical expert; In full control of process	Attention to the distribution (sample) of women & men; Consideration of gender-related factors in the questions asked and in data analysis
Maximizing use	Utilization-focused evaluation designs	Complicated; sometimes complex	Some stakeholder engagement; primarily key decision makers	Depends on primary users (from judge to collaborator). 'Situationally responsive' Directive but shared control	Attention to the distribution of gender re: decision making; Consideration of gender-related factors in analysis
Social justice	• Participatory (P-PE; T-PE) • Empowering • Transformative • Collaborative • Democratic • Developmental	Complex	Maximizing stakeholder engagement, participation	• Negotiator, facilitator, collaborator, educator, technical advisor/ consultant, advocate, critical friend/coach • Evaluator shares/devolves power	Attention to equality and quality of gender participation Consideration of gender-related factors in analysis
Gender equity	FE	Complex	Maximizing stakeholder engagement, participation; with gender/feminist lens	Social change agent: negotiator, facilitator, collaborator, educator, technical advisor/consultant, advocate	Specific focus on gender equity throughout evaluation process

jeopardize the broader aims of a project would clearly be counterproductive (Brisolara & Seigart, 2007). Patton (2002, as cited in Brisolara and Seigart, 2007) reminds us that evaluation frameworks are often mixed, and that a feminist model can contribute to an evaluation even though it may not be dominant.

Finally, it is important to acknowledge that a table, by definition a summary of information, oversimplifies a situation or approach, and should be understood as such. For example, a feminist evaluator could use some combination of all these approaches, depending on the situation. Patton (2008, pp. 211–212) emphasizes the importance of the evaluator being "situationally responsive," asking some fundamental questions about a given situation in order to respond appropriately. One adapts to the circumstances and people involved. I draw upon both in thinking about how to inform our understanding about differing approaches as they related to feminist evaluation.

I use an example of a grade 10 life skills program as a base for each model and apply a feminist lens to each as a way of enhancing the breadth and quality of an evaluation. The "Context" column in Table 3.2 draws on the Cynefin framework (Snowdon & Boone, 2007; see Figure 3.1).[6] Snowdon and Boone developed this framework to guide organizational decision making and Patton (2010) has adapted it to the evaluation context.

In *simple* situations, evaluation can be quite straightforward; for example, one measures the difference before and after an intervention. A controlled, predictable environment is assumed and clear cause-and-effect relationships are easily discernible. There is a high degree of agreement about what the problem is and what the solution should be. The evaluator assesses the facts of a situation, categorizes them, and draws conclusions based on established practice.

In a *complicated* context, there may be more than one right answer and though there may be a clear cause-and-effect relationship, it may not be entirely evident (Snowdon & Boone, 2007). An evaluator must analyze a situation and look at the pros and cons of different options or possibilities. The context is not as controllable as in a simple situation, but nonetheless has some degree of predictability.

Complex situations are unpredictable and in constant flux. Data are incomplete and there is no right answer; rather, over time, patterns can be discerned and a path forward emerges. In complex contexts, there are many opportunities for creativity and innovation; therefore, instead of attempting to impose a given method or draw conclusions too quickly, evaluation practice is emergent. Evaluators focus on identifying the initial conditions, monitoring and documenting what emerges, providing timely feedback, facilitating reflective practice among stakeholders, and embedding evaluative thinking in the process (Patton, 2010, p. 110).

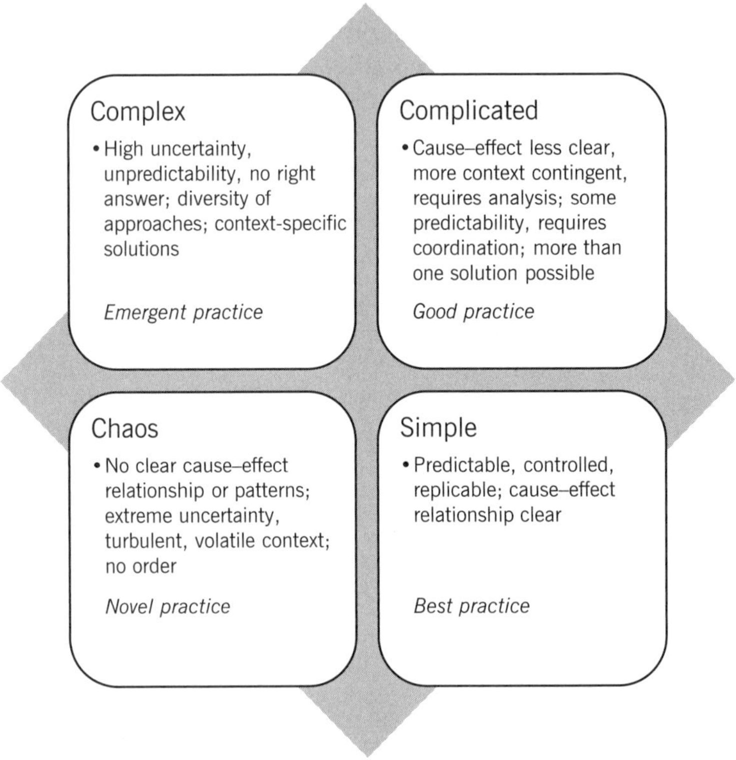

Complex
- High uncertainty, unpredictability, no right answer; diversity of approaches; context-specific solutions

Emergent practice

Complicated
- Cause–effect less clear, more context contingent, requires analysis; some predictability, requires coordination; more than one solution possible

Good practice

Chaos
- No clear cause–effect relationship or patterns; extreme uncertainty, turbulent, volatile context; no order

Novel practice

Simple
- Predictable, controlled, replicable; cause–effect relationship clear

Best practice

FIGURE 3.1. Modified Cynefin framework. Based on Snowdon and Boone (2007).

In *chaotic* situations, searching for right answers is pointless. There is no time for input; someone must take charge and decide what to do. The most important thing is to act immediately to "stop the bleeding" and establish some kind of order. An evaluator has a limited role here, other than to make immediate recommendations or even decisions, if leadership is otherwise lacking (Cousins, Whitmore, & Shula, 2012, citing Snowdon & Boone, 2007).

Below I elaborate briefly on each model and what a feminist lens might add.

Models Focused on Precision, Measurement, and Objectivity

If the primary focus of an evaluation is to measure a program effect with precision and (reputed) objectivity,[7] an evaluator could choose an experimental or quasi-experimental design. These assume a fairly simple context, and stakeholders are engaged only as "subjects," with no input into or control over the process. The evaluator's role is one of observation, as a detached technical expert; she or he is in full control of the process. Bamberger and Podems (2002) offer examples from international development contexts. An evaluation of gender and time-use impacts of the fresh-cut flower export industry in Ecuador, for example, "assessed the impact of women's employment on the allocation of paid and unpaid labor within the household" (p. 91). Afterward, the authors note that "a feminist analysis might also have examined how women used the time saved from domestic chores. Did they use it for leisure and social relations, education, quality time with their family, other income generating activities or simply to rest? They might also have asked if women's greater economic power helped remove other barriers to their empowerment (for example, social constraints on women's ability to travel outside the home)" (p. 92).

In the example of a life skills program for grade 10 students, a feminist lens would pay specific attention to the distribution of male and female students in both treatment and control groups and consider gender-related factors in the analysis. For example, evidence suggests that teenaged girls are more mature and thus could score higher than boys on certain measures (Colom & Lynn, 2004; Tanner, 1971). Thus the evaluator would examine more closely results that indicate gender differences.

Models Focused on Maximizing Use

If the primary focus of an evaluation is maximizing the use of evaluation results, then one selects a utilization-focused design. These are more likely to be appropriate in complicated or complex contexts. There is normally some stakeholder engagement, primarily of those in decision-making positions. The evaluator role can vary enormously, depending on the primary users and the purpose of the evaluation. For example, if the most likely users are funders or officials, the evaluator's primary role is that of judge; if the users are program staff and participants, the evaluator is in a more consultant role; if the evaluator is working primarily with a group of diverse stakeholders, she or he acts mostly as a facilitator (Patton, 2008, pp. 210–211). The evaluator is normally directive (in a very broad sense) but shares control.

In the example of a life skills program for grade 10 students, the utilization-focused evaluator, using a feminist lens, would also take particular note of the gender distribution among decision makers, and consider gender-related factors analyzing the data: who actually makes the decisions (overtly and with more subtle influences) and how do they play out over time in terms of their effects on females and males.

Models Focused on Social Justice

Many evaluation approaches focus, in one way or another, on social justice, among them participatory approaches, empowerment evaluation, transformative evaluation, collaborative evaluation, democratic evaluation, and developmental evaluation. Patton (2002) elaborates a set of "critical change criteria" common to all of these:

> increasing consciousness about injustices, identifying the nature and sources of inequalities and injustices, representing the perspective of the less powerful, making visible the ways in which those with more power exercise and benefit from power, engaging those with less power respectfully and collaboratively, building the capacity of those involved to take action, identifying potential change making strategies, praxis and embedding the evaluation in a clear historical and values context. (p. 103)

These approaches assume that one of the best ways to prevent the imposition of personal biases in the evaluation context is to engage stakeholders in all phases of the process, from initial discussions about conducting an evaluation, through design, implementation, reporting, and follow-up action. They are normally involved in complex situations, and seek to maximize stakeholder engagement and participation.

The evaluator plays a wide variety of roles, from technical advisor to facilitator, consultant, negotiator, collaborator, educator, and at times advocate. Empowerment evaluation (EE) sees the role primarily as a "critical friend or coach." The evaluator shares power/control of the process and either from the outset or more gradually devolves control to stakeholders, depending on the situation (Cousins & Whitmore, 1998). A feminist lens would keep a sharp eye out for gender dimensions in stakeholder participation (not only how many women and men are active, but more subtle aspects of participation—such as who listens, who talks, whose influence is evident and how) and consider gender-related factors in analyzing the data.

In the example of a life skills program for grade 10 students, social justice evaluators would seek to maximize the active engagement of stakeholders, especially the students. The feminist evaluator would pay particular attention to gender balance and participation, and whether this actually resulted in equity in terms of outcomes. If girls, for example, participate equally, but the final decisions still reflect boys' priorities, this outcome needs to be more deeply examined.

Models Focused on Gender Equity

Finally, evaluations with a gender equity focus, primarily feminist evaluation, are fully grounded in feminist values/principles with attention and commitment to the empowerment, personal or social, of women or some change as a result of the evaluation process (Pillow, 2002, p. 16). As with all social justice approaches, the feminist evaluator roles and purposes need to be explicit and formally negotiated with stakeholders (Patton, 2008, p. 182). This process (of negotiation) raises the issue of when (or not) to use the "f" word. (See the section below, entitled "Issues," for further discussion of this topic.)

Feminist evaluations are most likely found in complex situations. Though the evaluator roles are similar to those of social justice approaches, most feminist evaluators seek to maximize stakeholder engagement with special attention paid to the role of women. The word "most" is used here, as feminists using positivist approaches do not engage stakeholders, build capacity, or seek to share power with them. Rather, as stated earlier, the evaluator's use of a feminist lens is based on a deep understanding of women's oppression and the systemic biases and assumptions upon which it is based. This plays out in what is studied, the questions asked and how they are phrased, what behaviors are observed, what gets counted, what is left out and most importantly, how the data are interpreted (e.g., see Gilligan, 1982).

A gender lens with grade 10 students would focus on gender equity throughout the evaluation process. This would start with the initial conception of the program, its purposes, and expectations around outcomes. The feminist evaluator would keep gender equity issues front and center, informing the program design (the initial [and often unacknowledged] philosophical assumptions, what content and skills get included, what gets left out), the process of implementation, emphasizing gender relations (how girls and boys participate, raising awareness of inappropriate and appropriate behaviors and language as they arise, introducing feminist content, asking provocative questions, challenging androcentric bias, bringing in reflexive exercises, and interactive activities such as simulations, role plays, etc.). Outcome measures could include a variety of instruments and activities to gauge the learning (content), attitudes, and behavioral changes around gender equity. A number of issues emerge from this discussion.

Emerging Issues

How to Negotiate among Roles?

Each of these roles is fluid, and dynamic, and thus the evaluator is constantly having to shift among them or to combine them in creative ways. How, then, does the feminist evaluator choose among the various roles? The evaluator doesn't get out a checklist and decide that "today, or in this situation, I'm going to be . . . the technical expert." She or he will play all of those roles in any given situation, and will find herself or himself shifting from one to the other as the need arises. So, for example, a feminist evaluator may be working with school administrators on a survey of drug usage among teens. Here she or he is primarily a technical expert (designing a valid survey, how to frame questions, etc.), but she or he is also an educator, posing provocative questions (e.g., probing the role of male vs. female teachers in working with teens around drug use), a collaborator (working closely with not only the administrators, but with teachers and students in framing the questions and being sure that both males and females are equally represented), and even an advocate when it comes to supporting use of the results. Thus, the feminist evaluator may well play all of these roles in one way or another throughout an evaluation. As always, it will depend on the situation. In a large-scale study, for example, she or he is most likely to be in the technical expert role, but in conversations with the stakeholders will also be an educator and collaborator. In a situation where the evaluator is working with a small group of stakeholders who are interested in participatory approaches, she or he will emphasize the facilitator role.

The roles an evaluator plays will also depend on personal and professional characteristics, strengths, limitations, and her or his own proclivities. Some evaluators are comfortable with a facilitator role where control is shared and the process fluid and unpredictable. Others prefer the role of technical expert, where she or he is likely to have more control and the process is thus more predictable. An evaluator needs to have reflected upon who she or he is, what she or he does best, and when she or he pursues an opportunity or not. No one person is likely to be equally comfortable with all roles; it's a matter of emphasis. Knowing when to get help and team up with others is critical. An evaluator who is an excellent facilitator, and strong with qualitative methods, for example, may want to bring a quantitative methodologist onto the team.

One must always maintain awareness of feminist goals, however, and scrutinize a survey for hidden bias. For example, Gilligan (1982) examined not only the questions asked by Kohlberg, but also the whole framework and set of assumptions about what constituted moral behavior. If men are in the group, the feminist evaluator will pay attention to who speaks and who is silent and work to ensure equal participation. (This may be true in a group of all women as well.) She or he will always work through a feminist lens, however, posing questions to raise awareness yet being cognizant of cultural restrictions. This must be done with caution, however, in certain contexts. For example, urging women in certain cultures to speak out publicly, or even to participate, could be dangerous for them (Hendricks & Bamberger, 2010).

The feminist evaluator works to unpack structural issues that reinforce oppression. In their work on sanitation in rural communities in India, for example, Kar and Chambers (2008) discovered that custom dictated that women were not allowed to defecate in the open fields in the daytime. They could relieve themselves in private (in their hut, in a bucket) or outdoors only before dawn or after sundown. This could have serious health implications, to say nothing of their comfort or lack thereof. Providing a simple outhouse allowed women to go to the toilet at any time, and provided everyone some privacy. This has implications for the evaluator roles and how she or he does the work. In the sanitation project, the top-down (technical expert) approach had not worked (authorities installed latrines, but people continued to use the open fields). Kar and Chambers (2008) approached the situation from the bottom up, using participatory rural appraisal (PRA) techniques (educator, technical expert), collectively mapping the defecation areas (educator) and asking questions such as Where and when do the men go? And where and when do the women go? (facilitator, educator), discussing the health implications (educator), and collectively deciding what to do (collaborator, activist). The success rate has been impressive, as measured by latrines built and actually used, and health outcome statistics.

Power

The power and authority of the evaluator cannot be dismissed, as the position itself brings with it a certain status and expectation of leadership and responsibility. Key questions to be asked are: Whose interests are being served by the intervention? How are these interests reflected in the statement of objectives, rationale, structure, content, and process (VanderPlatt, 1995, p. 93)?

While appropriately sharing personal experiences and information helps to build trust, the evaluator must be aware of maintaining professional boundaries (Hesse-Biber & Leavy, 2007). In working to balance power and authority, the feminist evaluator shares her or his own biography with stakeholders. Hesse-Biber and Leavy (2007, p. 128) raise similar issues for feminist researchers. "Sharing identities and stories breaks down power and authority invested in the role of the researcher." One must be careful not to get too personal with the participants, however, as this can provide a false illusion that there is no power or authority. It might make respondents more vulnerable, encouraging them to reveal even more intimate details (Hesse-Biber & Leavy, 2007, p. 128). "Giving back interpretation and findings to the researched may be only a 'feel-good measure,' and may forego her intellectual responsibility of inter-pretation to gain rapport and approval from respondent" (Hesse-Biber & Leavy, 2007, p. 128).

In setting an agenda, evaluators exert power, however unconsciously or subtlety that may be manifest. Psyche Williams-Forson uses food to describe an episode illustrating how power and privilege work in silence(s). She advises us to "be attentive to the ways in which an evaluator can help to reconstruct or reshape power relations" (Forson, 2010). Her comment reminds me of the time I served lunch to the women participants in the single-expectant mother program (described earlier in this chapter; see Whitmore, 1990). While I used what I assumed were common fare (salad, cheeses, bread), the women looked for hot dogs and chips. The only item on the table that they could even relate to was the carrot sticks! In this case, they were not at all silent, and had no problem making their likes/dislikes known.

Language is power; the words the evaluator uses can clarify or mys-tify. The single expectant mothers very quickly let me know when I used "them big professor words" as we crafted the final report. Sometimes those "big words" could be my little words. For example, they considered the word *specific* to be "a big professor word."

But What about the Rigor?

Isn't all this "mushy," or, even worse, biased? Evaluators are (or should be) technical experts, objective and skilled at examining the merit and worth of a program. There has been extensive discussion of this issue in the literature—What is the appropriate role and objective of an evaluator? There is no question that the evaluator's role in ensuring rigor is essen-tial; how she or he does this is the topic of continued debate. While no consensus has been reached, there is general agreement that evaluations can legitimately have many objectives and thus the evaluator may have multiple roles (Donaldson & Scriven, 2003). All address rigor, though dif-ferently.

Do We Use the "F" Word in Naming the Role?

One question is whether or not to be explicit about one's feminist approach and the consequent role. Should we use the word *feminist* in discussions of our role with stakeholders or evaluands? This could be seen as an ethical issue—one of honesty—but involves risks and responsibilities as well. Are we being truthful when we avoid using the label? The "f" word, as we know, can evoke strong reactions, and misunderstandings, so when should we not "name" it while still using a feminist lens? (Seigart & Brisolara, 2002; Walby, 2011).

Labels can be restrictive, however; words can limit who and what we are. The conundrum is this: the practitioner who names her- or himself a "feminist" may limit the scope of work available; the academic, on the other hand, will want to use the label as she or he needs critique and peer-review in order to grow and learn. Labeling oneself as feminist can be educative, helping others to understand what/who a feminist evaluator is and what she or he does. At the same time, it gives her or him a community that provides support, learning, and colleagues with whom to talk and exchange ideas.

The feminist role can be played by a range of people. Who decides who gets to play this role? Surely, we want all evaluators to use feminist values, whatever the label or role. Though this would be mainstreaming, the option is to have a small cadre of people identified as feminist evaluators who will only play this role, and that would seem quite limiting. Feminist evaluators have to weigh the advantages and disadvantages of labeling themselves and what they do (Walby, 2011). Perhaps more inclusive language needs to be found, since feminist evaluation is about social justice in all its forms; being a feminist doesn't exclude other values—on the contrary. Some suggest the word *transformative*, as this provides an umbrella term on human rights (Mertens, 2009).

It is important to recognize that, in spite of the pervasiveness of gender criteria in such mainstream organizations as the World Bank, USAID, CIDA (Canadian International Development Agency), and so on, some remain unaware of gender issues and would see the role of a feminist evaluator as irrelevant. Caution is needed, however, when working cross-culturally. Engineers building roads in Africa may assume that everyone benefits equally, when women and men are impacted quite differently. A road can significantly change the routines and lifestyles of a village. For example, roads bring in trucks, with lonely drivers who look for services (of all kinds) on a stopover. They also bring imported goods that may displace local produce.

Insider–Outsider Issues Related to Role

In all approaches, the location of evaluators—inside or outside an organization or the evaluand—is a key consideration. An inside or internal evaluator is generally employed by the evaluand; an outside evaluator is an independent consultant and may or may not be employed by a university or an evaluation organization. The roles of the evaluator will have to be discussed and agreed upon, regardless of whether one is inside or outside the organization.

Internal evaluators support organizational development and learning (Love, 2005). If an evaluator is employed by an organization that identifies itself as feminist, she or he still needs to spend time discussing with stakeholders their understanding of the evaluator role and then clarifying specifically what will be expected in terms of the purposes, process, and outcomes of an evaluation.

If independent (or outside) evaluators who identify themselves (overtly or not) as feminist are approached by an organization that may not identify itself as feminist, a more thorough process may be needed. An initial discussion about the evaluator's underlying feminist values will be needed, as will an explanation of the extent to which these are compatible with the evaluand's principles. Assuming agreement, then details of role and expectations would follow. For example, Beardsley and Miller (2002) examined their experience as outside evaluators of a women's substance abuse education program. The evaluators first held face-to-face discussions with key members of the program, who subsequently formed a core evaluation team. The initial team meetings focused on developing a feminist group process and set of principles upon which all could agree. Overall, the authors conclude, "the staff was empowered from the beginning by becoming, with the evaluator, a collaborative feminist evaluation team" (p. 60).

Sometimes an evaluator can be both an insider and an outsider. Truman (2002) describes a collaboration with a gay men's health collective in conducting a large-scale needs assessment of gay men's health issues in northwestern England, particularly focused on identifying "hidden" aspects of the population. The author, though based in a university, was also known to individual members of the collective. This gave her an "insider status" and thus a degree of trust that allowed her to work closely with them in devising a design (especially a sampling strategy) that would reflect the diversity of the population in question.

Insider/outsider issues go beyond this, however. One is also inside or outside of a particular cultural, racial, or class grouping, for example. Can a feminist evaluator (or any evaluator for that matter) effectively negotiate certain boundaries, such as those of race and class? Can a white middle-class woman, for instance, effectively work with black working-class women or men? Being black is hardly monolithic, any more than being white; race is intertwined with other differences such as class, ethnicity, and cultural backgrounds. An example from my own experience illustrates this point. As the evaluator for a program serving single expectant mothers from

Spryfield, a working-class section of Halifax, Nova Scotia, I was interviewing program participants with a view to hiring them as co-evaluators (this was to be a participatory evaluation). I assumed that meeting them (and their children) in their own homes would make the encounter more informal and relaxed, and that we'd just "get to know each other." What I failed to realize was the impact of the class difference between us—I was a social work professor and they were welfare recipients. While this might not have been an issue for me, I was oblivious to their negative history with social workers, who, in their experience, snoop into their lives and have the power to give (or take away) essential resources. From their perspective, I was "way up there" (as they later told me in a debriefing session after the evaluation had been completed). However nice and friendly I may have been, my motivation was questioned and I was assumed to be "checking out" their living situations. Worst of all, I took notes (just as I had been trained to do), nor did it occur to me to show them what I had written down. This only heightened their mistrust! It took many months of working together to undo the damage (Whitmore, 1994).

As emphasized by Hesse-Biber and Leavy (2007, p. 143), I needed to have been sensitive to our differing social statuses and openly discussed them. In an evaluation process, one's insider/outsider status is fluid and can change in the course of a single encounter. It is important to note, however, that the evaluator's role/status can be shared with stakeholders on some issues (white mother with black mothers) but not so easily with others (growing up in very different, class-based neighborhoods).

The Demand for Good "People Skills"

The roles discussed in this chapter require more than a set of skills/techniques to be checked off on a list of capacities. They involve the evaluator as a whole person, including her or his personal values, beliefs, attitudes, knowledge, and skills. As noted earlier, the skills and techniques needed to work effectively with stakeholders are not normally taught in evaluation training programs. Rather, they are learned in programs such as social work, and sometimes nursing and clinical psychology, where the expectation is that, in order to do their work, practitioners must know how to build relationships and gain people's trust. Not surprisingly, these tend to be (predominantly) women's professions. Beardsley and Miller (2002, p. 69) pick up this theme: "Ironically, the feminist evaluator serves in a traditional female role, coordinating relationships, encouraging interactions, supporting others' ideas, and validating the entire process. And just as women's traditional caregiving role is essential to the continuation of such divergent institutions as the economy and the family, so also is this role to be valued as essential to the empowerment of individuals involved in a feminist program evaluation."

Part of good people skills involves a generous dose of humility, knowing what we don't know, recognizing others' knowledge/skills, and welcoming their collaboration with us. At the same time, we need to acknowledge our mistakes, gracefully and, as appropriate, with humor.

Have Fun!

"If I can't dance, I don't want to be part of your revolution."[8] "I did not believe that a Cause which stood for a beautiful ideal, for anarchism, for release and freedom from convention and prejudice, should demand the denial of life and joy" (Goldman, 1970, p. 56, as cited in Whitmore et al., 2011, p. 152).

We should not dismiss the importance of fun in this work (Whitmore & McKee, 2001; Whitmore et al., 2011; see also "The Kit" [www.ysb.on.ca/ The kit]). Feminists are stereotypically seen as having no sense of humor. Not true, of course, but important to keep in mind. A feminist evaluator does best who enjoys meeting people and being challenged. For many, good humor is necessary for just hanging in there and doing the difficult work. Long hours without some laughter tends to burn people out, or they just drop out. "If it isn't fun, youth probably won't want to do it," concluded a participant in a youth center project (Jamieson & Wichman, 2011, p. 104). Similarly, the Calgary Raging Grannies, taking full advantage of their age and stage in life, attribute part of their success to using humor to get their serious message across (Montgomary, 2011). While not made in the context of formal evaluations, these comments were made (by group participants) in response to the question: How do you know you are making a difference?

Technology

Kistler (2011) raises the question of social networking and the evaluation community. She points out that increasing use of social media is changing the evaluation field and how evaluators operate. Gone are the days of identifying program components that define success and then hone in on how to reify and replicate them. Social media challenge us with new types of programmatic goals, geographically and temporally dispersed stakeholders, rapidly changing technology, data proliferation and measuring what matters, and technical expertise requirements (p. 568). How do we "measure" results when the process involves a series of clicks or tweets? Or, as Kistler notes, perhaps the exchange process—of building awareness, of feeling a sense of belonging—is the result (pp. 568–569).

What is the impact on the feminist evaluator role? So far (in this chapter), the discussion of role has implicitly assumed face-to-face interaction (unless one is doing a survey or analyzing secondary data); hence the importance of "people skills." While I would certainly argue that those skills are still (and always will be) necessary, they take on quite different manifestations in social media. Social media definitely invite the incorporation of new voices and expertise—quite compatible with the feminist role. A feminist evaluator can be quite comfortable with the "cultural shift" inherent in social media, including increased communication throughout the evaluation, engaging in more two-way forms of communication rather than traditional forms of reporting, developing strategies that situate stakeholders at the center of decision making, and involving them in data exploration and interpretation (Kistler, 2011, p. 570). An ethos of participatory, collaborative, and developmental approaches is well attuned to feminist evaluation. This is a medium that invites collaboration, and the role of advisor or guide rather than expert (Kistler, 2011, p. 571).

So far so good. But, new tools and strategies are needed for the networked environment, especially for "digital immigrants" (those born before the digital revolution), who need to learn a new language and a different mode of operating. Feminist "digital natives" (born with digital gadgets in their cribs) are/will be essential players, as the evaluator role shifts.

Some Final Thoughts

The prospect of achieving women's equality in the world is an exciting, if formidable, goal. Many people continue to dedicate their lives to realizing it and evaluators committed to this goal can play their part in the process. The key is for evaluators to first become aware of women's oppression, learn about its many manifestations, develop the knowledge and skills necessary to incorporate a feminist lens into their work, and then to take whatever action they can in the context of the evaluation.

The many roles described above require complex thinking, high levels of skill, a clear understanding of what using a feminist lens means, and a commitment to ongoing learning. It presents exhilarating, if daunting possibilities for the feminist evaluator to play a role in contributing to a more just world.

NOTES

1. See Mathison (Chapter 2, this volume) for a detailed discussion of the similarities and differences between research and evaluation.
2. Examples of team-building techniques include "getting to know each other" exercises, sharing expectations (hopes and fears), and such "mundane" things as sharing meals.
3. Heather Menzies is a Canadian author whose works include *Whose Brave New World?* and *No Time: Stress and the Crisis of Modern Life*.
4. Specific team-building exercises are beyond the scope of this chapter, but there are numerous resources on how to do this. See, for example, Chambers (2002) and Coover, Deacon, Esser, and Moore (1985).
5. "Herstory" refers to history (reinterpreted as "his story") written from a feminist perspective, emphasizing the role of women or told from women's points of view (*Wikipedia.org/herstory*).
6. "Cynefin" is a Welsh word (pronounced "coon-ev'in") meaning "habitat, acquainted, accustomed or familiar, being both noun and adjective, and thus requiring context to understand its meaning in any given instance" (Patton, 2010, p. 106).
7. There is extensive discussion in the literature around this issue. See, for example, Droitcour and Kovar (2008) and Scriven (2008).
8. Attributed to Emma Goldman (1931/1970), based on a passage in *Living My Life*.

REFERENCES

Ahmed, D. A. A., Lewando-Hundt, G., & Blackburn, C. (2011). Issues of gender, reflexivity and positionality in the field of disability. *Qualitative Social Work, 10*(4), 467–484.

Bamberger, M. J., & Podems, D. R. (2002). Feminist evaluation in the international development context. *New Directions in Evaluation, Issue 96. Feminist evaluation: Explorations and experiences* (pp. 83–96). San Francisco: Jossey-Bass.

Beardsley, R. M., & Miller, M. H. (2002). Revisioning the process: A case study in feminist program evaluation. In S. Brisolara & D. Seigart (Eds.), Feminist evaluation: Explorations and experiences. *New Directions for Evaluation, 2002*(96), 57–70.

Belenky, M. F., Clinchy, B. M., Goldberger, N. R., & Tarule, J. M. (1986). *Women's ways of knowing: The development of self, voice, and mind.* New York: Basic Books.

Brisolara, S., & Seigart, D. (2007). Feminist evaluation research. In S. N. Hesse-Biber (Ed.), *Handbook of feminist research: Theory and praxis* (pp. 277–295). Thousand Oaks, CA: Sage.

Chambers, R. (2002). *Participatory workshops: A sourcebook of 21 sets of ideas and activities.* London: Earthscan.

Christie, C. A., & Vo, A. T. (2011). Promoting diversity in the field of evaluation: Reflections on the first year of the Robert Wood Johnson Foundation Evaluation Program. *American Journal of Evaluation, 32*(4), 547–564.

Coffman, J. (2007). "What's different about evaluating advocacy and policy change?" *Evaluation Exchange, 13*(1).

Collins, P., & Hopson, R. (2007). Building leadership development, social justice and social change in evaluation through a pipeline program. In J. W. Hanuum, W. Martineau, & C. Reinelt (Eds.), *The handbook of leadership development evaluation* (pp. 173–198). San Francisco: Jossey-Bass.

Colom, R., & Lynn, R. (2004). Testing the developmental theory of sex differences in intelligence on 12–18 year olds. *Personality and Individual Differences, 36*(1), 75–82.

Coover, V., Deacon, E., Esser, C., & Moore, C. (1985). *Resource manual for a living revolution: A handbook of skills and tools for social change activists.* Philadelphia: New Society.

Cousins, J. B., & Whitmore, E. (1998). Framing participatory evaluation. In E. Whitmore (Ed.), Understanding and practicing participatory evaluation. *New Directions for Evaluation, 1998*(80), 5–23.

Cousins, J. B., Whitmore, E., & Shula, L. (2012). Arguments for a common set of principles for collaborative inquiry in evaluation. *American Journal of Evaluation, 34*(1), 7–22.

DeVault, M. L., & Gross, G. (2007). Feminist interviewing: Experience, talk and knowledge. In S. N. Hesse-Biber (Ed.), *Handbook of feminist research: Theory and praxis* (pp. 173–197). Thousand Oaks, CA: Sage.

Donaldson, S. L., & Scriven, M. (2003). *Evaluating social programs and problems: Visions for the new millennium.* Mahwah, NJ: Erlbaum.

Droitcour, J. A., & Kovar, M. G. (2008). Multiple threats to the validity of randomized studies. In N. L. Smith & P. R. Brandon (Eds.), *Fundamental issues in evaluation* (pp. 65–88). New York: Guilford Press.

Forson, P. W. (2010, November 24). On food as a window into power and privilege. AEA365. Retrieved from *www.aea.org*.

Gilligan, C. (1982). *In a different voice: Psychological theory and women's development.* Cambridge, MA: Harvard University Press.

Goldman, E. (1970). *Living my life.* New York: Dover Publications. (Originally published 1931)

Guthrie, K., Justin, L., Tom, D., & Foster, C. (2005, October). *The challenge of assessing policy and advocacy activities: Strategies for a prospective evaluation approach.* Retrieved from *uploadedfiles/Publications/Evaluation/challenge_assessing_policy_advocacy.pdf.*

Hendricks, M., & Bamberger, M. (2010). The ethical implications of underfunding development evaluations. *American Journal of Evaluation, 31*(4), 549–556.

Hesse-Biber, S. N. (Ed.). (2007). *Handbook of feminist research: Theory and praxis.* Thousand Oaks, CA: Sage.

Hesse-Biber, S. N., & Leavy, P. L. (2007). *Feminist research practice.* Thousand Oaks, CA: Sage.

Hesse-Biber, S. N., & Piatelli, D. (2007). From theory to method and back again:

The synergistic praxis of theory and method. In S. N. Hesse-Biber (Ed.), *Handbook of feminist research: Theory and praxis* (pp. 143–153). Thousand Oaks, CA: Sage.

Hood, D. W., & Cassaro, D. A. (2002). Feminist evaluation and the inclusion of difference. In D. Seigart & S. Brisolara (Eds.), Feminist evaluation: Explorations and experiences. *New Directions for Evaluation, 2002*(96), 27–40.

Hood, S., Hopson, R., & Frierson, H. (Eds.). (2005). *The role of culture and cultural context: A mandate for inclusion, the discovery of truth and understanding in evaluative theory and practice.* Greenwich, CT: Information Age.

House, E. R. (1993). *Professional evaluation: Social impact and political consequences.* Newbury Park, CA: Sage.

Humble, M. (n.d.). *A quick guide to gender analysis in health and population projects.* Prepared for Management Sciences for Health (MSH), Boston, MA.

Innovation Network. (2008). Speaking for themselves: Advocates' perspectives on evaluation. A study commissioned by the A.E Casey Foundation and the Atlantic Philanthropies. Retrieved December 10, 2012, from *innonet.org/advocacy*.

Jamieson, S., & Wichman, L. (2011). The youth project, heroes and outlaws: Stories of success. In E. Whitmore, M. G. Wilson, & A. Calhoun (Eds.), *Activism that works* (pp. 92–112). Halifax, Nova Scotia: Fernwood.

Kar, K., & Chambers, R. (2008). *Handbook on community-led total sanitation.* London: Plan UK.

Kistler, S. J. (2011). Technology, social networking and the evaluation community. *American Journal of Evaluation, 32*(4), 567–572.

Kohler-Riessman, C. (1987). When gender is not enough: Women interviewing women. *Gender and Society, 1*(2), 172–207.

Love, A. (2005). Internal evaluation. In *Encyclopedia of evaluation* (pp. 206–207). Thousand Oaks, CA: Sage.

Mathison, S. (2005). Culturally responsive evaluation. In *Encyclopedia of evaluation* (pp. 96–102). Thousand Oaks, CA: Sage.

Mertens, D. M. (2009). *Research and evaluation in education and psychology: Integrating diversity with quantitative, qualitative and mixed methods* (3rd ed.). Thousand Oaks, CA: Sage.

Miller, C. (2004, May). *Measuring policy change: Assessing the impact of advocacy and influencing work* (Unpublished report). Ottawa, Ontario, Canada: C. Miller, Independent Consultant for One World Action.

Miller, V. (1994). *NGO and grassroots policy influence: What is success?* Washington, DC: Institute for Development Research and Just Associates.

Montgomary, S. (2011). Calgary raging grannies: Affective and effective. In E. Whitmore, M. G. Wilson, & A. Calhoun (Eds.), *Activism that works* (pp. 64–79). Halifax, Nova Scotia: Fernwood.

Moss, P. (2007). Emergent methods in feminist research. In S. N. Hesse-Biber (Ed.), *Handbook of feminist research: Theory and praxis* (pp. 371–389). Thousand Oaks, CA: Sage.

Patton, M. Q. (2002). Feminist, yes, but is it evaluation? In D. Seigart & S. Brisolara (Eds.), Feminist evaluation: Explorations and experiences. *New Directions for Evaluation, 2002*(96), 97–108.

Patton, M. Q. (2008). *Utilization-focused evaluation* (4th ed.). Thousand Oaks, CA: Sage.

Patton, M. Q. (2010). *Developmental evaluation: Applying complexity concepts to enhance evaluation use.* New York: Guilford Press.

Pillow, W. S. (2002). Gender matters: Feminist research in educational evaluation. In S. Brisolara & D. Seigart (Eds.), Feminist evaluation: Explorations and experiences. *New Directions for Evaluation, 2002*(96), 9–26.

Riessman, J., Gienapp, A., & Stachowiak, S. (2007). *A guide to measuring advocacy and policy.* Prepared for the Annie E. Casey Foundation by Organizational Research Services. Retrieved December 11, 2012, from *organizationalresearch.com* and *accf.org.*

Rosser, S. V. (2007). The link between theory and methods: Feminist experimental research. In S. N. Hesse-Biber, *Handbook of feminist research: Theory and praxis* (pp. 223–256). Thousand Oaks, CA: Sage.

Scriven, M. (2008). A summative of RCT methodology: And an alternative approach to causal research. *Journal of Multidisciplinary Evaluation, 5*(9), 11–24.

Seigart, D., & Brisolara, S. (Eds.). (2002). Feminist evaluation: Explorations and experiences. *New Directions for Evaluation, 2002*(96), 1–114.

Sielbeck-Bowen, K. A., Brisolara, S., Seigart, D., Tischler, C., & Whitmore, E. (2002). Beginning the conversation. In S. Brisolara & D. Seigart (Eds.), Feminist evaluation: Explorations and experiences. *New Directions for Evaluation, 2002*(96), 109–113.

Simmons, A., Reynolds, R. C., & Swinburn, B. (2011). Defining community capacity building: Is it possible? *Preventive Medicine, 52,* 193–199.

Snowdon, D., & Boone, M. E. (2007). A leader's framework for decision making. *Harvard Business Review, 85*(11), 68–77.

Stuart, C., & Whitmore, E. (2006). Using reflexivity in a research methods course: Bridging the gap between research and practice. In S. White, J. Fook, & F. Gardner (Eds.), *Critical reflection in health and social care* (pp. 156–171). Berkshire, UK: Open University Press.

Tanner, J. M. (1971). Sequence, tempo and individual variation in the growth and development of boys and girls aged 12–16. *Daedalus, 100*(4), 907–930.

Thompson-Robinson, M., Hopson, R., & SenGupta, S. (Eds.), (2004). In search of cultural competence in evaluation: Towards principles and practices. *New Directions for Evaluation, 2004*(102).

Truman, C. (2002). Doing feminist evaluation with men: Achieving objectivity in a sexual health needs assessment. In S. Brisolara & D. Seigart (Eds.), Feminist evaluation: Explorations and experiences. *New Directions for Evaluation, 2002*(96), 71–82.

VanderPlatt, M. (1995). Beyond technique: Issues in evaluating for empowerment. *Evaluation, 1*(1), 81–96.

Volkov, B. B. (2011). Beyond being an evaluator: The multiplicity of roles of the internal evaluator. In B. B. Volkov & M. E. Baron (Eds.), Internal evaluation in the 21st century. *New Directions for Evaluation, 2011*(132), 25–42.

Walby, S. (2011). *The future of feminism.* Cambridge, UK: Polity Press.

Ward, K. J. (2002). Reflections on a job well done: Well? In S. Brisolara & D.

Seigart (Eds.), Feminist evaluation: Explorations and experiences. *New Directions for Evaluation, 2002*(96), 41–56.

Whitmore, E. (1990). Empowerment in program evaluation: A case example. *Canadian Social Work Review, 7*(2), 215–229.

Whitmore, E. (1994). To tell the truth: Working with oppressed groups in participatory approaches to inquiry. In P. Reason (Ed.), *Participation in human inquiry* (pp. 82–98). London: Sage.

Whitmore, E. (1998). "We need to rebuild this house": The role for empowerment in an evaluation of a Mexican farmer's cooperative. In E. T. Jackson & Y. Kassam (Eds.), *Knowledge shared: Participatory evaluation in development cooperation* (pp. 217–230). West Hartford, CT: Kumarian.

Whitmore, E., & McKee, C. (2001). "Six street youth who could . . ." In P. Reason & H. Bradbury (Eds.), *Handbook of action research: Particupative inquiry and practice* (pp. 396–402). London: Sage.

Whitmore, E., Wilson, M. G., & Calhoun, A. (Eds.). (2011). *Activism that works.* Halifax, Nova Scotia, and Winnipeg, Manitoba: Fernwood.

Wilson, M. G., & Whitmore, E. (2000). *Seeds of fire: Social development in an era of globalism.* Halifax, Nova Scotia: Fernwood/New York: Atlas.

CHAPTER 4

A Transformative Feminist Stance

Inclusion of Multiple Dimensions of Diversity with Gender

Donna M. Mertens

We must meet our obligations to the world's women and children. We must do so not just to achieve MDG3 [Millennium Development Goal 3]. We must do so because healthy women are the answer to solving many of the world's most complex and pressing problems: poverty, hunger, disease, and political instability.
—UNITED NATIONS DEPUTY SECRETARY-GENERAL ASHA-ROSE MIGIRO (2011)

Introduction

Deputy Secretary-General Migiro's statement serves to both raise the issue of how women and girls can be viewed as a single entity and to ask why it is important to address their important dimensions of diversity. The United Nations (UN) is a leader in supporting ethical and pragmatic reasons to address the needs of women around the world and the need to do so with recognition of their heterogeneity. Women who live with poverty, hunger, disease, and political instability have significantly different life experiences than women of privilege. Hence, I argue that evaluators who work in communities with a goal of furthering human rights for women and the people who share their life spaces need to be aware of and able to implement approaches to evaluation that are responsive to the bases of differential experiences, including geographic regions; economic levels; religion; race/ethnicity; disability; deafness, refugee, immigrant, or indigenous status; tribal affiliations; and sexual identity. This argument has relevance for both domestic and international evaluators.

Addressing diversity in the context of programs specifically focused on women makes visible tensions within the feminist and evaluation communities, for example, use of the word *feminist* versus *gender-focused*, differences in the meaning of feminism in different contexts, and concerns about diluting the focus on women when other dimensions of diversity are included. Podems (2010) addressed the tension in the international development community around the avoidance of a feminist label for evaluations and the use of a gender-focused label as a more politically acceptable choice in the eyes of donor agencies. Podems reminds us that the choice of language has deeper implications in that gender-focused evaluations map women's position in comparison with men, while feminist evaluations challenge women's societal positioning as a result of power differences and critically examine issues of discrimination and oppression on the basis of gender.

I respect those who criticize feminist scholars for not representing their perspectives, for example, bell hooks (1990) and Patricia Hill Collins (2000), who call for black feminism, and Latina scholars Solorzano and Delgado Bernal (2001), who write about Latina feminist theoretical perspectives. I also respect those who make a choice to not label their work "feminist"; however, I argue that inclusion of the wisdom garnered through feminist scholarship should not be sacrificed for political correctness. Rather, evaluations that focus on women and girls should reflect the fact that "gender bias exists systematically and is manifest in the major institutions in society. . . . Feminism examines the intersection of gender, race, class, and sexuality in the context of power" (Mertens, 2005, p. 154). Rather than diluting the impact on gender as a variable, inclusion of diverse dimensions of diversity in reference to women-centered activities provides a means to address the needs of specific subgroups of women.

Feminist scholars recognize that relevant dimensions of diversity beyond gender need to be considered, as is found in this definition of feminist evaluation:

> Feminist evaluation includes judgments of merit and worth, application of social science methods to determine effectiveness, and achievement of program goals as well as tools related to social justice for the oppressed, especially, although not exclusively women. Its central focus is on gender inequities that lead to social injustice. It uses a collaborative, inclusive process and captures multiple perspectives to bring about social change. (Mertens, 2010a, p. 61)

The mention of "especially, although not exclusively women" in the above definition does not explicitly address diversity found within the targeted community in evaluations, nor does it provide guidance as to how to appropriately include women who are oppressed because of a combination of factors, such as economic status, disability, or race. However, the definition does suggest that feminist evaluation has a role to play in stimulating discussion of the potential exclusion of women's concerns in programs that are not specifically focused on women, as well as the need to bring a feminist lens to programs that do focus on women. To this end, a broader umbrella is needed that covers not only gender, but the many other characteristics of women and oppressive societal structures that limit their life opportunities and those of their families. The transformative paradigm is one such philosophical umbrella that prioritizes issues of human rights and social justice and is commensurate with feminist theory, as well as with other theoretical frameworks that have evolved from oppressed communities.

The Transformative Paradigm

The transformative paradigm is a set of philosophical assumptions that serves as a framework to guide the thinking of evaluators who position themselves within an explicitly value-oriented approach that is informed by the goals of increasing social justice and the furthering of human rights. The transformative paradigm is commensurate with feminist theory in that it focuses on power differentials on the basis of dimensions of diversity that are associated with more or less access to privilege, including gender. It can be succinctly described as a framework that

> is applicable to people who experience discrimination and oppression on whatever basis, including (but not limited to) race/ethnicity, disability, immigrant status, political conflicts, sexual orientation, poverty, gender, age, or the multitude of other characteristics that are associated with less access to social justice. In addition, the transformative paradigm is applicable to the study of the power structures that perpetuate social inequities. Finally, indigenous peoples and scholars from marginalized communities have much to teach us about respect for culture and the generation of knowledge for social change. (Mertens, 2009, p. 4)

The transformative paradigm builds on Guba and Lincoln's (2005) contribution to the scholarly community's understandings of the meaning of a paradigm in the evaluation context. Guba and Lincoln describe four major philosophical belief categories that constitute a paradigm:

1. The axiological assumption refers to the nature of ethics.
2. The ontological assumption refers to the nature of reality.
3. The epistemological assumption refers to the nature of knowledge and the relationship between the knower and that which would be known.
4. The methodological assumption refers to the nature of systematic inquiry.

The transformative paradigm (Mertens, 2009, 2010a; Mertens & Wilson, 2012), made up of these four philosophical assumptions, provides a framework for exploring the use of a social justice lens in evaluation. The transformative paradigm's philosophical assumptions are commensurate with evaluating programs that address the needs of women in their full diversity. These include:

1. Axiological beliefs that reflect explicit concern with human rights, social justice, discrimination, oppression, and power differences.
2. Ontological beliefs that call for the recognition of power in the identification and privileging of various versions of reality with a conscious effort to identify those versions of reality that either support or hinder the pursuit of social justice.
3. Epistemological beliefs that address issues of cultural competence, respect, and establishment of appropriate relationships with the diverse stakeholders, with particular focus on those whose voices have traditionally been excluded.
4. Methodological beliefs that support the use of culturally appropriate methods that provide data viewed as credible by all stakeholders and that link that data to social action.

The Transformative Axiological Assumption

The transformative axiological assumption includes the following concepts: respect for cultural norms, furtherance of social justice and human rights, reciprocity, and recognition of community strengths. This assumption is in accord with the United Nations' declarations and resolutions that recognize the rights of women (1979), racial minorities (1969), children (1990a), migrant workers (1990b), people with disabilities (2006a), and indigenous peoples (2006b). The United Nations' actions on behalf of marginalized groups provide a partial listing of the relevant dimensions of diversity that evaluators need to consciously address in their work. Gender is one basis of discrimination, but there are many more. Relevant dimensions of diversity are contextually dependent; hence, the need to identify the dimensions that are relevant within each evaluation study. The transformative paradigm can be useful in raising questions about the dimensions of diversity, in addition to gender, that are relevant within an evaluation contest.

The transformative axiological assumption suggests that we need to have active engagement with members of the communities in which we work to have sufficient knowledge of their cultural norms and how to behave in respectful ways. If we position ourselves as working toward social justice and human rights, how does that change our work as evaluators? What do we do differently than if we did not set these principles as primary definers of the ethics of what we do? The UN (1948) did approve the Universal Declaration of Human Rights to recognize the need to attend to the rights of all people and then added the Convention on the Elimination of All Forms of Discrimination against Women (CEDAW) to specifically focus on the rights of women. However, in recognition that everyone was not being afforded their rights, they also passed the aforementioned declarations of rights for indigenous peoples, people with disabilities, refugees and immigrants, and children. How do these multiple dimensions of diversity come into the ethical discussion of evaluations that focus on gender equity?

The transformative evaluator would give considerable reflection to these questions:

- What are the ethical principles that guide my work? How does the use of a feminist lens guide my work?
- How do these ethical principles reflect issues of culture and power differences? How are issues of gender addressed in terms of power differences?
- How can this evaluation contribute to social justice and human rights?
- What rights does this program advance under CEDAW, the Millennium Development Goals, and other women's rights?
- If I accept that this is a desirable goal for the evaluation, what would I do differently in terms of methodology? (Mertens, 2010b, p. 5)

Flaskerud and Nyamathi (2000) provide an example of how these transformative axiological questions can be answered in an evaluation of an HIV education program for low-income Latina women. The evaluation was conducted using a feminist, community-based, collaborative model that is commensurate with the transformative axiological assumption in that the authors began their work by acknowledging that their ethical principles included building the participants' knowledge and skills with the objective of translating those knowledge and skills into the power to be active agents in improving their health and clinical care. The authors explicitly addressed issues of power differences in terms of their social positions and the position of the participants. They noted that all evaluators and participants were women (except for three advisory board members) and that they shared lower-class origins, immigrant status, and farm-laborer experiences. They did note that the evaluators and participants differed in terms of their access to resources and they tried to address this by "reimbursing participants, providing child care and snacks, and conducting the program in an available and trusted community setting" (p. 330).

The evaluation began with a 3-month period in which focus groups were used to bring to visibility the norms and beliefs of the women participants around the topic of AIDS causes, prevention, and treatment. The focus groups were conducted in Spanish by Mexican American women trained in group leadership in collaboration with the evaluators themselves. Three meetings of an advisory board composed of community leaders and experts in culture were held to discuss the interpretation of the focus groups' results.

The Transformative Ontological Assumption

The transformative ontological assumption holds that there are various versions of reality. It is the evaluator's responsibility to investigate the sources of these different versions and to highlight the consequences of privileging one version of reality over another. In evaluation contexts, this might be seen as persons in power who believe that people with disabilities are not capable of independent living. This might lead to keeping people with disabilities at home, rather than supporting them in terms of transportation, education, or employment. If the person with a disability is a woman, this version of reality might be even more strongly held such that women with disabilities are viewed either as an embarrassment to a family or being in need of extra protection as compared to men. However, women with disabilities may want to and be capable of being productive members of society. Thus, the investigation of the various versions of reality from the perspective of issues of power and privilege leads to uncovering those versions of reality that have the greatest potential to realize the goals of social justice and respect for human rights. In terms of critical self-reflection with regard to the ontological assumption, the evaluation would ask the following questions:

- To what extent will the evaluation be designed to reveal different versions of reality? How will the experiences of men and women be made visible in terms of their versions of reality?
- How will the evaluator determine those versions of reality that

have the potential to either support or impede progress toward social justice and human rights?

- What were the consequences of identifying these versions of reality? How will the cultural norms and beliefs that have the potential to silence women be addressed?
- How did this evaluation contribute to the change in understandings of what is real and provide potential to address discrimination and oppression of women?

The focus groups in the Flaskerud and Nyamathi (2000) study of HIV/AIDS in low-income Latino communities identified different versions of reality in terms of the women's beliefs about the transmission, prevention, and treatment of AIDS. The different versions of reality were used as a basis for the development of the educational intervention. For example, some women had accurate knowledge about the transmission of the disease; others believed that AIDS could be transmitted casually from mosquitoes, toilet seats, and swimming pools. Their beliefs about prevention were also diverse, ranging from the use of condoms to washing after sex. They were also unaware of the extent of the problem of AIDS in the Latino community. Thus, the program developers used these different versions of reality as the basis for the content to be included in the intervention, including specific information about AIDS in the Latino community. The women expressed fear of infection from their male partners, so the education program also incorporated HIV testing and information about how to use condoms and how to negotiate the use of condoms. The evaluators were aware of the need to balance negotiation skills with fear of violence that might result from the women's advocacy for condom use with their partners. In the Latino community, cultural constraints arise related to the use of condoms from "religious prohibitions against birth control, value of children, and the association of condoms with sex workers or secondary partners" (p. 334).

The Transformative Epistemological Assumption

The transformative epistemological assumption recognizes the need for an interactive link between the evaluators and the full range of stakeholders in order to be responsive to the axiological and ontological assumptions that precede this assumption. Furthermore, evaluators need to be capable of uncovering the relevant dimensions of diversity, as well as interacting and supporting appropriate interaction strategies with all members of the stakeholder groups. This assumption raises questions about the skills needed in order to interact appropriately in the diverse cultural contexts in which we find ourselves as evaluators. This epistemological assumption is particularly germane to feminist evaluations because of the traditions in many cultures that silence women.

The American Evaluation Association's (2011) statement on cultural competency provides guidance in terms of this concept: "Cultural competence is a stance taken toward culture. [It] is not a discrete status or simple mastery of particular knowledge and skills. A culturally competent evaluator is prepared to engage fully with communities to capture important cultural and contextual dimensions."

Operating from a transformative epistemological stance directly addresses the need to examine competencies related to working within culturally complex communities in respectful ways. The transformative paradigm contributes these questions to this discussion:

- What are the skills necessary to engage in evaluations that promote social justice and human rights in terms of the types of relationships needed to accomplish this work successfully? How does the evaluator take the positioning of women in a cultural context into account?
- What is the nature of the relationship between the evaluator and the stakeholders? What are the implications of the evaluator's gender in terms of relating to the stakeholders?
- What evidence is there that the evaluator addressed issues of power differentials explicitly and that the voices of the least powerful are accurately expressed and acted upon? What strategies can be used to enhance the opportunity for women's voices to be heard in contexts in which they are traditionally silenced?
- How did the evaluator establish a trusting relationship with stakeholders? (Mertens, 2010b, p. 6)

Flaskerud and Nyamathi (2000) reported the use of a variety of strategies to establish relationships between themselves, the community workers, and the participants in order to address issues of trust and diversity within the community. The collaborative model they used meant that the participants and evaluators worked together as equals and shared responsibility for developing the evaluation questions, the intervention, and the evaluation of the intervention. The participation of the women in the focus groups was possible because of the adaptation of methods to be responsive to the particular cultural group:

> Language and low literacy levels had to be taken into consideration for all educational materials. Fears of deportation were widespread. The women believed that if they were discovered to be infected with HIV, they would be deported. Trust and confidentiality, therefore, became

of utmost importance in the project. The women were also poor . . . and reimbursement for participation was essential. Constraints of space and the women's hesitancy about having their blood drawn resulted in a decision to use finger-stick HIV-antibody tests for the initial screening. (pp. 331–332)

In addition to these measures, members of the community were hired as assistant investigators and were trained to interview the participants, in order to have shared ethnicity, language, culture, and social positioning.

The Transformative Methodological Assumption

The transformative methodological assumption suggests the need for an interactive link with communities as a starting point for methodological decision making and actions. The transformative paradigm's methodological assumption is commensurate with adopting a cyclical approach to evaluation that begins with clarification of values and involvement of communities. These initial methodological stages constitute qualitative moments in data collection that inform subsequent decisions about appropriate next steps in methods. These decisions might lead to quantitative or qualitative or mixed methods; however, they will be rooted in what is considered to be culturally appropriate practices. The results of each cycle of data collection will be vetted through members of relevant communities and used to inform the next steps of the data collection process. Such an approach allows for an extension of how evaluators might address "Are we doing the right things?" in a way that allows for responsive changes if the evaluation uncovers evidence that the versions of reality that were used to frame the definition of the "problem" or the intervention are not those that provide fruitful avenues for advancing social justice and human rights.

The UN's evaluation framework as it applies to gender-focused evaluation is most salient in the evaluation of UNIFEM-sponsored programs and initiatives.[1] The United Nations Development Fund for Women (commonly known as UNIFEM) had a mission to foster women's empowerment and gender equality. They used a rights-based approach to strengthen women's economic security and rights; combat violence and HIV and AIDS; and promote gender equity in governance in both conflict and nonconflict situations. UNIFEM used guidance from the United Nations Evaluation Group (UNEG; 2005) for human rights and gender equality in evaluation.

Evaluation in UNIFEM was guided by six key principles: "women's empowerment and gender equality, human rights, people-centered development, UN system coordination on gender equality, national ownership and managing for results on women's empowerment and gender equality" (2009, p. 3). It also abided by key evaluation standards: "participation and inclusiveness; utilization focused and intentionality; transparency, independence and impartiality; quality and credibility; and ethical" guidelines (2009, p. 3).

Evaluation in UNIFEM was defined by the UNEG Norms for Evaluation as

> an assessment, as systematic and impartial as possible, of an activity, project, programme, strategy, policy, topic, theme, sector, operational area, institutional performance, etc. It focuses on expected and achieved accomplishments, examining the results chain, processes, contextual factors and causality, in order to understand achievements or the lack thereof. It aims at determining the relevance, impact, effectiveness, efficiency and sustainability of the interventions and contributions of the organizations of the UN system. An evaluation should provide evidence-based information that is credible, reliable and useful, enabling the timely incorporation of findings, recommendations and lessons into the decision-making processes of the organizations of the UN system and its members. (2009, p. 3)

To this end, UNIFEM and its successor organization, UN Women, used gender analysis tools as an integral part of their evaluation strategies. Gender analysis is described as follows:

> The term "gender analysis" is used to describe a systematic approach to examining factors related to gender. It involves a deliberate effort to identify and understand the different roles, relationships, situations, resources, benefits, constraints, needs and interests of men and women in a given socio-cultural context. (International Training Centre of the International Labour Organization, 2009, p. 16)

Gender analysis focuses on the identification of variables that contribute to gender inequalities so they can be addressed. This might include differences in conditions, needs, participation rates, access to resources and development, control of assets, decision-making powers, and so on between women and men. Gender analysis raises the questions as to the need for different measures for men and women and how gender equality presents at a variety of levels in the programs (e.g., grassroots, service delivery systems, and the highest political levels).

By the inclusion of gender analysis as a tool in evaluation, UN Women provides a mechanism to address inequities on the basis of gender. If this tool is placed within an evaluation conducted from a transformative stance, then it becomes part of a cyclical process of examining relevant dimensions of diversity in addition to gender that need to be addressed in order to advance social justice and human rights. There is compatibility between the evaluation framework as it is conceptualized within UN Women and the use of a transformative lens to plan and implement evaluations. When such a lens is brought to the evaluation, additional questions are raised that have the potential to increase the power of UN Women's evaluations toward achieving their goals. Evaluators can reflect upon the following questions to guide their thinking:

- How was a cyclical design used to make use of interim findings throughout the study? How were the voices of women from diverse groups included in establishing the focus and data collection plans for the evaluation? To what extent did evaluators engage with the full range of stakeholders to gather quantitative and/or qualitative data that enhance their understandings of the community? Were the data disaggregated by gender and other relevant dimensions of diversity?
- To what extent were the methods used responsive to the specific needs of the different stakeholder groups? How were the needs of diverse groups of women addressed in order to give them access to full participation?
- How were the methodologies designed to enhance use of the evaluation findings to support the pursuit of social justice and human rights? How did the methodological lens contribute to identifying inequities on the basis of gender and other relevant dimensions of diversity? (Mertens, 2010b, pp. 7–8)

A cyclical approach was used in the Flaskerud and Nyamathi (2000) study. As mentioned previously, the study began with focus groups that were used to determine the different versions of reality that were held by the participants. These evaluation data were used as a basis for the development of the intervention that was culturally responsive in the content and the methods used in the intervention. For example, the information about HIV/AIDS was presented in the form of comic books and *telenovela* videos. Evaluation during the process of the program implementation was facilitated by the use of trained community members to interview the participants. The data collected during the implementation illuminated several topics that were used to make modifications to the intervention. For example:

1. One issue that came to light from the evaluation data was that many of the participants were reusing syringes without proper cleaning. The evaluators had assumed that instruction on cleaning

syringes should focus on repeated use of syringes for illegal drug injection. They saw very little evidence of such use, and therefore proposed deleting this from the training. However, the community researchers revealed that over 90 percent of the participants reused syringes to inject medications such as antibiotics that they had purchased over the counter in Mexico. The developers added a segment to the training on the proper cleaning of syringes with bleach and made bleach available to the participants.

2. The use of condoms did not initially increase, except for younger, unmarried women. The program developers decided that they needed to repeat the importance of the preventive effect of condom use every month. This resulted in a significant increase in the use of condoms; however, the increase continued to be primarily for younger, unmarried women. Married women who wanted to avoid pregnancy also increased their use of condoms.

Theoretical Lenses

The transformative paradigm is commensurate with thinking that emerges from the use of multiple theoretical lenses, including feminist theories, rights-based theories, critical theory, critical race theory, disability rights theory, queer theory, and indigenous theories (Mertens & Wilson, 2012). Using the appropriate combination of these theoretical perspectives leads to asking questions that are related to the dimensions of diversity that are relevant to a particular context and designing the evaluation to be responsive to these relevant dimensions.

The Intersection of Transformative Assumptions and Theoretical Lenses

The transformative assumptions serve to explicitly address the need to address diversity within groups of women and girls in contextually appropriate ways. For example, the axiological assumption is linked to methodological decisions that can be informed by active engagement with community members in order to understand the relevant dimensions of diversity in that context. Being aware of feminist theories, critical race theories, indigenous rights theories, and others provides a means to make inquiry about the dimensions of diversity that need to be considered, as well as to interrogate issues of power differentials and discrimination that present challenges in the evaluation. Evaluators can plan their evaluation methods to encompass strategies to identify the cultural norms within communities that relate to gender and other dimensions of diversity such that they can identify those that are supportive of, or deleterious to, the pursuit of human rights and social justice. They can plan with community members how to support those norms that support human rights and social justice and challenge those that sustain an oppressive status quo. They can build strategies into the evaluation that facilitate the creation of conditions that have increased potential to leave the community, including the women and girls, better off than before they began the evaluation. Strategies such as increased knowledge, capacity or changes in policies or practices can be considered and discussed within the stakeholder groups in ways that recognize the need for authentic engagement and cultural appropriateness.

Examples of how to do this can be seen in the Flaskerud and Nyamathi (2000) study in that they recognized that cultural beliefs that served as barriers to the use of condoms needed to be made visible and challenged. As noted previously in this chapter, the women's beliefs that inhibited the use of condoms included the religious prohibition of the use of birth control and the societal belief that condoms were used by sex workers. In order to challenge these beliefs, the intervention was developed to include the teaching of negotiation skills so women could be protected from HIV/AIDS infection.

The condition of women and girls with disabilities provides an example of how the intersection of the transformative paradigm and social justice-oriented theoretical lenses can bring greater understanding in evaluation studies. Gender, disability, and race intersect in interesting ways. In the United States, boys are twice as likely as girls to be identified with a disability (U.S. Department of Education, 2003). Incident rates for males are much higher for autism, serious emotional disturbance, learning disabilities, and speech impairments. Differences by gender become more complicated with consideration of race/ethnicity. Black males are more likely to be identified as mentally retarded or emotionally disturbed than either white males or females, or black females. For an evaluator who is engaged to evaluate a special education identification and placement program, having this knowledge is not sufficient. The evaluator will gain added insights by applying a transformative paradigm and the lenses of feminist theories, critical race theories, and disability rights theories. Additional insights for new evaluators can be gleaned from examples of studies that employ a transformative feminist lens. For example, the Flaskerud and Nyamathi (2000) study illustrates many strategies that evaluators can use to combine the use of feminist theories and critical race theories. Evaluators can explore additional ideas for combining transformative theories such as feminist, critical race, and disability rights by answering the questions presented in the following section.

Based on feminist theories, the evaluation that would emerge from such a critical stance might ask questions such as:

- Is the picture of incidence of disabilities by gender an accurate picture?
- Is there overidentification of boys, and, if so, what variables contribute to overidentification?
- Do girls manifest the indicators of disabilities differently than boys do?
- Does this lead to the underidentification of girls and consequent failure to provide the supportive services necessary for girls to achieve success in school and later life pursuits? (Mertens, 2012).

Based on critical race theory, the evaluator might ask:

- Who has the power to make decisions about the identification of students' disabilities and what is their understanding of the racial/ethnic cultures that are relevant?
- Is the picture of disabilities for students of color an accurate picture?
- Is there overidentification of black males because of cultural differences or other variables?

Disability rights theories add questions related specifically to the definition of disabilities and the means of identifying and placing children, such as:

- What are the definitions of the disabilities that are used for identification and placement?
- What culturally specific behaviors might contribute to inappropriate identification and classifications?
- What measurement instruments are used to make decisions and are relevant cultural groups involved?

Shettle (2009) examined the status of women with disabilities in the international development community and identified a number of dimensions of diversity that required additional attention, not least of which is the type of disability. Disabilities include those with physical impairments that require wheelchairs to those who have learning disabilities and require additional support in education and employment. Even within the disability categories, the nature of the disability that influences the types of accommodations necessary can range from fairly mild to quite severe. In addition to these characteristics, women with disabilities also include variations in terms of sexual identities and orientations, whether they are young or old, whether they are refugees or immigrants. They are often viewed as marginalized populations within marginalized populations.

In the developing world, education is often devalued for women and girls, and girls with disabilities are in double jeopardy when it comes to opportunities for an education (Shettle, 2009). Given scarce resources in high-poverty areas combined with the additional skills necessary to effectively teach students with disabilities, it is not surprising that girls and women with disabilities are at the lowest levels of education. This lack of education has implications for their abilities to obtain meaningful employment and enjoy independence and self-control over their life choices. Shettle identified the following concerns that are relevant for evaluation of programs that focus on women and girls:

1. Women with disabilities that also belong to other minority and marginalized groups face a compounded effect of the unique challenges of each group, which further entrenches the exclusion they face.
2. Girls with disabilities are less likely to have access to health care services, education, and assistive devices compared to boys with disabilities.
3. Aging with disabilities receives little attention in the development agenda. This affects issues such as health, economic status, safety, and care facilities for women with disabilities in advanced age.
4. Women refugees with disabilities face unique challenges due to inaccessible facilities and camps.

Given the recognition of these critical dimensions of diversity associated with groups of women and girls domestically and internationally, and given the harsh consequences of current practices of denial of access to essential life experiences and opportunities, it behooves evaluators to adopt a transformative stance that provides guidance for the creation of evaluations that encompass the range of diversity that is found in these populations.

Conclusions

Women and girls are a diverse lot. Attention to relevant dimensions of diversity in the evaluation context increases the potential to bring attention to the needs of individuals and communities in which these women and girls live. The transformative paradigm provides a philosophical umbrella that provides a framework for thinking about the dimensions of diversity in programs for women and girls from the axiological assumption's emphasis on social justice and human rights. The ontological assumption calls for a recognition of different versions of reality and the social and contextual variables that lead to those versions. It also demands the use of a critical lens in interrogating those versions of reality to determine which are more supportive of the furtherance of human rights and which are more likely to sustain an oppressive status quo. Epistemologically, the evaluator needs to be able to establish a trusting relationship with stakeholders that is respectful and supportive and allows for authentic engagement with all stakeholders, including those from marginalized communities in their full range of diversity. Methodologically, evaluators need to devise ways to include members of the community into the development, implementation, and use of the evaluation. Cyclical approaches that allow for ongoing feedback and community interaction provide opportunities to make changes that allow program developers and service providers to better address the needs of the diverse population of women and girls in their programs. This pathway is not without challenges; however, it does provide hope that evaluators can broaden their feminist lens to be inclusive of women and girls so that relevant dimensions of diversity are added to gender throughout the process of evaluations.

NOTE

1. UNIFEM was merged with other UN initiatives that address the needs of women in late 2010. Nevertheless, the UNIFEM policies and practices that were produced in that earlier timeframe have relevance for this discussion and so are included here.

REFERENCES

American Evaluation Association. (2011). AEA Public Statement on Cultural Competence in Evaluation. MA: Author.

Collins, P. H. (2000). *Black feminist thought: Knowledge, consciousness, and the politics of empowerment*. New York: Routledge.

Flaskerud, J. H., & Nyamathi, A. M. (2000). Collaborative inquiry with low-income Latina women. *Journal of Health Care for the Poor and Underserved, 11*(3), 326–342.

Guba, E. G., & Lincoln, Y. S. (2005). Paradigmatic controversies, contradictions, and emerging confluence. In N. K. Denzin & Y. S. Lincoln (Eds.), *The Sage handbook of qualitative research* (3rd ed., pp. 191–216). Thousand Oaks, CA: Sage.

hooks, b. (1990). *Yearning: Race, gender and cultural politics*. Boston: South End.

International Training Centre of the International Labour Organisation. (2009). *Training module: Introduction to gender and development*. Turin, Italy: Author.

Mertens, D. (2005). Feminism. In S. Mathison (Ed.), *Encyclopedia of evaluation* (p. 154). Thousand Oaks, CA: Sage.

Mertens, D. M. (2009). *Transformative research and evaluation*. New York: Guilford Press.

Mertens, D. M. (2010a). *Research and evaluation in education and psychology: Integrating diversity with quantitative, qualitative, and mixed methods* (3rd ed.). Thousand Oaks, CA: Sage.

Mertens, D. M. (2010b). Social transformation and evaluation. *Evaluation Journal of Australasia, 10*(2), 3–10.

Mertens, D. M. (2012). Special education and gender. In J. A. Banks (Ed.), *Encyclopedia of diversity in education* (pp. 2062–2064). Thousand Oaks, CA: Sage.

Mertens, D. M., & Wilson, A. T. (2012). *Program evaluation theory and practice: A comprehensive guide.* New York: Guilford Press.

Migiro, A. R. (2011, March 8). *Investing in women and entrepreneurship: Solutions to addressing MDG3.* Presentation made to the United Nations Office for Partnerships and the U.S. Chamber of Commerce's Business Civic Leadership Center, U.N. Headquarters, New York, NY.

Podems, D. (2010). Feminist evaluation and gender approaches: There's a difference? *Journal of Multidisciplinary Evaluation, 6*(14). Retrieved from *http://survey.ate.wmich.edu/jmde/index.php/jmde_1.*

Shettle, A. (2009). *Women with disabilities in development: Intersecting invisibility, intersecting realities.* Washington, DC: Global Partnership for Disability and Development.

Solorzano, D. G., & Delgado Bernal, D. (2001). Examining transformational resistance through a critical race and latcrit theory framework: Chicana and Chicano students in an urban context. *Urban Education, 36*(3), 308–342.

UNIFEM. (2009). *UNIFEM evaluation policy.* New York: Author.

United Nations. (1948). *Universal declaration of human rights.* United Nations, New York. Retrieved February 11, 2008 at *www.un.org/Overview/rights.html.*

United Nations. (1969). *The international convention on the elimination of all forms of racial discrimination.* United Nations, New York. Retrieved February 11, 2008 at *www.ohchr.org/english/law/pdf/cerd.pdf.*

United Nations. (1979). *The convention on the elimination of all forms of discrimination against women (CEDAW).* United Nations, New York. Retrieved February 11, 2008 at *www.un.org/womenwatch/daw/cedaw/text/econvention.htm.*

United Nations. (1990a). *Convention on the rights of the child.* United Nations, New York. Retrieved February 11, 2008 at *www.ohchr.org/english/law/pdf/crc.pdf.*

United Nations. (1990b). *International convention on the protection of the rights of all migrant workers and members of their families.* United Nations, New York. Retrieved February 11, 2008 at *www.un.org/millennium/law/iv-13.htm.*

United Nations. (2006a). *Convention on the rights of persons with disabilities.* United Nations, New York. Retrieved December 20, 2010 at *www.un.org/disabilities/default.asp?id=259.*

United Nations. (2006b). *Declaration on the rights of indigenous peoples.* United Nations, New York. Retrieved March 21, 2007 at *www.un.org/esa/socdev/unpfii/en/declaration.html.*

United Nations Evaluation Group. (2005). *Norms for evaluation in the UN system.* New York: United Nations.

United States Department of Education. (2003). *29th Annual Report to Congress on the Implementation of the Individuals with Disabilities Education Act.* Washington, DC: Author.

WEB-BASED RESOURCES

Disability Rights International
www.disabilityrightsintl.org

Provides resources regarding persons with disabilities; it has a special section on advocacy for the ratification of the UN Convention on Rights of Persons with Disabilities.

Global Partnership for Disability and Development
www.gpdd-online.org

The GPDD is an alliance of disabled people's organizations, government ministries, bilateral and multilateral donor agencies, UN agencies, NGOs, and national and international development organizations to promote the economic and social inclusion of people with disabilities in developing countries.

Harvard Law School Project on Disability
http://hpod.org/activities/events-detail/disability-and-race

Provides research and evaluation resources related to disability and race, ranging from education, poverty, housing, and civil rights.

United Nations Entity for Gender Equality and the Empowerment of
    Women
www.unwomen.org

Contains documents related to how the UN is working to achieve the Millennium Development Goals (MDG), with specific emphasis on how addressing MDG3 (related to women and girls) needs to be considered in relation to all the other MDGs.

Office of Special Education and Rehabilitative Services
www2.ed.gov/about/offices/list/osers/osep/index.html

Provides information about infants, toddlers, children, and youth with disabilities (ages birth–21 years), including support for research and statistical data on the demographics of the special education population in the United States.

CHAPTER 5

Feminist Evaluation for Nonfeminists

Donna Podems

Introduction

Programs that aim to change the lives of women, the disempowered, and the "poorest of the poor" are implemented in developed and developing countries all over the world. Often attached to these programs are evaluations that intend to improve, judge, or create knowledge from program activities. A program evaluation, according to Robert Stake (2004), is "the pursuit of knowledge about value" (p. 16). Few evaluation approaches assert their values as openly as feminist evaluation, and while every evaluation approach pursues knowledge laden with its own, often implicit, values, hardly any come under as heavy criticism as feminist evaluation.

Not a feminist? This chapter explores how feminist evaluation can be useful—even for nonfeminist evaluators—by discussing the key challenges that often prevent the use or consideration of feminist evaluation, providing a practical description of feminist evaluation, and demonstrating effective use of feminist evaluation by a nonfeminist with an evaluand that is not about women. Thus this chapter describes how a practitioner would implement, draw from, or be guided by feminist evaluation, not by how a feminist would implement evaluation. This is an important distinction.

Challenges to the Use of Feminist Evaluation

Program evaluations often explore an intervention within some aspect of society and with a particular focus on specific human beings. Rarely simple, these situations are often complicated, and in many instances complex, and more often than not a combination of the three. Designing an appropriate evaluation that will provide empirical information in a multifaceted political, social, and cultural environment, in a timely fashion and within budget, is challenging at best. Understanding a plethora of approaches enhances an evaluator's potential to develop a cultural-, social-, and technical-appropriate evaluation.

One approach often disregarded by evaluators is feminist evaluation, a somewhat new approach that lies outside of mainstream evaluation (Seigart & Brisolara, 2002). This chapter encourages evaluators to explore and consider feminist evaluation as an additional approach that would bring value to an evaluator's range of knowledge and skills, and to join in bringing feminist evaluation into the mainstream.

Confusion over Who Defines Feminism, What Defines a Feminist, and Who Applies the Feminist Label

Numerous definitions and understandings of feminism exist; this complicates how people understand feminist evaluation (Podems, 2010). When I first mention feminist evaluation, rarely do people first ask me about the approach. Rather, I find that often people make assumptions about what feminism is (and is not) and are not often willing or interested in engaging in a discussion about feminism. After all, I am most likely there to discuss evaluation, not feminism. Therefore, the initial challenge I face is not defining feminism; it is accepting that people have preconceived notions and that they bring those assumptions to bear on what they think is feminist evaluation. The first challenge, then, is to resist the attempt to discuss feminism (unless invited to do so) at an academic or theoretical level. Rather, a focus on feminist evaluation (discussed below) is often more useful, though a quick explanation of the common threads found in all feminisms (e.g., a belief that men and women should have equal access to opportunities, in all spheres of life) may be judicious.

A related challenge to the initial inquiry to feminist evaluation is, Does one need to be a feminist to implement feminist evaluation? Before I address this question, I discuss what defines a feminist and equally important, who, if anyone, gets to decide that someone is a feminist. For instance, if I define feminism in a particular way, and someone else meets those criteria, do I have a right to label her or him a feminist even if she or he proclaims not to be one?

In practical terms, some feminist values appear to overlap with values rooted in other ways of thinking. For example, feminists believe in a woman's right to own property and not be abused by men. Many people who do not identify as feminists also hold such beliefs. This is the next complexity: in the multifaceted world in which we live a person is often guided by more than one value system. While feminism (a specific definition or our chosen interpretation of that definition) may influence a feminist's thinking, more than likely this thinking and its resulting actions are also guided by other overlapping or additional value systems (e.g., religious or cultural beliefs) in their lives. This brings us back to the question, Does someone else have the right to label a person a feminist if she or he appears to have feminist values, or does a person have to claim to be (or not be) a feminist? I proudly identify as a feminist, and as a feminist I work toward social transformation. However, others may think that I do not have feminist values since, for instance, I like it when a man opens a door for me.

Do you need to be a feminist in order to implement feminist evaluation? While identifying as a feminist may be an advantage because a person is comfortable using the word, in my experience it is not critical to using or drawing on feminist evaluation. In order to bring feminist evaluation into the mainstream it is important to dissolve this widely held belief that you need to be a feminist to implement feminist evaluation. I suggest that it is not important to identify as a feminist (or even to know much about feminism) if this approach, or elements of it, appear to provide value to an evaluation's appropriateness, credibility, and feasibility. While I argue that a person does not need to be a feminist, or identify as a feminist, in order to implement, be guided by, or draw from feminist evaluation, there are people who would not be likely aspirants to use the approach, such as a misogynist or perhaps a philistine.

This same argument is not to be confused with how to label feminist evaluation. Here I would suggest that if an evaluation is labeled "feminist evaluation" it does need to address the core tenets of feminist evaluation (described in this chapter and by Brisolara, Chapter 1, this volume). However, given that very few evaluation methodologies are "pure" (i.e., only draw from one evaluation approach), I do not consider this a conundrum. Most likely an evaluation that draws from or is guided by feminist evaluation also incorporates other approaches, which are described within an evaluation's methodology, and do not always result in a label for the evaluation explicitly linked to a specific approach.

The next section discusses another key challenge that I face when applying this approach: confusing feminist and gender approaches.

Lack of Concrete Examples

Another key challenge to using feminist evaluation is a misunderstanding of what is or qualifies as feminist evaluation. This may be related to the lack of published examples. There is a dearth of feminist evaluation illustrations in academic journals, books, and published papers, particularly when compared with the many examples of feminist evaluation's doppelganger: gender-responsive approaches.

Why are there so few published examples of feminist evaluation? Several reasons have been identified. Denise Seigart (2005) provides two of them; she claims that feminist evaluation is a rather new approach in the evaluation field and also suggests that evaluators are hesitant to formally label their approach as feminist. A third point was noted earlier in this chapter; there is rarely a "pure" approach when evaluating a programme. An evaluator who authors an evaluation article may choose a label that, while still appropriate, is more encompassing or recognizable (and perhaps more palatable), such as an "impact evaluation."

A fourth related point is that there are few published examples of other mainstream approaches incorporating or embracing feminist evaluation; this is one way that other newer research and evaluation approaches have gained notice and respect. Take, for example, mixed-methods evaluation. In evaluation, this is a relatively new concept that has gained tremendous momentum over the past decade. While books and other scholarly discussions on mixed-methods approaches are readily available, there are few that describe how to use mixed methods guided by feminist evaluation (Hodgkin, 2008). While the lack of published examples of how to use feminist evaluation to guide evaluators remains a challenge, this chapter and this volume seek to address this situation and contribute to the field.

The Name

The label provokes a challenge. As Sielbeck-Bowen, Brisolara, Seigart, Tischler, and Whitmore (2002) note, the word *feminist* invokes multiple types of responses. Using a word that may cause offense, or at the very least provoke people, often militates against an academic or practical discussion of the approach itself. Other more commonly known evaluation approaches tend to use rather soothing or engaging words (e.g., utilization, empowerment, goal-free) that do not immediately elicit defensive responses; at the very least such titles neutralize the emotional response to the second part of their title, the word *evaluation*.

Including "feminist" and "evaluation" in the same title is a challenge. Both words often elicit initial apprehensive or other strong emotions (Patton, 2008). In order to address this challenge I often find that when I use a feminist evaluation approach, removing the feminist label helps. For example, introducing various feminist evaluation ideas while not using the word *feminist* can (and in my experience has) result in an approach that produced a useful process, a process that led to evaluation findings that the primary user found appropriate and informative. Applying feminist approaches and not using the label "feminist" can allow for use of the approach without the potential backlash, or its nonuse. However, not identifying feminist elements of an evaluation approach as hailing from feminist evaluation has consequences.

First, "hiding" uses of feminist evaluation does not provide examples of feminist evaluation that others can learn from, as noted earlier in the chapter. For instance, published examples of feminist evaluation would allow for others to understand how feminist evaluation is used as a stand-alone model or with other approaches. Second, not publishing examples of feminist evaluation does not allow the model to be externally critiqued based on its approach, and therefore evolve and improve over time.

Thus not labeling an evaluation as "feminist evaluation" or identifying its influence when used in combination with other approaches contributes to the challenges identified in this chapter's introduction regarding feminist evaluation. On the other hand, not using the feminist label may facilitate the actual use of the approach. While presenting a conundrum, using a feminist evaluation approach or using an element of it but not labeling it as such may often be far more realistic. Deciding whether or not to use or refer to the feminist label may depend on the evaluator's reason for using feminist evaluation; Is it to further a feminist agenda through evaluation? Or is it to develop a credible evaluation and evaluation process? The two may not be mutually exclusive. Let me offer a final comment on labels: while academic journals and books habitually encourage labels and descriptions, in my experience, it is not as common in practice that evaluators clearly label their evaluation approach.

While the next section introduces some key challenges to using feminist evaluation in a developing-country context, many of these challenges overlap with the challenges mentioned above, with a slightly different twist. At the same time, some challenges mentioned in the next section are also issues that I have faced when discussing or attempting to apply feminist evaluation in developed countries.

Challenges in the International Development (or Developing Country) Context

When working in developing countries and introducing feminist evaluation, the discussion almost always revolves around the notion that feminism is a Western concept, so why would it be appropriate in a non-Western developing country? I would like to address this issue with several points. First, the use of gender frameworks in the development context is not often (if ever) challenged based on its use of the term "gender," yet published gender-framework approaches are mostly developed by donors based in developed (Western) countries (Bessis, 2001).

Second, program evaluation itself is a Western concept. Most program evaluation approaches that are found in today's academic journals and books have been developed in the West, or developed by an author situated in the West, and applied in the development context. For instance, Michael Patton's *Utilization Focused Evaluation* is the only evaluation approach publicly endorsed by the African Evaluation Association—a Western approach by a Western theorist. David Fetterman's *Empowerment Evaluation* is widely known and used in southern Africa; this is another Western approach by another Western thinker. Other examples of evaluation approaches developed by Western evaluators and often drawn upon in the developing-context setting include Donna Mertens's Transformative approach, Realist Evaluation, Outcome Based Evaluation, and Goal-Free Evaluation. While used in the developing countries, these approaches rarely elicit this criticism. Perhaps they should.

I would like to root the next discussion in this argument and examine if it is the feminist label that brings strong reactions or is it the actual approach? For this discussion I would like to raise several distinct arguments. In my experience, few evaluators or donors understand or can explain feminist evaluation, yet most are familiar with gender approaches. Moreover, as noted above, there are few published examples of feminist evaluations. Therefore, it is highly unlikely that the approach is shied away from because evaluation practitioners and donors have enough experience or knowledge to determine that the approach is inappropriate or not useful. Therefore there must be another reason, which may be the feminist label.

While the feminist label and the lack of understanding about what feminist evaluation is raises two possibilities for feminist evaluation not being viewed as a popular approach, a third potential reason for the common reaction to feminist evaluation could be its value-laden label (feminism) combined with the perceived lack of evaluative guidance in feminist evaluation. However, other words commonly used in developing countries also lack clarity and appear to be value-laden, and these words are not often viewed by most as contentious. For example, numerous donor agencies and nonprofit organizations (NPOs) promote the idea of empowerment. This is rarely defined—What does it mean to empower someone? If we empower someone, then is someone else disempowered, and if so how then is that empowerment? Who exactly are we empowering if we empower "poor people"? In what sense are we empowering them? Are these versions of empowerment culturally-specific or appropriate? Can one be empowered in one way and still lack empowerment in another? This provides just one example of often used but rarely defined terms that are readily acceptable to most evaluation practitioners in the developing-country context, and a popular word used by many international donors.

As there is a lack of empirical evidence that identifies the reasons for the slow uptake of feminist evaluation, these arguments are based on my experience.

Acknowledging the Challenges and Moving Forward

Key to addressing the challenges mentioned above is engaging with the discussions below. First, we need to understand feminist evaluation; What exactly is meant by this approach? Then, given that gender approaches are often confused with feminist evaluation, I present a concise discussion of the more common gender approaches. The gender framework section is not meant to be a comprehensive discussion; rather, this section contrasts how feminist evaluation and gender framework histories resulted in distinct and yet faintly intertwined approaches.

Implementing a gender approach is not necessarily (and often not in my experience) the same as implementing a feminist evaluation, and choosing to use or draw from a gender approach has its feminist criticisms. As a result, understanding both approaches is key to addressing many of the challenges mentioned in this chapter. Further, engaging in this discussion will form the basis from which to begin to discuss whether feminist evaluation offers a useful approach to feminists and nonfeminists alike.

Feminist Evaluation

Clarifying Concepts: Gender and Sex

Before clarifying the differences between feminist evaluation and gender approaches, it is important to clarify concepts used by both: "gender" and "sex." Each time I fill out a survey that asks for my gender and provides the choice of male or female (rarely have I seen the category "other" offered), I want to provide this category and write, by my U.S. socialization I would define myself as 75% female and 25% male. Of course, what they are asking about (I am pretty sure) is my biological sex.

In the 1970s, the term "gender" was popularized as an analytical term. Anne Oakley (1982) was one of many feminist theorists who began to use "gender" to describe those characteristics of men and women that are socially and not biologically determined. Other feminist theorists used the terms "sex" to describe anatomical differences between females and males and "gender" to refer to the socially constructed relationships between women and men (Barrett & Phillips, 1992; Scott, 1986). In feminist evaluation and gender approaches the word *sex* is used as an analytic category to make a distinction between males and females. There are also critics of these two categories as some literature argues that male and female categories are also limiting (Hood & Cassaro, 2002). In international development, the term "gender" also has its critics. As Cornwall, Harrison, and Whitehead summarize, "Diluted, denatured, depoliticized, included everywhere as an afterthought, 'gender' has become something everyone knows that they are supposed to do something about" (Cornwall, Harrison, & Whitehead, n.d., p. 1).

Roots and Growth of Feminist Evaluation

Understanding the difference between feminist evaluation and gender approaches will help an evaluator to understand how to use them separately, when to incorporate them into other approaches, and when—if at all—to apply them. Feminist evaluation's particular history and growth untangles it from gender approaches.

Feminist evaluation is rooted in feminist theory and research. Denise Seigart (2005) put forward the idea that the women's movement influenced feminist theory and feminist research, and encouraged researchers and evaluators "to question what it means to do research, to question authority, to examine gender issues, to examine the lives of women, and to promote social change" (pp. 154–155). Feminist evaluation draws heavily on a feminist research argument that a story written based on a man's experience is missing half of the picture; adding a woman's perspective enables a researcher to more fully construct a picture of reality (Connelly, Li, MacDonald, & Parpart, 2000). Over the years (and described in very broad leaps), feminist research has moved from feminist empiricism, to standpoint theory, and finally to postmodern feminism. Postmodern feminism makes defining feminist evaluation slightly challenging (Flax, 1990). As other sections in this book describe feminist theory and the feminist evaluation approach in more detail, I'll frame the rest of my chapter by providing a succinct overview in order to compare and contrast feminist evaluation with gender approaches.

Defining Feminist Evaluation

Part of the challenge in using feminist evaluation is defining it, particularly when feminist evaluation can be described as "fluid, dynamic, and evolving" (Seigart & Brisolara, 2002, p. 2). Unlike most gender approaches, feminist evaluation does not provide a framework. Rather, feminist evaluation theorists tend to describe the theory as flexible and do not advocate a precise approach; rather, feminist evaluation is often defined as a way of thinking about evaluation (Beardsley & Hughes Miller, 2002; Hirsch & Keller, 1990; Hughes, 2002; McRobbie, 1982).[1] Feminist evaluation does not stand alone; not all mainstream evaluation approaches provide frameworks. For example, Robert Stake (2004), when writing about Responsive Evaluation, also notes that he provides a way of thinking about evaluation and not a formula.

Equally challenging are the multiple definitions (and variations) of feminism, as noted earlier in this chapter. Seigart (2005) describes postmodern feminism as an approach that encourages the exploration and acknowledgment of multiple perspectives and realities in the process of research and "avoids the creation of grand narratives or theories" (p. 155). Hood and Cassaro (2002) further explore and define feminist approaches to research by stating: "Feminism as a paradigm for social inquiry falls under the genre of critical theory. It utilizes poststructuralist notions that challenge assumptions of universal concepts and essential categories and acknowledges that 'reality' is socially constructed" (p. 28).

In defining feminist evaluation, I use the term "feminism" with the following understanding: "A common belief that guides feminism is that gender bias exists systematically and is manifest in the major institutions in society. . . . Feminism examines the intersection of gender, race, class, and sexuality in the context of power" (Mertens, 2005, p. 154).

What guidance is provided by a feminist evaluation perspective? Six fundamental beliefs are often used to guide this approach (Patton, 2002; Sielbeck-Bowen et al., 2002). Sielbeck-Bowen et al. (2002) defined these six tenets as follows:[2]

- Feminist evaluation has as a central focus the gender inequities that lead to social injustice.
- Discrimination or inequality based on gender is systemic and structural.
- Evaluation is a political activity; the contexts in which evaluation operates are politicized; and the personal experiences, perspectives, and characteristics evaluators bring to evaluations (and with which we interact) lead to reflect a particular political stance.
- Knowledge is a powerful resource that serves an explicit or implicit purpose.
- Knowledge should be a resource of and for the people who create, hold, and share it. Consequently, the evaluation or research process can lead to significant negative or positive effects on the people involved in the evaluation/research. Knowledge and values are culturally, socially, and temporally contingent. Knowledge is also filtered through the knower.
- There are multiple ways of knowing; some ways are privileged over others. (pp. 3–4)

The concept of knowledge is mentioned in three of the six core beliefs, suggesting that an evaluator who develops or draws from feminist evaluation would place a heavy emphasis on exploring knowledge. This can be interpreted and applied in slightly different yet similar ways.

Elizabeth Minnich (1990) and Michael Patton (2002) explain that feminist approaches recognize and give voice to multiple ways of knowing, including integrating reason, emotion, and experience. For example, when conducting or being guided be a feminist evaluation, an evaluator would recognize that human interactions contain emotions and intuition and that these provide a legitimate source of knowledge (Hughes, 2002). In a slightly different light, an evaluator would seek to identify and differentiate social, political, and cultural contexts that privilege some ways of knowing over others (Sielbeck-Bowen et al., 2002; Stanley & Wise, 1993). For instance, an evaluator would actively seek out people from different social groups or political viewpoints, each of whom may bring new and insightful data. Finally, an evaluator would analyze the data and attempt to identify alternative explanations to men's (or those in power) understanding of reality and way of knowing (Gilligan, 1982; Stanley & Wise, 1993).

Other evaluation approaches are not silent on this topic. In fact, several evaluation theorists suggest the importance of involving people who are affected by the evaluation process and who may not necessarily be members of the most powerful or influential group (Cousins & Whitmore, 1998; House, 1993; House & Howe, 1999; Patton, 1997). What feminist evaluation brings to this discussion is emphasizing the importance of valuing and hearing the multiple voices that diverse women bring to the discussion.

Another key point for feminist evaluation is that the practitioner recognizes that evaluation is a political activity which is tied up in the need to be a reflexive researcher. Most evaluators would acknowledge that all evaluations are political. For instance, Thomas Schwandt (2000) writes that evaluations are "moral–political rather than a technical undertaking" (p. 229). Other evaluation theorists also recognize evaluation as a political activity (House & Howe, 1998, 1999; Mertens, 1999; Patton, 2008). Guided by feminist evaluation, an evaluator is reminded to contextualize the research politically and sociopolitically with an emphasis on how gender and other influential discourses influence each person's experience (Olesen, 2000).

Recognizing that evaluation is political also encourages self-recognition of how our own political values influence the process and encourages an explicit recognition. Although qualitative research (Jewiss & Clark-Keefe, 2007; Ryan, Greene, Lincoln, Mathison, & Mertens, 1998) and the American Evaluation Association's (2004) *Guiding Principles for Evaluators* call for self-reflection, feminist evaluation insists that the evaluator explicitly recognize that she or he is neither value-free nor dis-interested, and that she or he is a political being. Feminist evaluation asks evaluators to be explicit regarding their issues, values, and interests at the evaluation's onset (Hood & Cassaro, 2002; Olesen, 2000; Thompson, 2001; Truman, 2002). This reflexivity is intricately linked to every aspect of feminist evaluation design, including the evaluator's ability to ensure power sharing with the people, project, or program being evaluated (Patton, 1997, 2002, 2008).

A feminist evaluation encourages an evaluator to view her- or himself as an activist. Feminist evaluation processes and findings should attempt to bring about change (Olesen, 2000). The approach allows for and actively encourages an evaluator to explicitly use the process and its findings to further the cause of a particular group. Often, a driving force for implementing feminist evaluations is to positively impact the provision of increased social justice for women and other exploited and disadvantaged people, and to hear previously unheard and marginalized voices, regardless of their origin. Few other evaluation approaches address this issue so concretely. One that does so is Donna Mertens's (1999) transformative theory. She advocates ensuring that the rights of the previously excluded are addressed and may result in credible information concerning interventions; "transformation can only occur if this information is used to inform policies that effectively address the inequities that create the need for social programs" (p. 12).

When conducting an evaluation, I am rarely afforded the opportunity for a dialogue that allows for such theoretical discussion. Therefore, when using feminist evaluation in any context, I suggest that providing a simple, all-encompassing definition may prove useful in starting a conversation. I further suggest that the best place to start a feminist evaluation conversation with potential interested evaluation users is not to define feminism (as discussed in the introductory part of this chapter) but rather to draw on Michael Patton's (2008) commonly accepted broad description of feminist evaluation. He defines feminist evaluation as an approach that places a strong emphasis on processes that involve participation, encourage empowerment, and advance social justice agendas (Patton, 2008).

Gender Approaches to Evaluation

In contrast to feminist evaluation, gender approaches have a separate history, their own core beliefs, and often bring a specific implementation approach. During my 20 years as an evaluator who focuses on women and human rights issues, not once was I ever asked to implement a feminist evaluation. For evaluations conducted in parts of Asia and Africa, I have been asked to serve as the "gender-attentive" person on multiple evaluation teams, to conduct gender-focused evaluations, and even to apply specific gender frameworks on particular programs. I draw on an interesting example from an experience serving as a gender evaluation expert for an international donor organization that focuses on improving the lives of women. At the bequest of this international organization, I was asked to recruit gender specialists to evaluate programs aimed at bettering the lives of women. I was given strict instructions to never use the word feminism, even in the context of exploring whether or not potential candidates had experience with feminist evaluation.

So what is this gender approach and how does it differ from feminist evaluation? The next section provides a succinct introduction to several gender approaches. The intent is to provide basic information that allows for a focus on comparing it with feminist evaluation and suggesting how the two can be used together. The section is not meant to be an exhaustive review of gender evaluation approaches.

A Brief History of Gender Approaches

The gender approach has a distinctly different history than that of feminist evaluation. In the 1950s and 1960s, interventions designed for women in the developing world were based on a human rights context, and often took a welfare approach (e.g., providing handouts and services, such as clothes and family planning). The approach did not challenge women's status or patriarchal structures, and therefore, as Moser (1993) suggests, this approach remained fashionable well into the 1990s. I would argue that gender approaches were still fashionable in 2011, as a rapid review conducted over several months late in 2010 sampled more than 25 international multilateral and bilateral North American and European donor websites and identified multiple projects using a gender evaluation approach. But let's step back to 1970.

The 1970s brought recognition that women were an important part of a country's growth, particularly in relation to areas traditionally managed by women in developing countries: population and food. Boserup's (1970) *Women's Role in Economic Development* encouraged donor organizations to recognize women as an integral part of any intervention[3] aimed at changing some aspect of people's lives. In 1985, the United Nations made this a formal recognition (Pietilä & Vickers, 1990; Tinker, 1990).

The 1970s brought three main gender approaches to program design, and in a certain way a new approach to evaluation, that aimed at changing women's lives: (1) women in development, (2) women and development, and (3) gender and development. Each approach focuses on women as an analytical and operational research category. Each was developed by and with the sponsorship of Western donors.

Women in Development and Women and Development

The women in development (WID) approach is a liberal approach that emphasizes a focus on poverty. Influenced by the modernization paradigm, the WID approach suggested that underdevelopment was explained by obstacles that could be dealt with pragmatically. The WID approach asserts that women were not efficient in what they were currently doing and therefore interventions were aimed at making women more efficient (Gardner & Lewis, 1996; Ostergaard, 1992). A common approach for evaluating WID interventions included a statistical measurement of women's lived experiences (Connelly et al., 2000).

Women and development (WAD) interventions emerged as the result of dissatisfaction with WID (e.g., the latter approach ignored women's reproductive role), and emerged as a critique of the modernization theory. Influenced by a Marxist approach, WAD-influenced programs are designed based on the assumption that development is a process through which the rich got richer and the poor got poorer. With this in mind, WAD interventions drew a theoretical link between women's position in society and structural changes. Intervention strategies were focused on a developing country's economic, political, and social structures. Evaluations of WAD programs then examined changes in the macrocontext and assumed that if the macrocontext improved, women's lives would also improve.

Gender and Development

Informed by the experiences of and analyses by Western socialist feminists who advocated for WID and WAD, a gender and development (GAD) approach emerged with its roots in socialist feminism and feminist anthropology. A major shift from WID and WAD, GAD replaces women as the analytical category with gender relations. A GAD approach focuses on the interconnection of gender, class, and race and the social construction of their defining characteristics. Like feminist evaluation, some GAD approaches draw lightly on feminist theory and research. For instance, relationships between women and men are explored and, drawing on feminist theory, this approach assumes that gender relations are socially constructed patterns of behavior. This assumption then becomes a part of GAD research decisions and analysis (Bamberger & Podems, 2002; Connelly et al., 2000; Jacobson, 1994).

In addition, a GAD evaluation framework investigates women's material conditions and class position, explores existing patriarchal structures, and identifies ideas that define and maintain women's subordination. GAD gives specific attention to oppression of women in the family by entering the so-called private sphere and also views women as agents of change in the development process. GAD programs would also acknowledge the importance of strengthening women's legal rights, such as the reform of inheritance and land laws (Bamberger & Podems, 2002; Connelly et al., 2000; Jacobson, 1994).

Originally outlined in *Gender Roles in Development Projects: A Case Book* (Overholt, Anderson, Cloud, & Austin, 1984), the Harvard framework is a much-used GAD approach that provides specific data-collection categories. First, an activity profile answers the question of who does what, including gender, age, time spent, and location of the activity. Next, an access-and-control profile identifies the resources used to carry out the work identified in the activity profile. It also encourages data collection regarding access to and control over resource use by men and women. Finally, the Harvard framework provides an approach for mapping factors that influence gender differences in the above two profiles and the project cycle analysis, which examines a project or intervention in light of gender-disaggregated information (Overholt et al., 1984).

Another GAD approach makes further distinctions. Caroline Moser (1993) and Maxine Molyneux and Deborah Steinberg (1995) put forward the theory that there are two types of interests: (1) practical gender interests and (2) strategic gender interests—a distinction that influenced the eventual development of Moser's framework. In her framework, found in her book *Gender Planning and Development Theory, Practice and Training* (1993), Moser provides a systematic and transparent approach to examining practical and strategic gender needs.

Practical gender interests are those defined by women acting to promote perceived practical needs that they have as a part of their given gender role in the sexual division of labor. For example, practical gender needs arise out of concrete conditions; these are immediate perceived needs, such as the need to provide food, shelter, education, and health care. *Strategic gender interests* are derived from a critique of male domination and arise out of an analysis of women's subordination and require changes in the structures of gender, class, and race that define women's position in any given culture. Strategic interests include attaining the goal of gender equality and tackling the issue of women's subordination; therefore they are "often labeled feminist" (Moser, 1993, p. 39).

A GAD framework appreciates the reality that interventions may have different impacts on women and men; therefore data need to be collected from both sexes if the project is aimed at "humans." In addition, most GAD-based frameworks suggest that patriarchal relationships are socially constructed rather than biologically determined. They also often assume that patriarchy exists in a variety of different cultural and economic settings to oppress women. GAD evaluation frameworks encourage the collection of data that examine inequalities in income, work roles, reproductive roles, education, and several other socially constructed concepts and that use gender as an analytical category (Jahan, 1995; Moser, 1993). Moser's (1993) approach brings in a feminist way of viewing women by suggesting that different women experience oppression differently, according to their race, class, colonial history, culture, and position in the international economic order. Although there is a minor focus on understanding the interaction between men and women, the major focus is primarily on women.

Most would agree that gender approaches are perceived as less threatening than feminist evaluation since gender approaches do not overtly seek to challenge the social, political, or power status quo (Longwe, 1995; Ogundipe-Leslie, 1994). Longwe (1995) provides one perspective on how gender and feminist approaches are often viewed in the international development setting. She suggests that since most development agencies work with patriarchal host governments, they would not risk upsetting this relationship by suggesting an evaluation guided by feminist theory and research. Most gender approaches do not bring these same ideals or potential challenges to the patriarchy. Given that they most likely do not seek to change the status quo they are often more acceptable to those in power (Longwe, 1995).

Criticisms of Gender Approaches and Feminist Evaluation

In the international development context, gender approaches are more popular and often more accepted than a feminist evaluation approach. For evaluators working anywhere in the world, the gender approach may appear "appropriate" when designing an evaluation that involves human beings. The short descriptions above provide insight into how various gender approaches offer a variety of ways to incorporate women's issues and gender issues into a program or an evaluation. Many practitioners and evaluation users find these approaches practical, effective, and informative. There are numerous published articles that testify to their usefulness.

Nonetheless, before embracing gender approaches and leaving feminist evaluation behind, it is a good idea to be familiar with the most common feminist criticisms. Feminist criticism of gender approaches provide particular and significant points. These should be considered when determining whether or not to use or incorporate a gender or feminist approach into your evaluation design, or ultimately deciding to use neither.

A feminist perspective points out that WID programs seek to increase women's productivity in relation to the national and global economies with little consideration to how this may influence a woman's daily life. Therefore, an evaluation of a WID intervention would focus on determining if that intervention brought about a change in the national or global economies and, if the shift demonstrates an increase in those, the data would suggest that the intervention appeared effective. What is not generally explored is the effect that the intervention made upon the woman's life. Reasonably, it could be assumed that this intervention made her life more difficult by adding increased responsibilities and work to her already full day. However, we will not know if this has happened because the WID-focused evaluation would not likely explore this potential reality. While a general feminist critique of WID, WAD, and gender approaches is that they fail to challenge male-dominated power structures (McClean, 2000), others may see this as a strength of the approach.

Moreover, the WID- and WAD-influenced evaluation approaches often only evaluate women as a homogeneous class, not distinguishing between racial, ethnic, or other differences (Mohanty, 1997). In the international development context, Mohanty points out that many gender evaluations use the term "third-world woman" as an analytical category. Mohanty contends that using this term presents an artificial picture that all third-world women are the same. Moser (1993) contends that women experience oppression differently, according to their race, class, colonial history, culture, and position in the international economic order. The practical differences between a woman who lives below the poverty line, is a single mother of one, and is illiterate from a woman living below the poverty line who supports seven children and has a basic education are many. Further, women with the same attributes living in different developing countries would more than likely bring differences that influence how an intervention affects their lives. Gender approaches also appear to ignore lesbian, bisexual, transgender, transvestite, and transsexual categories, whereas feminist evaluation would not exclude these groups (Podems, 2010).

Therefore, a relatively common assumption is also a common criticism: the assumption that what works for one group of people must work for another (Connelly et al., 2000). Evaluations designed on the basis of feminist evaluation theory would tend to acknowledge and value these differences, not considering "women" to be a homogeneous category. Moser's (1993) framework acknowledges some of these differences, whereas most gender evaluation frameworks tend to ignore them. Expanding this thought, no group is truly homogeneous: the "poorest of the poor," "businessmen," or even "men." In designing, implementing, and evaluating programs aimed at improving the lives of people, drawing on these discussions may positively influence the evaluation design.

The question is then what happened to the feminist ideals in these approaches aimed at improving the lives of women? Bamberger and Podems (2002), Jahan (1995), and Reid (1995) suggest that these approaches to improving the lives of women resulted from economic pressure rather than feminist pressure, and from development agencies (patriarchal structures) rather than feminist influences.

Unlike gender approaches that are often described, criticized, and debated, few people openly criticized feminist evaluation based on its methodological or epistemological approach in published literature. While this could be due to the lack of published feminist evaluation articles and examples as noted earlier in this chapter, the reality is that this lack of published criticism exists.

Gender approaches appear to have benefited from wide criticism; various versions of gender approaches have emerged and address some of the criticisms faced by earlier approaches. It is my hope that this chapter, and this volume, will broaden people's knowledge of feminist evaluation and bring about scholarly criticism from a theoretical standpoint and practitioners' criticism from field-based experience. Engaging with these criticisms will help to identify weaknesses, thereby challenging and strengthening the feminist approach.

Key Distinctions for Practitioners: Applying Feminist and Gender Approaches

There are practical differences between evaluations that draw primarily on feminist evaluation and those that use a gender approach. In the preceding section, I mentioned that gender approaches do not challenge (or in any way dispute) women's position in society. If an evaluation is needed that only records the differences between men and women in different ways, a GAD approach may be appropriate. Feminist evaluation challenges and attempts to strategically improve women's lives, while most GAD approaches tend to map them. Therefore, feminist evaluation would be used to guide the evaluation methodology if the evaluation questions seek to understand *why* differences exist between men and women (Moser, 1993) and to bring about social change.

In addition to making women more efficient in their current roles, some development interventions assume that equality with men is one goal of an intervention aimed at women. An evaluation influenced by gender approaches is useful if this assumption is not (and should not) be challenged. As noted by Maitrayee Mukhopadhyay, gender approaches have become a "technical fix" and an approach that is ahistorical, apolitical, and decontextualized, and that "leaves the prevailing and unequal power relations intact" (in Cornwall et al., n.d., p. 4). A feminist evaluation would take a more activist approach and through its evaluation design explore the possibility that perhaps not all women want what men have, nor do all women have the same wants, needs, and desires as men, or even other women.

Let's take a practical example. A widespread development intervention is one that focuses on women gaining access to the previously male-dominated workforce. Using the Harvard framework as the guiding approach, the evaluation would examine whether or not, as a result of this intervention, women did acquire access to and control of that resource. Enhancing the evaluation approach with the Moser (1993) framework would expand our evaluation methodology and bring in additional categories to explore, such as a woman's strategic and practical gender needs. If the approach were further influenced by feminist evaluation, then additional questions and analysis regarding the assumptions regarding what this particular group of women wanted and how the intervention met those needs would be included. The evaluation design would most likely seek to identify how the intervention succeeded in identifying and addressing structural barriers. Finally, the evaluation's empirical findings would then be used to initiate change.

Some evaluation practitioners prefer different levels of guidance on how to practically apply a specific evaluation approach. Feminist evaluation offers broad guidance that encourages an evaluator how to think about an evaluation, and how to use that reflection to inform the evaluation's design, data collection, and communication of findings. Gender approaches often provide more concrete guidelines and prescriptive methods for data collection and analysis.

More specifically, feminist evaluation encourages evaluators to be reflexive; recognize that evaluations are neither value-free nor disinterested; consider and value different ways of knowing; hear multiple voices; stress the need to give voice to women within different social, political, and cultural contexts; and advocate for marginalized groups. Feminist evaluation encourages evaluators to be open to changing the evaluation design should important variables or questions emerge from the data. Feminist evaluations *do not* provide frameworks. In contrast, most GAD approaches provide a specific approach or framework that details how to collect and examine specific gender data.

In terms of practical application, feminist evaluation and gender approaches can be quite complementary, with feminist evaluation effortlessly integrating gender approaches as a part of the evaluation design. For example, feminist evaluation uses the concept of gender as an analytical category and easily incorporates various gender approaches. Further, some theoretical underpinnings overlap. For instance, most gender approaches and feminist evaluation agree that "values and knowledge are culturally, socially and temporally contingent" (Sielbeck-Bowen et al.,

2002, p. 6). Each approach brings its own strengths to the table that can positively influence an evaluator's way of thinking about how to design evaluations that investigate interventions that aim to change the lives of people, regardless of whether an evaluator identifies as a feminist or not.

Case Narrative

During my 20 years of conducting program evaluations in developing countries I have had many appropriate opportunities to incorporate feminist and gender approaches into my evaluation designs. I do not always use these approaches, or explicitly use them; I am guided by their potential usefulness, feasibility, and ultimately their credibility with the evaluation's primary intended users.

The following case narrative demonstrates the usefulness and challenges posed by mainly using a feminist evaluation guided by a Utilization-Focused approach. I chose this particular example because it is not an explicitly obvious choice for a feminist or gender approach. By reflecting on this case narrative, I want to demonstrate that feminist evaluation is not limited to evaluating women's projects or feminist evaluators; this case does not focus on women and was implemented with my nonfeminist colleague. As we worked with the program staff to define the evaluation questions, it became apparent that feminist evaluation would provide a good way to gather credible data and provide a useful evaluation.

Background

In the early 1990s, in Botswana,[4] a nonprofit organization (NPO) established itself on the physical grounds of a rather underfunded government mental institution. The NPO had three goals that they initially shared with me. These included to (1) provide basic services to the mental patients otherwise not provided by the hospital, (2) improve the physical surroundings, and (3) improve staff morale. The aim of the evaluation was to provide the NPO with data that they could use to improve their program, demonstrate successes, and engage the hospital management in supporting or, at the very least, not preventing the NPO from their work. The relationship between the NPO and the hospital was, at best, civil and at worst, downright hostile. This was the NPO's first evaluation.

Matching the Evaluation Approach to the NPO

As I drove through the hospital's gates I had an eerie feeling. The grounds were overgrown with weeds and surrounding buildings were in much need of repair. There did not appear to be any people and the high fences that surrounded the hospital had multiple rows of electric fencing and razor wire. Once on the grounds I drove for about 10 minutes before I encountered the NPO's building, a stately old Victorian house that was in slightly better shape than the rest. I was welcomed with tea and invited to sit in their one-room office decorated with metal chairs and old wooden desks, colorful posters, and worn curtains. There were a few laptops and piles of items that appeared to be donated clothes and household items. Run by an all-volunteer staff on a shoestring budget for nearly 20 years, the three core management staff said that they did not know much about evaluation, had little money for it, and yet they valued an objective review of their NPO's work. They earnestly wanted to understand what they did well and to know how they could improve their program. They also mentioned at this point that they wanted to use the information to convince the hospital that the NPO provided a useful service to patients and staff.

With few documents to review such as project reports, field reports, program theory, or logic documents, or even a website, these initial informal yet focused chats over tea, and a lengthy review of the NPO's large newspaper scrapbooks provided a descriptive history of the NPO. In the scrapbook, the newspaper and magazine articles documented their advocacy work over the past 20 years, including their very public challenges and achievements.

The initial interviews provided more detail, which led to a clear description of the NPO, how it worked, what it did, what the organization intended to achieve, and clarified their organizational values. These values appeared to fit with a feminist evaluation approach. These are described in the next section.

Introduction to the NPO

What became evident early on in the evaluation process was that the NPO did more than their three stated objectives. The NPO also served as an advocate for patient and hospital staff rights. Their approach combined advocacy for basic human rights and meeting patients' and staff's various basic needs; the approaches appeared to be seamlessly intertwined.

Several of the NPO's activities demonstrated their value for human dignity for a marginalized population. For example, many patients lacked appropriate clothing. The NPO's one-roomed clothing and goods shop provided donated clothes at a minimal cost to new patients, to outpatients that needed decent clothes to apply for jobs, and for patients newly released that were returning home. The NPO's shop also sold slightly used goods (and some new) that were donated, allowing patients to purchase affordable gifts for their friends and families when they returned home on holiday or for short visits such as for a family birthday or wedding. The small funds generated from this activity supported a tea room and a beauty salon that offered services at an affordable cost to the patient. The NPO also provided interactive sports and handicraft sessions and implemented projects that aimed to improve the hospital's infrastructure.

Thus the activities ranged from those that demonstrated valuing mental patients as human beings and bringing them dignity (e.g., haircuts, clothing) to activities that provided fun and some smaller skills (e.g., handicrafts and sports), to an overall approach that advocated for patient's rights (e.g., safer rooms to sleep in, private rooms that offered more dignified intake sessions for new patients). Human rights, compassion, and providing dignity to an otherwise unheard or overlooked population appeared to drive most of the NPO's activities.

As volunteers conducted their work, they often identified patient issues and developed ways to advocate for patients' rights. Several of the ad hoc initiatives resulted in a better environment for the patients. For instance, the NPO's advocacy role resulted in the hospital limiting the number of patients per room, providing safer outside surroundings for patients, and changing their approach to patient intake so that the process resulted in a more private, positive, and friendlier atmosphere. Interview data with volunteers further confirmed that the NPO valued their advocacy role for patients' rights and the ability to provide a more humane atmosphere.

The same approach appeared to be used for identifying staff needs. For instance, various NPO staff described how, while working in the hospital, they would recognize challenges faced by hospital staff that were not being addressed adequately by the hospital administration. Some examples included low staff morale, old and uncomfortable uniforms, and lack of basic equipment. For addressing low staff morale, the NPO offered small gestures such as providing holiday parties, staff recognition days, and other staff events that resulted in the staff feeling appreciated. Hospital staff, in particular the nursing staff, confirmed these findings.

The NPO identified two reasons why they chose to address staff issues. First, as with the patients, the NPO attempted to meet a need of a not very powerful (and often unheard) group. Secondly, the NPO theorized that "happy" staff would lead to better treatment of patients.

A complicating factor for the NPO, and the evaluation, was that the hospital management did not always appear to welcome the NPO's activities. While the hospital management tolerated their existence, they also provided barriers to block the NPO from achieving additional potential results. The hospital management staff refused formal evaluation interviews (they did speak to us at one meeting; this is discussed later) and severely limited our access to patients and staff.

This NPO appeared to be doing work that no one else was doing, wanted to do, or would do in their absence. While evaluating the project presented numerous challenges (such as lack of access to key stakeholders, few written internal documents, limited evaluation budget, and a short time frame), we were afforded the opportunity to make a difference to the NPO and the hospital staff, which in turn could potentially make a significant change in the lives of the mental patients, a truly disempowered people. We designed an evaluation that was strongly influenced by feminist evaluation and drew on other approaches that then led to an evaluation process that resulted in credible and useful findings. Key elements of this approach are described in the next section.

The Role of Feminist Evaluation

Every critical decision point in the evaluation—including the decision to do the evaluation—was influenced by feminist evaluation. For the purpose of this chapter, only the key evaluation elements influenced by feminist evaluation are discussed, with a brief acknowledgment of other approaches that influenced the evaluation approach.

Self-Reflection

Prior to this evaluation I had not had any experiences with the mentally ill in a personal or professional capacity. After much self-reflection, I discerned three reasons for undertaking the evaluation. First, I was curious (Was the NPO doing what it thought it was doing?). Second, I had a strong desire to help the NPO (while they informed me that their tiny evaluation budget ruled out many evaluators wanting to do the evaluation, their eagerness for an evaluation was inspiring). Third, I had a keen interest in promoting the rights of the disempowered (which at the onset I viewed as the mentally ill, but while conducting the evaluation I realized that the disempowered voices also belonged to the hospital staff and to the NPO itself in its attempt to represent the mentally ill). I was neither value-free nor disinterested in the work of the NPO, or the mentally ill. I recognized that a well-designed evaluation that produced empirical data would have the potential to influence potential change at many levels. My nonfeminist colleague went through a similar reflection and reported similar reasons for taking part in the evaluation.

This self-reflection influenced the evaluation design in several ways. First, we feared that our biases or even perceived biases would result in, well, biased findings. Therefore, in order to strengthen our findings, we continuously questioned the process and our results. During the evaluation process we took an hour or more each day to reflect on, examine, and record any decisions we had made and to question any initial findings. This reflection process then informed what we continued to explore or reexamine. Planned reflection processes had proven useful in other evaluation contexts, greatly strengthening the evaluation process (Podems, 2007). We believe that these reflection sessions resulted in a strengthened evaluation and improved our evaluation skills.

Role as an Activist

A feminist evaluation approach encourages an evaluator to view her- or himself as an activist. From the onset of the evaluation we both strongly recognized this as our potential role. We also viewed the process and its findings as a way to strengthen the NPO's ability to advocate for the rights of the mentally ill patients and the hospital staff. Given the strength of our data that demonstrated the usefulness of the NPO, we also viewed it as our role to advocate for the NPO's continued existence in the hospital. How we did this is explained later in the chapter.

Interviews

Because we intended to hear and represent previously unheard and marginalized voices, in this case the NPO, the hospital staff, and the patients, we designed different interview tools to gather and record these often unheard voices. We carefully designed questions that used appropriate language for each group and limited the length of the instrument. The instrument design was theoretically guided by a feminist approach (e.g., we focused questions with particular attention to ensuring it encouraged a conversation), practically influenced by drawing on Moser's GAD approach (e.g., we explored the strategic and practical needs of the different groups), and while gender frameworks encourage us to gather data gathering by sex, we also allowed for a wider recognition of differences in our data collection and our analysis. We explicitly recognized that these were not homogeneous groups (e.g., female nurse, male patient) and differences about each person might result in different experiences and perceptions.

We used our interviews to probe the volunteers about additional differences that may result in the patient experiencing the NPO's activities and services in a different manner. One key finding revolved around the access to clothing. Some volunteers stated that they had some cases where the male patients would rather dress in clothes intended for women. However, the hospital staff actively encouraged them to clothe patients according to their appropriate gender. This is one example that demonstrated how not assuming that all women (or all men) experience the

NPO services in the same way; it is assumed that men who wanted to purchase the clothing intended for women and turned away experienced the NPO service differently than those who were able to purchase clothes they wanted. We provided this evaluation finding to the NPO during the evaluation process, an action that was influenced by Utilization-Focused Evaluation. In retrospect, this illustrated how using a feminist lens (and to some extent queer theory) led to a small finding that could potentially positively touch the lives of this marginalized subgroup.

However, the data-gathering process had some challenges during implementation.

One roadblock for the evaluation process was our lack of access to patients. We were never granted permission by the hospital management to interview them. This posed a serious challenge to an evaluation that intended to represent often unheard voices—it is difficult to represent a previously unheard voice that we were never able to hear. Thus, our only interviews were with the NPO management and volunteers that interacted with the patients.

While we had few interviews, the NPO management and the volunteers delivering the services provided in-depth responses. For example, despite our initial efforts to keep the interviews short in respect of their time constraints, most volunteers and management staff provided lengthy and often multiple interviews. This may have been a result of the interview tool's design, which encouraged a conversational approach to interviewing.

Observation Data

Observation provided another data-gathering approach that also had challenges. We had restricted observation to certain activities where potential contact with patients was minimal. For example, we were allowed to view the store that sold clothes to the patients and observe the volunteers that provided haircuts and tea. But we were not allowed to ask question or interact in any way while patients were in the room. This constrained our data collection significantly and left us reliant on focused observational data-gathering tools.

Drawing on the Harvard and Moser framework, we gathered data from these limited observations that specifically focused on issues of access (e.g., which patients accessed these services, what times were the services available), and influenced by feminist evaluation we modified the tool so that we also focused on the behavior of the volunteer (e.g., the person holding a more powerful position). For instance, did the volunteer's behavior appear to encourage or limit the patient's interaction or ability to access the service? What was it about the volunteer's behavior that encouraged, or discouraged, a respectful interaction? While we were searching for observable power dynamics between the patients and volunteers that may have influenced the patient's experience, at times we also had the opportunity to observe interactions between hospital staff and volunteers.

Additional Finding: The Unheard Voice

During the evaluation process, we realized that for this evaluation the "unheard voice" was also the NPO's voice—it was unheard by the hospital management. Toward the end of the evaluation process the hospital management invited us to a meeting, opening a space to engage with (but not interview) the hospital management. At this point we had strong data that demonstrated the value of the NPO (as perceived specifically by the hospital's nursing staff and the NPO's volunteers, and informed by our observational data). At this meeting we were able to bring these empirical findings to the hospital management's attention while at the same time gathering some insight into the hospital's perspective on the NPO.

How we provided feedback to the hospital was influenced by Donna Mertens's (1999) transformative theory that, like feminist evaluation, addresses the need to hear previously unheard voices (p. 12). During our data collection and analysis process, these approaches encouraged us to question social inequity and social justice in the hospital and analyze how power influences relationships (e.g., between the hospital management and the NPO). This understanding enabled us to have an effective strategy in how to use our evaluation results to encourage action (e.g., focused dialogues that used the evaluation data) between the hospital and the NPO. Every unique and often up-until-this-point unheard voice (which in this case was the NPO and the hospital's nursing staff, not the patient voice as originally envisioned) added insight and significance to the findings and their actual and potential use.

A result of the evaluation was the potential for a more productive relationship between the hospital and the NPO, which will likely enhance patients' experiences at the hospital. What encouraged the use of the evaluation findings was that the NPO and the hospital administration had a common starting point: they were both there to serve the patient, and the evaluation findings provided empirical data to encourage that dialogue.

On Acknowledging Evaluation Influences

While feminist evaluation heavily influenced this evaluation, I would be remiss if I did not briefly mention other evaluation theorists, in addition to those noted above, who influenced the evaluation design. These included Ernest House (1998) and House and Howe (1999), who encourage an evaluator to consider social democracy and to only advocate using empirical data, and Michael Patton (2008), who encourages evaluation use and other various human rights approaches. As noted at the introduction of this section, this is not an exhaustive explanation of our approach; rather, it attempted to explain elements that were heavily guided by feminist evaluation.

Sharing Our Methodology with the NPO

Throughout the evaluation we never mentioned the type of evaluation approaches that we were using, nor were we asked. When we offered to share the approach with the NPO management, they responded that they were mainly concerned with who we interviewed and that our interview and observational processes did not offend the hospital staff or its patients. I suggest that this is a significant yet anecdotal point; in my experience it is rare that an evaluation client asks about an evaluation approach (beyond methods) and as a result, what underpins the design and other decisions is often left largely unchecked.

We chose a feasible and appropriate approach that aimed to be sensitive to the NPO's data needs, and provided empirical findings that could be used to make a difference for the lives of patients, hospital staff, and the NPO. At the same time, as an evaluation team that had both a feminist and nonfeminist, we also chose an approach that mirrored our own explicit values.

Qualifications for Using Feminist Evaluation

While I suggest that an evaluator does not need to be a feminist to be guided by, draw from, or implement feminist evaluation, several prerequisites do exist. A key prerequisite to using feminist evaluation is to be able to understand what it is. This includes how it overlaps and yet differs from gender approaches. A second broader prerequisite is to understand when to use the approach, how to practically apply the approach, and how to introduce the approach, if at all, to your evaluation team and the user of the evaluation findings. A final prerequisite is that the values that underpin feminist evaluation must resonate with your own personal values.

Conclusion

Feminist evaluation should not be exclusively for those that identify as feminists; the belief that only feminists conduct feminist evaluation keeps the approach out of mainstream evaluation and prevents nonfeminists from exploring its potential use in their own evaluation activities. Choosing a feminist evaluation approach, like choosing any evaluation approach in any part of the world, needs to be done with careful consideration of multiple factors. Feminist evaluation should be applied based on its cultural, social, and technical appropriateness to a given context and should lead to a feasible, useful, appropriate, and credible evaluation.

The challenges that I face when I attempt to implement, use, or draw from feminist evaluation are not insurmountable. At the same time labeling an evaluation as a "feminist evaluation" brings its own challenges and considerations. Can an evaluation guided by only a few elements of feminist evaluation still be labeled feminist evaluation? I suggest that being aware of methodological choices and making appropriate process and design decisions are more important than the "final" label. On the other hand, I also suggest that published examples of feminist evaluation, or any evaluation that draws on feminist evaluation, will create a space for critique and improvement of the approach, and hopefully lead to its further use.

As feminist evaluation attempts to insert itself into mainstream evaluation in the West, it is also beginning to have a quiet influence in the development context. Those that argue that feminist evaluation is not appropriate in developing countries because "feminism" is rooted in Western thought could also use that same logic to argue the relevance of many program evaluation approaches. Some feminist evaluators may argue that feminist evaluation should keep women as its focus (and in a purest sense I agree); however, this chapter demonstrates that while women may be one focus, any evaluation that seeks to explore the voices of the disempowered may benefit from feminist evaluation.

NOTES

1. I emphasize that this section does not pretend to exhaust all feminist evaluation definitions, discussions, or explanations; rather, I provide accepted tenets central to feminist evaluation, which are now updated in this book.
2. These principles have been revised and are elaborated in the first chapter of this volume.
3. International development interventions refer to any project, program, activity, or intervention aimed at improving or changing the social and/or economic well-being of people living in a developing-world context. Examples of interventions include preventing HIV/AIDS and TB, increasing access to education for girls, or providing access to water to underprivileged people.
4. Location of the case study has been changed to protect the organization.

REFERENCES

American Evaluation Association. (2004). *Guiding principles for evaluators.* Fairhaven, MA: Author. Retrieved from *www.eval.org/Publications/Guiding-Principles.asp.*

Bamberger, M., & Podems, D. (2002). Feminist evaluation in the international development context. In D. Seigart & S. Brisolara (Eds.), Feminist evaluation: Explorations and experiences. *New Directions for Evaluation, 2002*(96), 83–96.

Barrett, M., & Phillips, A. (1992). *Destabilizing theory: Contemporary feminist debates.* Stanford, CA: Stanford University Press.

Beardsley, R., & Hughes Miller, M. (2002). Revisioning the process: A case study in feminist program evaluation. In D. Seigart & S. Brisolara (Eds.), Feminist evaluation: Explorations and experiences. *New Directions for Evaluation, 2002*(96), 57–70.

Bessis, S. (2001). The World Bank and women: Instrumental feminism. In S. Perry & C. Shank (Eds.), *Eye to eye: Women practicing development across cultures* (pp. 10–24). London: Zed Books.

Boserup, E. (1970). *Women's role in economic development.* London: Allen & Unwin.

Connelly, M., Li, T., MacDonald, M., & Parpart, J. L. (2000). Feminism and development: Theoretical perspectives. In J. Parpart, M. P. Connelly, & V. E. Barriteau (Eds.), *Theoretical perspectives on gender and development* (pp. 51–160). Ottawa, Canada: International Development Research Centre.

Cornwall, A., Harrison, E., & Whitehead, A. (n.d.). Introduction: Repositioning feminism in gender and development. *Repositioning Feminisms in Development.* IDS Bulletin, *35*(4).

Cousins, J., & Whitmore, E. (1998). Framing participatory evaluation. In E. Whitmore (Ed.), Understanding and practicing participatory evaluation. *New Directions for Evaluation, 80*, 5–23.

Flax, J. (1990). Postmodernism and gender relations in feminist theory. In L. J. Nicholson (Ed.), *Postmodernism and gender relations in feminist theory* (pp. 39–62). New York: Routledge & Kegan Paul.

Gardner, K., & Lewis, D. (1996). *Anthropology, development and the postmodern challenge.* London: Pluto Press.

Gilligan, C. P. (1982). *In a different voice: Psychology, theory and women's development.* Cambridge, MA: Harvard University Press.

Hirsch, M., & Keller, E. F. (1990). Conclusion: Practicing conflict in feminist theory. In M. Hirsch & E. F. Keller (Eds.), *Conflicts in feminism* (pp. 370–385). New York: Routledge.

Hodgkin, S. (2008). Telling it all: A story of women's social capital using a mixed-methods approach. *Journal of Mixed Methods Research, 2*(4), 296–316.

Hood, D., & Cassaro, D. (2002). Feminist evaluation and the inclusion of difference. In D. Seigart & S. Brisolara (Eds.), Feminist evaluation: Explorations and experiences. *New Directions for Evaluation, 2002*(96), 27–40.

House, E. R. (1993). *Professional evaluation: Social impact and political consequences.* Newbury Park, CA: Sage.

House, E. R., & Howe, K. R. (1998). The issue of advocacy in evaluations. *American Journal of Evaluation, 19,* 233–236.

House, E. R., & Howe, K. (1999). *Values in evaluation and social research.* Thousand Oaks, CA: Sage.

Hughes, C. (2002). *Key concepts in feminist theory and research.* London: Sage.

Jacobson, J. (1994). *The economics of gender.* Oxford, UK: Blackwell.

Jahan, R. (1995). *The elusive agenda: Mainstreaming women in development.* London: Zed Books.

Jewiss, J., & Clarke-Keefe, K. (2007). On a personal note: Practical pedagogical activities to foster the development of "reflective practitioners." *American Journal of Evaluation, 28,* 334–337.

Longwe, S. H. (1995). The evaporation of policies for women's advancement. In N. Heyzer, S. Kapoor, & J. Sandler (Eds.), *A commitment to the world's women: Perspectives on development for Beijing and beyond.* New York: United Nations Development Fund for Women.

McClean, M. (2000). Alternative approaches to women and development. In J. Parpart, M. P. Connelly, & V. E. Barriteau (Eds.), *Theoretical perspectives on gender and development* (pp. 179–190). Ottawa, Canada: International Development Research Centre.

McRobbie, A. (1982). The politics of feminist research: Between talk, text and action. *Feminist Review, 12,* 46–48.

Mertens, D. (1999). Inclusive evaluation: Implications of transformative theory for evaluation. *American Journal of Evaluation, 20,* 1–14.

Mertens, D. (2005). Feminism. In S. Mathison (Ed.), *Encyclopedia of evaluation* (p. 154). Thousand Oaks, CA: Sage.

Minnich, E. (1990). *Transforming knowledge.* Philadelphia: Temple University Press.

Mohanty, C. T. (1997). Under Western eyes: Feminist scholarship and colonial discourse. In N. Visvanathan, L. Duggan, L. Nisonoff, & N. Wiegersma (Eds.), *The women, gender and development reader* (pp. 79–86). Cape Town, South Africa: David Philip.

Molyneux, M., & Steinberg, D. L. (1995). Mies and Shiva's ecofeminism: A new testament? *Feminist Review, 49,* 86–107.

Moser, C. (1993). *Gender planning and development theory, practice and training.* New York: Routledge & Kegan Paul.

Oakley, A. (1982). *Sex, gender and society.* Bath, UK: Pittman Press.

Ogundipe-Leslie, M. (1994). *Re-creating ourselves: African women and critical transformations.* Trenton, NJ: African World Press.

Olesen, V. L. (2000). Feminism and qualitative research at and into the millennium. In N. Denzin & Y. Lincoln (Eds.), *Handbook of qualitative research* (2nd ed., pp. 215–255). Thousand Oaks, CA: Sage.

Ostergaard, L. (1992). *Gender and development: A practical guide.* London: Routledge.

Overholt, C., Anderson, M. B., Cloud, K., & Austin, J. E. (1984). *Gender roles in development projects: A case book.* West Hartford, CT: Kumarian Press.

Patton, M. (1997). *Utilization-focused evaluation: The new century text.* Thousand Oaks, CA: Sage.

Patton, M. (2002). *Qualitative research and evaluation methods.* Thousand Oaks, CA: Sage.

Patton, M. (2008). *Utilization-focused evaluation* (4th ed.). Thousand Oaks, CA: Sage.

Pietilä, H., & Vickers, J. (1990). *Making women matter: The role of the United Nations.* London: Zed Books.

Podems, D. (2007). Process use: A case narrative from southern Africa. In J. B. Cousins (Ed.), Process use in theory, research, and practice. *New Directions for Evaluation, 2007*(116), 87–97.

Podems, D. (2010). Feminist evaluation and gender approaches: There's a difference? *Journal of MultiDisciplinary Evaluation* [online] *6*(14). Access at *http://survey.ate.wmich.edu/jmde/index.php/jmde_1/article/view/199/291.*

Reid, E. (1995). Development as a moral concept: Women's practices as development practices. In N. Heyzer, S. Kapoor, & J. Sandler (Eds.), *A commitment to the world's women: Perspectives on development for Beijing and beyond* (pp. 113–125). New York: United Nations Development Fund for Women.

Ryan, K., Greene, J., Lincoln, Y., Mathison, S., & Mertens, D. (1998). Advantages and challenges of using inclusive evaluation approaches in evaluation practice. *American Journal of Evaluation, 19,* 101–122.

Schwandt, T. (2000). Further diagnostic thoughts on what ails evaluation practice. *American Journal of Evaluation, 21,* 225–229.

Scott, J. (1986). Gender: A useful category of historical analysis. *American Historical Review, 91*(5), 1053–1075.

Seigart, D. (2005). Feminist evaluation. In S. Mathison (Ed.), *Encyclopedia of evaluation* (pp. 154–157). Thousand Oaks, CA: Sage.

Seigart, D., & Brisolara, S. (2002). Editors' notes. In D. Seigart & S. Brisolara (Eds.), Feminist evaluation: Explorations and experiences. *New Directions for Evaluation, 2002*(96), 1–2.

Sielbeck-Bowen, K., Brisolara, S., Seigart, D., Tischler, C., & Whitmore, E. (2002). Exploring feminist evaluation: The ground from which we rise. In D. Seigart & S. Brisolara (Eds.), Feminist evaluation: Explorations and experiences. *New Directions for Evaluation, 2002*(96), 3–8.

Stake, R. (2004). *Standards-based and responsive evaluation.* Thousand Oaks, CA: Sage.

Stanley, L., & Wise, S. (1993). *Breaking out again: Feminist ontology and epistemology* (New ed.). London: Routledge.

Thompson, D. (2001). *Radical feminism today.* London: Sage.

Tinker, I. (1990). *Persistent inequalities: Women and world development.* Oxford, UK: Oxford University Press.

Truman, C. (2002). Doing feminist evaluation with men: Achieving objectivity in a sexual health needs assessment. *New Directions for Evaluation, 2002*(96), 71–82.

FIRST REFLECTION

Saumitra SenGupta
Denise Seigart
Sharon Brisolara

As we switch gears in our journey, let us pause for a moment and briefly review a few key concepts from Part I. The intent of this part was to lay a theoretical foundation before exploring the application of specific feminist approaches in evaluation and research. For those who are already immersed in feminist evaluation and research, many of the concepts and theories laid out in Part I were an opportunity to reacquaint, refresh, and refocus. For others who have been interested in pursuing feminist approaches but are not as familiar with the tenets, we hope the first five chapters have provided some new learning, and, perhaps, opened the door to new terminology such as "reflexivity" and "axiology." We can identify six key areas of theoretical understanding that emerged from Part I: diversity of approaches, using a social justice lens, the impact of feminist theories at different levels of research and evaluation, the roles of the feminist evaluator or researcher, a transformative paradigm, and the distinctions and commonalities between research and evaluation in light of feminist approaches.

One fundamental facet of feminist approaches to research and evaluation that emerges from Chapter 1, by Brisolara, is the diversity within feminist theories from which researchers/evaluators are likely to find themselves drawing as they label their work "feminist." A central theme that emerges is the centrality of gender in one or more phases of research or evaluation including conceptualization, operationalization, reporting, and follow-up. At the same time an important aspect that is noted by Brisolara and discussed in detail by Mertens (Chapter 4) is the nonexclusivity of the gender dimension in feminist evaluation or research.

This is a critical take-home point from the theoretical background discussion. Yes, gender takes a central role in the feminist articulation of theory and practice, but it is considered in the context of other demographic, cultural, contextual, and situational variables. Mertens asks the question, "How do these multiple dimensions of diversity come into the ethical discussion of evaluations that focus on gender equity?" Brisolara similarly posits, "Gender inequities are one manifestation of social injustice. Discrimination cuts across race, class, and culture and is inextricably linked to all three." In Part II, Sielbeck-Mathes and Selove (Chapter 6) present examples of program implementation and evaluation in which they articulate the challenges faced by feminist evaluators to focus on gender issues when the ostensible program aims are "gender-neutral."

In recent years, the evaluation literature has blossomed with emphasis on each of these areas. Much of this literature has evolved around social justice and the role of evaluators in ensuring such—a point made at length by both Mertens and Whitmore (Chapter 3). Gender justice and gender equity are firmly entrenched in a larger social justice context. The privileging of information for research and evaluation and how this privileging is done constitute the essence of much of the discussion on the impact of feminist approaches by both Brisolara and Mertens. Both Hay (Chapter 8) and Nichols (Chapter 7) in their respective chapters in Part II focus on this issue with examples of their own works in international evaluation.

Brisolara (Chapter 1) provides a detailed account of the implications of incorporating a social justice lens with a feminist approach at different levels of research: ontological, epistemological, and methodological. How the research or evaluation is framed at each of these levels has profound implications for whether and how it becomes feminist. She also provides a historical context in which feminist approaches are seen as evolving; for example, in some instances feminist evaluators have relied on what would be considered a positivist approach to overcome misogynist obstacles to obtaining objective truth. Mathison's (Chapter 2) distinction between exploratory, descriptive, and explanatory research provides a good backdrop for why different methodologies may be called for depending on the context. For instance, gender inequity is often best demonstrated by presenting hard numbers such as income differences or disparities in the incidence of gender-based violence. At the same time, the real impact of such disparities may remain immeasurable in a quantitative way. In-depth, qualitative ways of knowing may offer the best means of assessing the true impact.

The feminist evaluator role is multifaceted. Whitmore's Chapter 3 discusses this issue at length. She makes a personal connection to what it means to be a feminist evaluator and examines the roles she outlines in light of different evaluation models, including ones based on social justice and feminist inquiry. She makes an important point that feminist evaluation (and research) is likely to take place in complex situations that by necessity require different ways of knowing than pure positivist or quasi-experimental approaches provide.

Mertens's Chapter 4 on the transformative paradigm identifies the sources of complexities that feminist evaluators and researchers often face. One can argue that the central tenets of her axiological, ontological, epistemological, and methodological stances, that is, social justice, discrimination, oppression, power differentials, and cultural competence, are all concepts not easily captured by quantitative means alone. Whitmore (Chapter 3) describes evaluator roles as important in identifying and closely examining these issues whether the endeavor is labeled "research" or "evaluation." All four chapters in Part II offer examples of how these complex issues are unpacked in very diverse arenas, with practical toolkits and lessons learned.

Mathison's (Chapter 2) delineation between research and evaluation is an important one to guide us through Parts II and III as we delve into specific examples of feminist evaluation and research from around the world. Discussing a number of definitional aspects, she points out that social science research and program evaluation have a lot in common, yet possess very distinct characteristics and purposes. Mathison's review of the relationship between facts and values leads to a bigger question regarding learning the evaluand versus what to do with the evaluand, an essential question in action research. As the reader moves to Parts II and III, she or he will find that we have made an attempt to characterize and categorize the chapters as primarily belonging to either the evaluation or research domain. She or he will also discover that the chapters in the evaluation section, almost by necessity, describe their theoretical approaches in order to frame the evaluation examples they present. However, the distinctions in both content and focus between the chapters in Parts II and III also led us to categorize them separately.

Finally, Podems (Chapter 5) identifies the challenges of labeling her evaluation as feminist very clearly and cautions against falling into a lengthy discussion on feminism in introducing feminist evaluation. She draws some fundamental distinctions between who may or may not be labeled as "feminist" and how, regardless of such distinctions, many evaluators could be able to conduct a feminist evaluation. She also distinguishes between gender-based approaches to evaluation and feminist evaluation. This chapter should clarify for many of us who have often struggled with the understanding of the differences between the two approaches.

As we transition to Part II, we will discover at least three things. First, we cannot fail to notice a common theme running across the chapters, that of the challenges of using the term "feminist evaluation" and common reactions, from misunderstanding to fierce criticism, encountered by the authors in their respective evaluative endeavors. Second, we are going to see that the authors have employed rather different strategies and frameworks in addressing these potential challenges in conducting feminist evaluation. In the end, we will find that despite the diversity of challenges, strategies, and frameworks, a common pattern emerges that underscores how these authors have conceptualized and applied feminist evaluation principles, and the fundamental similarity in the core principles they have followed. We will see that very pragmatic and practical considerations can lead to better acceptance of feminist evaluation and potentially more useful evaluation findings and utilization thereof.

One type of challenge presented by Sielbeck-Mathes and Selove (Chapter 6) concerns the situation in which the evaluator wishes to conduct feminist evaluation but finds the evaluand lacking any particular gender focus or possessing a gender neutral theory of change. This chapter offers two main take-away points. First, it demonstrates that it is possible to apply a feminist evaluation framework in such a situation; and second, and perhaps more importantly, it argues that a feminist evaluation approach in such settings can lead to changes in future program planning and reorientation among program staff in listening to women's voices and understanding the particular issues impacting women's participation and outcomes.

While Sielbeck-Mathes and Selove turn to framing theory of communication and interaction between individuals and groups to implement a feminist evaluation framework, Nichols (Chapter 7) uses the time-tested ecological model and its intersectionality with feminist theories to evaluate the impact of initiatives to foster democracy in war-torn countries, using Angola as an example. The ecological framework allows the evaluator in this case to unpack a complex situation using Bronfenbrenner's levels of ecology, from individual to collective levels, which also changes how the gender focus is achieved at different levels.

Drawing on their Latin American experience, Salinas-Mulder and Amariles (Chapter 9) approach a complex situation with emphasis on the context, politics, and analysis of power relations in order to conduct feminist evaluation. They make a powerful case for attention to power relations in the program and evaluation contexts so that all stakeholders are respected, listened to, and represented. They caution against evaluation and research designs that use participants as information sources but not as valid and valuable evaluation audiences. The authors provide very practical tips for every stage of an evaluation that is relevant not only in diverse international development settings but in almost any context where feminist evaluation is conducted.

Like the chapter by Podems (Chapter 5) and that by Salinas-Mulder and Amariles (Chapter 9), Hay (Chapter 8) identifies strategies and characteristics of feminist evaluation in international development with South Asia as a backdrop, most using evaluation examples from India and Bangladesh. She examines the importance of the choice of methods, rigor, accountability, ways of detecting change, and use of evaluation results as distinct areas that characterize a feminist evaluation. She emphasizes paying attention to feminist principles at each evaluation stage and questioning the dominant paradigm as essential to conducting feminist evaluation. Hay recognizes that there is no single strategy or methodology to conduct a feminist evaluation. She underscores the idea that whether a feminist lens or standpoint was used in conducting the evaluation ultimately characterizes a feminist evaluation.

As we transition from Part II to Part III, we will come back to the common themes and strategies that run through the chapters in both these sections. However, one theme that starts emerging from Part II is examining issues from a feminist perspective and questioning current paradigms. Mertens uses the term "transformative paradigm" to advance Fourth-Generation Evaluation concepts to fit a feminist evaluation approach and advocates labeling feminist evaluation as such. Meanwhile Podems (Chapter 5), perhaps more than any other author in this volume, provides a lengthy discussion of the pros and cons of using the label "feminist" in characterizing an evaluation.

As feminist evaluators and researchers, we must recognize that we sit at a crucial juncture in acknowledging and valuing feminist approaches in our work. This is an evolving and shifting proposal, thanks to the hard work of these authors and many others in mainstreaming the concept. The questioning of the existing paradigms, their shortcomings and blind spots as they translate to epistemology and methods, and how they do or do not relate to social justice from a feminist standpoint is a legitimate enterprise. We hope Part I has set you, the reader, on that journey. Part II will continue the conversation, and familiarize you with the more practical, operational questions that Part I has raised for your practice.

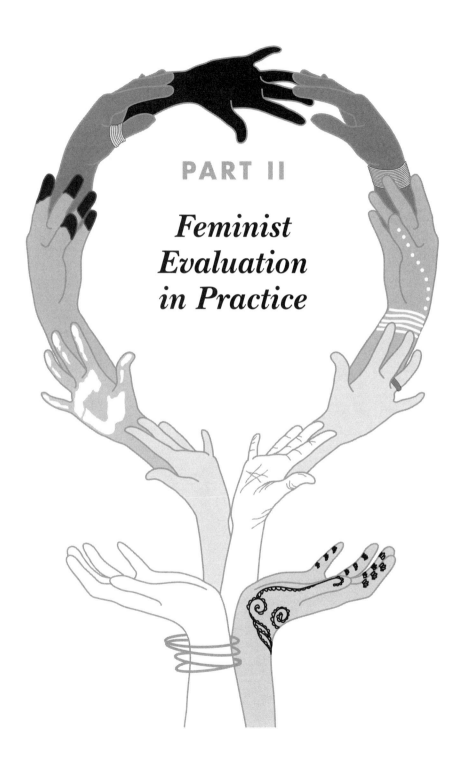

PART II

Feminist Evaluation in Practice

CHAPTER 6

An Explication
of Evaluator Values

Framing Matters

Kathryn Sielbeck-Mathes
Rebecca Selove

Introduction

In this chapter we use evaluation of three rural co-occurring mental
health and substance abuse treatment programs to describe our processes
of (1) identifying and articulating feminist values for ourselves; (2) thinking through how to frame important messages about trauma, substance
abuse, and treatment for women so they are communicated in a language
that is translatable and transferable; and (3) designing and responding to
the analysis process and findings so as to improve outcomes immediately
for women and in future programs. We focus on the second program to
illustrate the potential for feminist evaluation to deepen our awareness of
the value of attention to how we frame our work.

A key theme in this discussion is that in order to use the evaluation
process to bring about social change, we must translate feminist values
and evaluation findings into a language that is meaningful, compelling,
and actionable for those who will be funding and providing services.
While we may or may not use the word "feminist," the frame we use will
incorporate the principles on which the word was founded. Feminist here
aligns with third-wave feminism which embraces diversity and change. In
this wave, as in previous ones, there is no all-encompassing single feminist
theory. Third-wave feminism seeks to challenge or avoid what it deems

the second wave's "essentialist" definitions of femininity, which often assumed a universal female identity and overemphasized the experiences of upper-middle-class white women.

Appalachian Women's Perspectives

Appalachian Culture

Research on women's lives in rural Appalachian communities today reflects both change and strongly held traditions in structure and women's roles. On the one hand, rates of divorce, teen pregnancy, and unmarried cohabitation are rising. Birthrates, employment rates among women, and the number of female-headed households are now similar across metro and nonmetro areas (Brown & Lichter, 2004). On the other hand, rural women still marry younger and at a greater rate than their urban counterparts, place greatest value on their homemaking and mothering roles, and are less likely than their urban counterparts to terminate a pregnancy (McLaughlin, 1999). Among program females, 73% had been married during their lifetime, but only 21.5% were married at the time of enrollment, 88% were mothers, and 100% were involved in the criminal justice system with co-occurring mental health and substance abuse disorders.

Gender Roles

Further, past research suggests that social and environmental factors, particularly gender socialization, gender roles, and gender inequality account for many significant behavioral differences between women and men. Many of these differences are not biological or unchangeable; they are ascribed by society and relate to expected social roles. While there are numerous shared expected social roles for women (e.g., caregiver, nurturer, childbearer), there are a number of social roles strongly influenced and determined by external factors. Communities and societies create social norms of behavior, values, and attitudes that are deemed appropriate for men and women and the relations between them.

Co-Occurring Disorders among Appalachian Women

Review of the literature also reveals that Appalachian women who have co-occurring disorders often face more barriers to accessing treatment than do urban women because in addition to inadequate or the absence of services, they often have to deal with cultural norms that result in so much stigma and shame that they are forced to hide and/or deny their need for help. Our female program participants had all been involved with the criminal justice system because of their addiction and/or criminal behavior, and they were thus forced to come out of hiding in order to comply with mandates from the court or to meet requirements to maintain custody of their children.

While substance abuse and dependence may affect the legal status, child custody, employment, and housing situations of both men and women, many of these issues have a greater impact on women because of ascribed societal gender roles and the ways in which women derive their identities, particularly in rural Appalachian communities (Grella, 1997). Women in Appalachia with substance abuse problems who are seeking treatment also face significant barriers such as no public or private transportation, poverty, unemployment, and unsafe or unstable housing.

Barriers to Treatment and Stigma

Women face barriers to treatment related to childrearing responsibilities (Allen, 1995; Grady, Grice, Dustan, & Randall, 1993), and more limited incomes, education, and job skills in comparison to men (Arfken, Klein, di Menza, & Schuster, 2001; Ashley, Marsden, & Brady, 2003; Green, Polen, Lynch, Dickinson, & Bennett, 2002). Lack of transportation and the role-related desire for anonymity are believed to be key reasons why fewer Appalachian women participate in recovery support groups such as Alcoholics Anonymous and Narcotics Anonymous, which can be critical to long-term maintenance of sobriety. Further, beliefs related to fatalism, self-sufficiency, and distrusting outsiders can also be potential barriers to accepting treatment and recovery services (Martin, 2009).

The literature also indicates that the problem of addiction is rarely, if ever, a single-dimensional issue for women. Addiction is always a part of a larger portrait that includes a woman's individual history, and the cultural, social, and economic factors that create the context of her life. Therefore, when evaluating a substance abuse treatment program that includes women, it is essential to start from the premise that theory and practice must be based on a multidimensional perspective, which requires an understanding of, and sensitivity to, the context of women's lives both inside and outside of the program. According to Finkelstein, Kennedy, Thomas, and Kearns (1997), stigma is the *main* psychosocial issue differentiating the substance abuse of women from that of men.

Women who abuse substances contrast significantly with society's view of femininity and the roles of wife and mother. "Women often internalize this stigma and feel guilt, shame, despair, and fear when they are addicted to alcohol or other drugs. Women who are mothers also know that addiction may cause them to lose their children. Further, stigma and the threat of severe consequences often lead women and their families to minimize the impact of substance abuse by using denial" (Covington, 2008, p. 2). Viewed through a feminist lens, we can also understand reluctance to acknowledge their substance abuse as women's efforts to maintain the elements of their role that provide them with a degree of power in sometimes tenuous situations.

Experience of Trauma

In addition to their dependence on alcohol and/or drugs, two elements often shared by women with addiction regardless of their age, race, culture, or geographic location are the lack of healthy relationships and the experience of trauma (e.g., physical abuse, sexual abuse, emotional abuse, deep poverty, persistent racism) (Covington, 1999). These elements create multiple issues that are interrelated in women's lives and require an intentional focus when addressing addiction and recovery. Research in general has indicated that female involvement in substance abuse and dependency is more frequently associated with anxiety and depression, particularly due to physical and sexual abuse, than male substance abuse.

Women with a history of physical or sexual abuse are much more likely to develop substance abuse and mental health problems or co-occurring disorders than those without it (Brady & Ashley, 2005; Macmillan, 2001; Najavits, 1997; Rosenberg et al., 2001) and women with co-occurring disorders are more likely to be exposed to environments and relationships that are prone to violence (Harris, 1998). Also relevant to women enrolled in the program central to this discussion, nearly eight out of 10 female offenders with a mental illness report have been physically or sexually abused (Smith, 1998).

Nationally, physical or sexual abuse victimization is highly prevalent among women with co-occurring disorders—50–70% of women in psychiatric care have experienced victimization, and 55–99% of women (depending upon the population being studied) with substance abuse disorders have been victimized (Briere & Zaidi, 1989; Cascardi, Mueser, DeGiralomo, & Murrin, 1996; Najavits, 1997). Exposure to traumatic events with subsequent posttraumatic stress disorder (PTSD) can have a severe impact on individuals' health, health-care utilization, general functioning, and other aspects of their overall quality of life, and increases risk to addiction recovery (Covington, 2008). In comparison to a woman with a single psychiatric disorder, women with co-occurring disorders have increased rates of service use, family burden, HIV infection, noncompliance with medication regimens, increased rates of hospitalization, psychotic symptoms, incarceration, and homelessness (Kessler et al., 1997). Women with PTSD have higher odds of high school and college failure, teenage childbearing, marital instability, and unemployment than women without PTSD. Sadly, women with co-occurring substance abuse and mental health disorders who have experienced physical, sexual, and/or emotional abuse have not been well served by our existing service delivery systems (Amaro et al., 2007; Gatz, Brounstein, & Taylor, 2005), in part because most of them will not receive treatment that addresses both the impact of trauma and their current psychiatric and substance use disorders (Becker et al., 2005).

Overview of the Three Related Programs

In the Beginning

The program at the heart of this discussion was the second of three that addressed co-occurring mental health and substance abuse disorders in rural Tennessee among men and women involved in the criminal justice system. The first, called the Methamphetamine Treatment Program (MTP), was considered to be gender-neutral, with no specific attention to gender or trauma. The evaluation as conceptualized and implemented did not incorporate feminist principles, and outcome measurement emphasized quantitative methods over qualitative methods. During the analysis, we observed that women and men responded to the program in very different ways. While both men and women experienced improved outcomes overall, men improved at different rates and exhibited different outcome variables than women.

The Second Program

What we learned from evaluating MTP informed the evaluation design and questions for the second community-based program, Project FREE. Project FREE provided the context that sharpened our focus on how to integrate a feminist frame into the evaluation. Implementation included the same Matrix Model (which is explained later in this chapter) as was used in the first program, TIP 44, which provided guidelines for implementing programing among individuals with co-occurring substance abuse and mental health disorders, and an optional trauma-focused curriculum, Seeking Safety, as well as a global commitment to incorporate a trauma-informed approach.

Despite inclusion of a trauma-focused curriculum, trauma was not well documented during intakes, no gender-specific groups were offered, and therapists rarely referred women to the Seeking Safety program. Women who were referred rarely enrolled and/or completed the program. Of those participants in the substance abuse treatment program with a formal diagnosis of PTSD, *none* were enrolled in the trauma-focused curriculum.

However, conducting the analysis of outcome data with a feminist lens (i.e., examining differences in baseline and outcome data by gender, and interviewing providers and participants to better understand those differences) led to our awareness of limitations in the way we framed trauma at the outset of this project. Seventy-one percent of women enrolled in the program reported histories of past or current trauma. If the evaluation had been structured differently from the outset, perhaps by training program staff to be more aware of their assumptions about trauma-focused treatment, program staff may have recognized the prevalence of trauma and systematically referred women to the ancillary trauma-recovery Seeking Safety program more often, and women's recovery and mental health could have been significantly improved.

The Third Program

These observations and findings helped to inform the third program, Team Recovery, which, unlike the previous programs, included court-mandated involvement, gender-specific groups, comprehensive trauma screening, and the Seeking Safety program for every woman who screened positive. As explained in this chapter, these program elements were congruent with and facilitated integration of feminist principles, such as seeking to understand the lived experiences of women using evaluation to empower women, and addressing social injustice more fully into the frame that was used to present evaluation findings to staff and participants.

The Second Program as Planned

The following section provides more detail about Project FREE and the evaluation that helped to transform implementation and evaluation of a substance abuse treatment program for individuals with co-occurring substance abuse and mental health issues. Project FREE was a 3-year initiative funded by the Substance Abuse and Mental Health Services Administration (SAMHSA) that served seven rural south-central Tennessee counties. Program staff provided comprehensive substance abuse treatment services for men and women in the criminal justice system with co-occurring mental health and substance abuse disorders over a 3-year period. Because this project was implemented in a rural setting, several service components were added, such as transportation, community education, physical and mental health screenings, referrals to after-care services, and other community-based supports and opportunities. The program was intended to be gender-neutral and was implemented by two female and two male therapists. Each therapist conducted mixed-gender groups. Each person enrolled participated in a range of intensive services such as early recovery, relapse prevention, family/client education, individual therapy, aftercare, urine screening, and social support. Each of the three curricula utilized in the program is described briefly below.

The Matrix Model

The Matrix Model, a 16-week manualized (i.e., a sequenced and scripted guidance for provider interventions), comprehensive substance abuse treatment approach, emphasized client engagement using education and techniques designed to enhance the therapeutic alliance. The intent of the model is to guide participants to an intellectual and emotional state that helps them embrace treatment and abstain from alcohol and substance abuse, all within a safe, nonjudgmental environment. A key aspect of treatment was helping clients learn to self-monitor, specifically to help them bring into awareness any dysphoria, uncomfortable symptoms, thoughts, warning signs, high-risk situations, and/or subtle precipitating events that could result in relapse. Treatment was also designed to help clients gain skills in identifying their triggers to use substances, cope with daily pressures, and manage immediate problems.

Treatment Improvement Protocol

Treatment Improvement Protocol (TIP) 44 ("Substance Abuse Treatment for Adults in the Criminal Justice System"; Center for Substance Abuse Treatment, 2006) incorporates what is scientifically known about effectively treating substance use problems to ensure that each treatment component is supported by a strong evidence base. The program encompassed a full range of services including screening and assessment, treatment planning, counseling, intensive outpatient substance abuse treatment, family/individual substance abuse education, crisis intervention, relapse prevention, drug testing/monitoring, and case management and other recovery support services, as well as linkages with wraparound care (including primary and mental health care).

Seeking Safety

Seeking Safety is a short-term, 24-session manualized cognitive-behavioral treatment program specifically designed to address both trauma and substance abuse in either group or individual settings (Najavits, 1997). Sessions are structured and include basic education on substance abuse and PTSD, action skills to prevent drug use and control PTSD symptoms, cognitive restructuring with particular attention to maladaptive thoughts associated with substance abuse disorders and PTSD, and a focus on relationship issues and developing effective communication skills to build a healthy support network. Session topics are meaningfully connected to patient reports of unsafe behavior and coping skills.

The Matrix Model and TIP 44 were implemented consistently and with high fidelity throughout the life of the project. The Seeking Safety curriculum was available but program participants had the choice to opt in or opt out.

The Problem of Co-Occurring Disorders

Accurate insight into the lives of addicted women provides the feminist evaluator with greater ability to illuminate details and seemingly routine aspects of a woman's experience and create meaning, effectively convey a sense of understanding, and identify potential and realized breaches in social justice and equity. To expand this level of understanding, in addition to our review of the literature, we listened to the stories of female participants in our programs in rural Appalachia. Seeking to understand the realities and lived experiences of women aligns closely with our feminist values of equity, social justice, and empathy.

Women enrolled in Project FREE were from the lower socioeconomic class and maintained traditional female identities, viewing men as the "head of the household" and "in charge." Participants told us that an Appalachian woman tends to "stay married no matter what" and "takes her wedding vows seriously." Demographic studies of women living in rural Appalachian communities revealed that they were active participants in what they defined ideologically as the "man's world" (Shannon, Havens, Mateyoke-Scrivner, & Walker, 2009). Men primarily took care of the responsibilities outside the domestic sphere and women were responsible for taking care of their husbands/boyfriends, domestic tasks, and the children. Many times this included taking a job to "help make ends meet."

Attempts were made to interview women completing the Seeking Safety curriculum; however, because of employment, relocation, or other responsibilities, connections with the evaluator were never possible. Informal interviews were conducted with two women who had completed the Matrix Model only. The two women's stories had some relevant similarities. Both married very early and both experienced significant domestic violence and abuse that eventually led to an addiction to crack cocaine for "Sue" and to methamphetamine, marijuana, and alcohol for "Pam."

In both cases, the women's boyfriend/husband introduced them to substance use. When asked about the level to which discussions of past and present trauma were incorporated into her treatment program, "Sue" stated that they were "not allowed" to talk about their "dirty laundry" during group. "Sue" could not remember being asked to share, but stated that she did not talk about what was going on at home because she did not want the police involved and she also was concerned that information might be shared with the Department of Children's Services (DCS) and could impact custody of her children. Further, she took her wedding vows very seriously and she would not consider leaving her marriage for any reason.

Use of Mixed Methodologies

Both qualitative and quantitative data were collected and analyzed in order to gain insight into program strengths, weaknesses, areas needing improvement, and client outcomes. The outcomes were measured using three key data collection instruments: the GPRA Tool, Outcome Questionnaire–45 and the Short Form–12. All participants completed the baseline interview and 6-month follow-up assessment.

The Outcome Questionnaire 45–Version 2 (OQ-45.2; Lambert et al., 1996) is a 45-item questionnaire that measures overall mental health functioning and three subdomains: symptom distress (anxiety and depression), interpersonal relations, and social role performance. This instrument tracks outcomes and allows the clinician to assess progress during behavioral health treatment. Psychometric properties for validity and reliability of the questionnaire have been established (Lambert et al., 1996).

The Short Form Health Survey–Version 2 (SF-12v2; Ware, Kosinksi, Turner-Bowker, & Gandek, 2007) is a 12-item questionnaire used to measure seven domains of health and mental health functioning: general health, physical functioning, lack of bodily pain, mental health (anxiety and depression), vitality, social functioning, and the role of physical health and of emotional problems in limiting participation in activities or accomplishing what one would like. The instrument has acceptable psychometric properties related to validity and reliability (Ware et al., 2007).

In addition to administering standardized instruments to assess changes in client drug use, mental health, and physical health status, client feedback was collected using four open-ended questions administered during the follow-up interview. Questions included:

1. "What was the most important thing that you learned?"
2. "How have you used what you learned to keep from relapsing?"
3. "What would you have done if the program was not available to you?"
4. "How could the program have helped you to be more successful?"

Findings from Project Free

Program staff established positive relationships with clients, the community, and the criminal justice system (drug court, judges, probation officers, and law enforcement); assisted with finding funding opportunities; and applied for and were awarded a new SAMHSA grant to continue service provision for another 3 years in a neighboring underserved area after Project FREE ended. Analysis of participants' total OQ-45 (a measure of depression and anxiety) baseline scores compared to 6-month scores showed statistically significant improvement in mental health. However, Figure 6.1 reflects that women (dashed line) reported clinical levels of anxiety and depression at baseline (≥ 64) whereas men (solid line) did

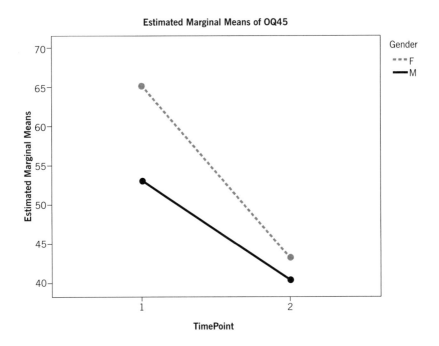

FIGURE 6.1. Estimated marginal means of OQ-45 scores.

not. Only seven women enrolled in, and just four of those completed, the 24-session Seeking Safety curriculum. When SF-12 scores of general health, physical functioning, physical role, bodily pain, vitality, social functioning, emotional role, and mental health were compared with the original program SF-12 scores, we observed significantly higher scores in every outcome except physical functioning. The four women who completed both the Matrix Model and Seeking Safety responded very positively to this integrated approach.

Figure 6.2 reflects the consistently higher scores across indicators when the Matrix Model-only outcomes were compared with the Matrix Model plus Seeking Safety outcomes. We do have to use caution when interpreting these results as there were only four women who completed the Seeking Safety curriculum. While we did not have a sample size to make a causal claim, the results were compelling enough to serve as an opportunity for discourse with the program staff.

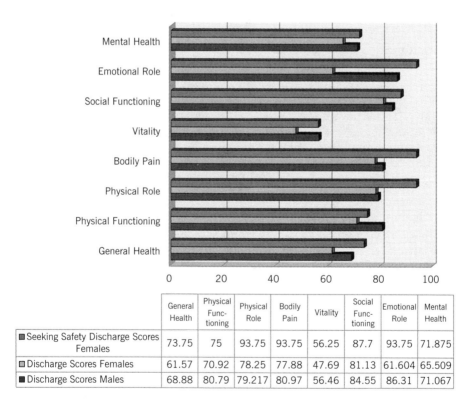

	General Health	Physical Functioning	Physical Role	Bodily Pain	Vitality	Social Functioning	Emotional Role	Mental Health
▨ Seeking Safety Discharge Scores Females	73.75	75	93.75	93.75	56.25	87.7	93.75	71.875
▢ Discharge Scores Females	61.57	70.92	78.25	77.88	47.69	81.13	61.604	65.509
▪ Discharge Scores Males	68.88	80.79	79.217	80.97	56.46	84.55	86.31	71.067

FIGURE 6.2. Comparison of SF-12 discharge scores (males vs. females matrix model only and matrix model + seeking safety).

These distinct differences observed between Seeking Safety female participants and treatment-as-usual participants led us to conduct a secondary data analysis of key community mental health indicators that further clarified our female program participants' realities. The majority of women enrolled in the program had histories of trauma (71% overall), with 51% reporting emotional abuse, 55.7% reporting physical abuse, and 42.9% reporting sexual abuse. Interestingly, only 12.7% of these women had a formal PTSD diagnosis recorded in their medical record. Despite these astounding statistics, less than 5% of women were enrolled in the Seeking Safety program specifically designed to address trauma.

Revising the Program from the Perspective of Feminist Evaluation

With the aim of enhancing quality and increasing the comprehensiveness of the evaluation, a feminist perspective and approaches were integrated during year 2 of the Project FREE grant. These approaches included seeking to understand the perspectives and lives of women enrolled in the program, particularly as they related to their histories, daily life, and their current position in society; understanding the problem from a feminist perspective; using mixed methodologies; and committing to change the status quo by communicating evaluation findings to program staff and funders, raising awareness related to the unique needs of women, pointing out disparities, and recommending changes in implementation strategies.

We initiated several discussions with program staff and administered a survey to program therapists in order to better understand their attitudes toward trauma among women and the efficacy of Seeking Safety. We learned that most therapists believed that because the Seeking Safety curriculum was not mandatory, and it required more time, self-reflection, and self-work, women were not self-motivated to enroll. Other reasons therapists reported for nonenrollment included lack of adequate/safe child care and reliable transportation, drug court requirements, work schedule, and long travel time.

These constraints might have explained some of the low enrollment; however, as feminist evaluators we suspected that other more socially constructed barriers were also present. We returned to the medical records for a closer document review.

Behavioral health treatment histories suggested that women were not directly connecting their mental health with their trauma histories. During intake assessments women shared their histories of physical and sexual abuse; however, the box aligned with emotional abuse was rarely checked. This disconnect may have reflected cultural norms of mind and body dualism, where emotional abuse was seen as less relevant or real than physical and sexual abuse.

However, when this finding was shared with program staff, they indicated the more likely explanation was that when conducting the intake assessments, therapists asked about physical and sexual abuse but failed to ask about emotional abuse, and thus the check box was left blank. This was not an intentional oversight or a conscious area of neglect; rather, it reflected something more systemic including their differing philosophies and training.

Identifying and Articulating Feminist Values

As feminist evaluators, universal professional values including honesty, integrity, accountability, tolerance, and respect for people influence the work that we do. These values are aligned with fairness, social justice, equity, and empathy regardless of political, social, economic, geographic, gender, ethnic, and age differences. We intentionally design evaluations in ways that increase the likelihood that the data we collect and analyze help us to understand the multiple realities and lived experiences of women as well as sensitize us to social structures that perpetuate inequity, oppression, social injustice, and the powerlessness of women. The ultimate aim is to generate knowledge that can be used to create change that makes a difference in the lives of women.

Key Tasks

Key tasks associated with feminist evaluation include (1) understanding the problem from the perspective of the individuals our programs are designed to serve, (2) studying the interior and external context of the program in order to understand the realities and lived experiences of women, and (3) identifying the invisible structures that can undermine even the most diverse, gender-responsive, trauma-informed program. Accomplishing these tasks requires suspension of the conviction that we are experts, authentic and respectful intention to learn from program participants and service providers about their view of barriers to their success, careful questioning of our own assumptions, and deep listening for different nuances in the way the problem is framed. This all requires a continual internal monitoring of our own subjectivity and the impact that we have in the evaluative context. Margaret Attwood (1986) eloquently justified this level of mindfulness when she wrote: "At each moment of our lives our every thought, value, and act from the most mundane to the loftiest takes its meaning and purpose from the wider political and social reality that constitutes and conditions us" (p. 139).

Using the Word "Feminist"

There are multiple understandings and uses of the word "feminist" in the evaluation literature and in larger cultural contexts. Use of the male perspective as the standard for normal is predominant, and the influence of this viewpoint is so pervasive that it often is unseen. One result is that substance abuse treatment programs labeled "gender-neutral" are actually male-based, and the male experiences of recovery are assumed to provide an adequate basis for program design for both men and women. At the same time, we know that gender is an important mediator of substance abuse treatment outcomes because the background characteristics, substance abuse patterns, needs, barriers, and personal stories of female substance users are different from those of males. Past research suggests that social and environmental factors, particularly gender socialization, gender roles, and gender inequality, account for many significant behavioral differences between women and men. Many of these differences are not biological or unchangeable; they are ascribed by society and relate to expected social roles.

As evaluators it is important to recognize that using the term *feminist* can undermine the intent of the work that we do. Depending upon one's culture/perspective, describing our approach to evaluation as *feminist* may suggest exclusion rather than inclusion to some audiences. Furthermore, systematic oppression can be totally invisible to women who have internalized it from the cradle. For example, Donna Mertens described working with evaluators from Africa who were designing evaluations to address the United Nations's priorities for women in Africa, and noted that they found feminist principles of evaluation (Sielbeck-Bowen, Brisolara, Seigart, Tischler, & Whitmore, 2002) informative, but were resistant to using the term *feminist*, preferring *gender-responsive* to describe their work. If the feminist evaluator's intent is to integrate feminist guidelines to frame the evaluation (i.e., placing women's realities at the center of evaluation planning and analysis, understanding the problem context from a feminist perspective, exhibiting a willingness to challenge the status quo, using mixed methods, and actively disseminating findings and advocating for and with female participants, as described by Ward [2002]), she or he must carefully consider whether utilizing the term "feminist" is beneficial. Evaluators must consider the specific culture within which a program is embedded in order to understand the perspectives of program staff and participants, as well as those to whom evaluation results will be disseminated, if shared meaning-making and identification of a common frame is the goal.

Gender as a Key Determinant

All inquiry begins with a question. Evaluation questions established at the beginning of Project FREE were based upon a practical interest in understanding the impact of treatment and therapy, as well as values aligned with feminist principles. These included identifying women at risk for inequity, particularly in terms of access to gender-responsive interventions that are sensitive to societal, cultural, demographic, and familial norms that could perpetuate disparity, disempowerment, and disenfranchisement. Initial evaluation questions were based upon very general treatment frames that were largely discipline-informed: substance abuse treatment providers believed that readiness and accountability for personal recovery determined outcomes regardless of gender, while mental health providers believed that providing guidance and support while helping people develop self-efficacy, learn about their addiction, understand the physiological impact of drugs on their brains/bodies, as well as identify personal strengths, were keys to recovery regardless of gender. As feminist evaluators, we believed that gender was a key determinant of women's mental health/substance abuse disorders and in many cases was also strongly linked to current or past trauma. The selection of treatment frames reflected assumptions associated with the values of the program staff and related to their training, experience, and worldviews/perspectives. Naturally, because the values and backgrounds of the service providers and the evaluator varied, assumptions about what constituted optimal treatment and outcomes varied as well.

Framing Theory and Its Implications

Framing Theory has evolved from three streams of study. The first, described by Dewulf et al. (2009) as the cognitive tradition, involves the concept of cognitive schemas as an explanation of memory. The second flow of meaning for frames reflects the thinking of Goffman (1974) and focuses on frames as recurring aspects of interactions. That is, socially and organizationally defined roles frame exchanges between people in ways that might not be obvious; however, the frames can have significant impact on the meaning and even amount of content they exchange. The third and perhaps most common use of framing is in the field of business and political communication as described by Fairhurst and Sarr (1996). Defining framing as "a quality of communication that causes others to accept one meaning over another," these organizational consultants focused on framing as strategic communication during which meaning is "co-constructed" to support a leader's agenda. More specifically, framing can contribute to "the construction of political consciousness" because it establishes certain ways of thinking about a topic or issue as the norm and excludes alternatives (Hardin & Whiteside, 2010).

Implications of Framing Theory include recognizing that the personal and professional histories of all individuals at the evaluation planning table influence their view of what a new program can offer, how it can be most effectively implemented, what outcomes are relevant, and how findings should be interpreted. Sheikh et al. (2011) observed that framing in health policy and systems research is "skewed" in favor of attention to factors such as organizational structures rather than political and social contexts, and relationships; furthermore, detailed descriptions of interventions are more prevalent than information about the preexisting organizations and culture within which the intervention will be delivered.

There is good reason to treat the values and biases animating the evaluation process and frame formulation as epistemic resources, helping us to discover and understand alternative aspects of the world and to see them from new perspectives, rather than as obstacles to the search for the "truth" (Haraway, 1991; Harding, 1986). A pluralism of theories, perspectives, values, and frames should be accepted as a normal feature of social science inquiry as long as interventions are improving outcomes equally regardless of gender. However, during the evaluation it became apparent that differences in frames led to intervention strategies that were out of alignment with women's needs in Project FREE. Had we worked more closely with the program staff to develop a frame that integrated feminist values, women might have experienced interventions more closely aligned with their unique needs and ultimately experienced better outcomes. Hardin and Whiteside (2010), in their articulate analysis of framing as a tool "in support of an activist research agenda," advocate close examination of assumptions and beliefs that might reflect the dominant culture throughout the research process. We can be strategic as feminist evaluators by asking about the viewpoint of women, especially female research participants, when we establish research questions, develop approaches to collecting data, assign meaning to the data, and consider alternative approaches to reporting results.

Discussion

We believe that our values of fairness, social justice, and gender equity heightened our sensitivity to invisible structures that negatively impacted women's access to gender-responsive treatment in this rural context. Because our female program participants were rural, marginalized, and poor, we recognized that the risk of injustice and mistreatment was significant.

> In the decades since World War II, the United States has emerged as the industrialized society with the greatest income and wealth inequality and a consequent increase in health disparities. The top quintile of Americans now command a greater share of wealth than at any time in 60 years, and almost one fourth of U.S. children live in poverty. Asymmetries of power, ideology, persistent racism and sexism, and problems of environmental justice are exacerbated by growing inequalities of income and wealth. (Hofrichter & Bhatia, 2010)

Despite our own connection with our personal values, we did not spend sufficient time understanding the differing values, language, perspectives, frames, etc., of the program staff, program manager, and project director, rather assuming we were interpreting trauma in the same ways and sharing the same values around the issue of trauma specifically and programing for women in general. In hindsight, focusing on this understanding should have held the same importance in the evaluation as measuring fidelity and outcomes. The decisions made by program staff were based upon their value systems, and their language reflected the frames that invoked those values. Our ways of communicating likewise reflected the frames that invoked our values. Thus our message was not interpreted as we had intended. This lesson has implications for how we frame important messages about feminist evaluation, its value, and its impact. In order to gain attention and respect for the adoption of feminist frameworks, principles, and values for conducting program evaluation, it is imperative that we frame our conversations to connect rather than compete, align rather than malign, and garner acceptance rather than objection.

Feminist evaluators realize that it is critical to understand their intersubjectivity in order to clearly explicate their personal values. This intimate connection with the values that determine one's perspective and worldview help to anchor conversations and information sharing that helps in finding common ground in principles such as equity, opportunity, equality, safety, and empowerment for all women. Shared values can help us to construct a shared way of communicating that can open doors—and minds—to more fruitful discussions about policy change that can lead to social and structural change.

Stating our values clearly and consistently gives our words authenticity. When we talk about feminist evaluation, and the feminist principles that we believe in and stand for, our values are reflected clearly in our language and our words are marked by authenticity. As cognitive linguist and political advisor George Lakoff (2004) wrote, "A position on issues should follow from one's values, and the choice of issues and policies should symbolize those values" (p. 17). Everyone, from the homeless to homemakers, from secretaries to heads of state, expresses their experience of the world through the language or lens of their values. Connecting through words, images, symbols, and stories grounded in values helps make solutions accessible and relevant to program stakeholders, service organizations, and funding agencies.

Linking an issue to a widely held cultural value helps start the framing process by appealing to program stakeholders and increasing their interest in learning more. Individuals' stated and tacit values are more important that any particular issue (sexism, racism, terrorism, war, economy, health care, education, etc.) (Lakoff, 2004). Our job as feminist evaluators is to clearly frame our own values, seek to understand the values of program stakeholders, and establish ways to communicate shared and divergent values in the process. This process can potentially help identify structural inequality that exists in the fabric of many organizations, institutions, governments, or social networks where embedded bias provides advantages for some members and marginalizes or produces disadvantages for others.

Once identified, a new frame can be established through consistent, repetitive, strong, and broad-based communication. Language and appropriate framing requires knowledge of the environment, cultural context, and value systems on multiple levels. This knowledge can then be linked to building trusting, honest relationships that are continuously evolving and intentionally opened to sharing meaning, understanding systems, and challenging the status quo. Developing this context for program evaluation typically does not happen automatically—it requires a commitment to shared meaning making throughout the evaluation process (not necessarily consensus or agreement on all points).

The programs we used to illustrate a feminist evaluation perspective involved providing substance abuse treatment for individuals, some with co-occurring mental health concerns, living in rural Appalachia. Each of these three overlapping dimensions of program participants' lives required specific attention to the experience of women, because women have had experiences that affect the ways they hear and see what the programs offer. In the context of Project FREE, conducting a feminist evaluation intentionally focused on women by (1) raising general awareness about trauma and the pervasiveness of it among females enrolled in the program; (2) describing the impact of the rural Appalachian context and culture on women's mental health and substance abuse in our reports, staff meetings, and one-on-one conversations; and (3) frequently sharing data about the gender differences in program outcomes and strongly recommending enrolling all women with trauma histories in the Seeking Safety program.

Feminist evaluators must consciously investigate how their personal values align, intertwine, and/or conflict with the values of key stakeholders as they define problems, identify target populations, design programs, measure outcomes, and report findings. Without this critical step, the evaluator is likely to ask the wrong questions, collect incomplete data, make inappropriate analysis decisions, and report findings that are not used to improve programing and the overall quality of life for women. Ultimately, such evaluations will side-step critical opportunities to frame important recommendations that have the potential to lead to social change.

Framing Theory helps explain why some evaluators do not choose feminist approaches to evaluation. They do not see how incorporating feminist principles into their work aligns with their personal values, or perhaps another dimension of their work has more weight (e.g., objectivity, rigorous evaluation designs, resource constraints, values of the funding agency). Evaluators' perceptions are largely determined by what they already know and associate with a particular issue. Our role as feminist evaluators is to introduce new information that can connect with common values so that new associations can be established that align with feminist principles and the value that their application can bring to evaluation.

In order to frame the value of feminist principles in evaluation, we need to think about creating messages that can reduce resistance to the integration of feminist principles. For example, a message describing social justice for women as a way to achieve healthy communities and equitable income distribution, complete with visual and/or statistical representations of how we see this happening, can be very powerful. In this way, the concepts of social justice for women, healthy communities, income, and equality are framed together.

Many of the communication challenges in feminist evaluation represent dominant frames that make it difficult for stakeholders, funding agencies, and/or other evaluators to hear your messages, much less value a feminist approach. If it seems as if you are not being heard . . . you probably are not. A feeling of frustration can be a signal that reconstruction of a shared meaning based upon shared values is necessary.

Recommendations

This chapter illustrates the importance of clarifying feminist values and methods, identifying their relevance for program evaluation, and using framing in the course of planning and conducting evaluations. Thus the first step for a feminist evaluator is to clarify her or his own mental model of the relationship of feminist values to the setting and topic within which evaluation is being planned. This reflects the cognitive approach (Dewulf et al., 2009) to frames, with an emphasis on words and phrases that represent and potentially convey the values that guide the evaluator's work.

With consideration for Bateson (1954), we suggest that the evaluator pay particular attention to his or her anticipated relationships with key stakeholders in the project, including evaluation and program staff and program participants. Planning includes reflecting on one's own feelings within imagined dialogues, and how the roles of staff, participants, and evaluators might be viewed from each other's perspectives. Next, we recommend that the evaluator seek opportunities to engage stakeholders in conversations about the project, during which the evaluator should listen for the metacommunication about the relationships, as well as about the congruence and dissonance regarding the feminist frame. This means that the evaluator understands that perceptions and responses to perceptions of power and authority, whether associated with formal roles or with personal histories and access to information, may be communicated outside of verbal content.

Like Chong and Druckman (2007), we recommend that evaluators use dialogues with key stakeholders to clarify the primary problems they jointly wish to address. By carefully listening and using framing strategies as described previously, evaluators should work with all stakeholders—funders, program staff, and potential participants—to identify the various understandings of what causes problems, including proximal and distal historical and spatial contributions to the problems. For example, women with a history of substance abuse and incarceration might or might not identify previous trauma experiences as being relevant to their current difficulties. Staff members might not realize that women within a small, isolated community are unlikely to consider utilizing a program that focuses exclusively on them, as this may be regarded as unfair to their families.

These conversations can also include identifying attitudes about who is responsible for what aspects of the problems and/or programs. Clarifying each stakeholder's frames for how best to address and resolve the problems is also important as a way of identifying common ground, as well as differences in perspective that will need to be negotiated or accommodated. This can be done by asking staff and participants about how they would design a good program, describe and publicize it, and what they think might be barriers to participant involvement. As Chong and Druckman (2007) note, (1) the relevance of a specific frame (such as a feminist perspective) can be enhanced by motivating individuals to consider it, and (2) making it more visible within a field of alternative frames.

Finally, Pillow (2002) and Ward (2002) respectively provided helpful reviews of themes that are common in feminist research, and guidelines for feminist evaluations that we have integrated in the following list of recommendations for evaluators who embrace feminist principles:

1. Gender is addressed as a significant variable. The evaluator intends to understand the perspective of women and the impact of the project context on women. Topics of importance to the women who are involved as participants or program staff are important to the evaluator. The impact of being male and not female, or being female and not male, in relationship to the study question is a topic of investigation.

2. The "daily lived experiences" (Pillow, 2002) of women are seen as highly important. A feminist evaluator is interested in the meaning and impact of what is routine, even those aspects of daily life that may be considered irrelevant to the project by women themselves.

3. The evaluator takes a proactive stance toward examining her or his relationship to the research topic and process of investigation. Her or his responses related to gender during the project are documented and studied as data.

4. From the outset of a project, a feminist evaluator is mindful and prepared for changing assumptions and procedures that perpetuate injustice and disempowerment. She or he intends to improve the lives of women through the evaluation process and use of data obtained in the course of the work. As a change agent, a feminist evaluator anticipates that there will be opportunities to change the status quo, and aims to develop collaborative relationships that can facilitate change. This goal includes involvement with women's advocates and community activists, as well as the participants in the program themselves.

5. A feminist evaluator recognizes that multiple methods for studying a topic or program of interest will allow a broader and deeper understanding of phenomena that need to be addressed in order to support social change. Reliable and valid quantitative and qualitative measures are essential.

6. It is imperative that a feminist evaluator take an active role in sharing information that is obtained during the course of her or his work with program participants, and with others who have authority and responsibility for service delivery and program policies.

By using similar frames and coordinated messages across feminist evaluation we can focus our messages, recommendations, and calls for action and social change to improve women's lives. It is our hope that over time our efforts to frame information about the process and outcomes of feminist evaluation will change perceptions, and we will see increased integration of feminist principles in program evaluation more broadly. The initial step, however, is to achieve a clear sense of where we need to go in order to facilitate enduring changes that positively impact women's outcomes. This can only be done by intentionally establishing a common language to describe a common goal.

> "Cheshire Puss," she [Alice] began rather timidly. . . . "Would you tell me, please, which way I ought to go from here?"
> "That depends a good deal on where you want to go," said the Cat.
> "I don't much care where," said Alice.
> "Then it doesn't matter which way you go," said the Cat.
> —LEWIS CARROLL (1865), *Alice's Adventures in Wonderland*

REFERENCES

Allen, K. (1995). Barriers to treatment for addicted African American women. *Journal of the National Medical Association, 87* (10), 751–756.

Amaro, H., Dai, J., Arevalo, S., Acevedo, A., Matsumoto, A., Nieves, R., et al. (2007). Effects of integrated trauma treatment on outcomes in a racially/ethnically diverse sample of women in urban community-based substance abuse treatment. *Journal of Urban Health: Bulletin of the New York Academy of Medicine, 84*(4), 508–522.

Arfken, C. L., Klein, C., di Menza, S., & Schuster, C. R. (2001). Gender differences in problem severity at assessment and treatment retention. *Journal of Substance Abuse Treatment, 20,* 53–57.

Ashley, O. S., Marsden, M. E., & Brady, T. M. (2003). Effectiveness of substance abuse treatment programming for women: A review. *The American Journal of Drug and Alcohol Abuse, 29*(1), 19–53.

Attwood, M. (1986). *The handmaid's tale.* New York: Random House.

Bateson, G. (1954). A theory of fantasy and play. *Psychiatric Research Reports, 2,* 39–51.

Becker, M. A., Noether, C. D., Larson, M. J., Gatz, M., Brown, V., & Giar, J. (2005). Characteristics of women engaged in treatment for trauma and co-occurring disorders: Findings from a national multisite study. *Journal of Community Psychology, 33*(4), 429–443.

Brady, T. M., & Ashley, O. S. (Eds.). (2005). *Women in substance abuse treatment: Results from the Alcohol and Drug Services Study (ADSS).* DHHS Publication No. SMA 04-3968. Rockville, MD: Substance Abuse and Mental Health Services Administration, Office of Applied Studies.

Briere, J., & Zaidi, L. Y. (1989). Sexual abuse histories and sequalae in female psychiatric emergency room patients. *American Journal of Psychiatry, 146,* 1602–1606.

Brown, J. B., & Lichter, D. T. (2004). Poverty, welfare, and the livelihood strategies of nonmetropolitan single mothers. *Rural Sociology, 69,* 382–401.

Carroll, L. (1865). *Alice's Adventures in Wonderland*. Available at *http://manybhoks. net/_scripts/download-ebook.php*.

Cascardi, M., Mueser, K. T., DeGiralomo, J., & Murrin, M. (1996). Physical aggression against psychiatric inpatients by family members and partners. *Psychiatric Services, 47*, 531–533.

Center for Substance Abuse Treatment. (2006). TIP 44. Retrieved January 21, 2013, from *http://store.samhsa.gov/product/TIP-44-Substance-Abuse-Treatment-for-Adults-in-the-Criminal-Justice-System/SMA09-4056*.

Chong, D., & Druckman, J. N. (2007). Framing theory. *Annual Review of Political Science, 10*, 103–126.

Covington, S. (1999). *Helping women recover: A program for treating addiction* (with a special edition for the criminal justice system). San Francisco: Jossey-Bass.

Covington, S. S. (2008). Women and addiction: A trauma-informed approach. *Journal of Psychoactive Drugs* (SARC Suppl.), *5*, 377–385.

Dewulf, A., Gray, B., Putnam, L., Lewicki, R., Aarts, A., Bouwen, R., et al. (2009). Disentangling approaches to framing in conflict and negotiation research: A metaparadigmatic perspective. *Human Relations, 62*, 155–293.

Fairhurst, G. T. & Sarr, R. A. (1996). *The art of framing: Managing the language of leadership*. San Francisco: Jossey-Bass.

Finkelstein, N., Kennedy, C., Thomas, K., & Kearns, M. (1997). *Gender-specific substance abuse treatment*. Alexandria, VA: National Women's Resource Center; Center for Substance Abuse Prevention/Substance Abuse and Mental Health Services Administration.

Gatz, M., Brounstein, P., & Taylor, J. (2005). Serving the needs of women with co-occurring disorders and a history of trauma: Special issue introduction. *Journal of Community Psychology, 33*(4), 373–378.

Goffman, E. (1974). *Frame analysis: An essay on the organization of experience*. New York: Harper & Row.

Grady, K., Grice, D. E., Dustan, L., & Randall, C. I. (1993). Gender differences in substance use disorders. *American Journal of Psychiatry, 150*, 1707–1711.

Green, C. A., Polen, M. R., Lynch, F. L., Dickinson, D. M., & Bennett, M. D. (2002). Gender differences in outcomes in an HMO-based substance abuse treatment program. *Journal of Addictive Diseases, 23*, 47–70.

Grella, C. E. (1997). Effects of gender and diagnosis on addiction history, treatment utilization and psychosocial functioning among a dually diagnosed sample in drug treatment. *Journal of Psychoactive Drugs* (SARC Suppl.), *1*, 289–295.

Haraway, D. (1991). Situated knowledges. In *Simians, cyborgs, and women* (p. 188). New York: Routledge.

Hardin, M., & Whiteside, E. (2010). Framing through a feminist lens: A tool in support of an activist research agenda. In P. D'Angelo & J. A. Kuypers (Eds.), *Doing news framing analysis: Empirical and theoretical perspectives* (pp. 312–330).

Harding, S. (1986). *The science question in feminism*. Ithaca, NY: Cornell University Press.

Harris, M. (1998). *Trauma recovery and empowerment: A clinician's guide for working with women in groups*. New York: Free Press.

Hofrichter, R., & Bhatia, R. (2010). *Tackling health inequities through public health practice: Theory to action*. New York: Oxford University Press.

Kessler, R. C., Crum, R. M., Warner, L. A., et al. (1997). Lifetime co-occurrence of DSM-III-R alcohol abuse and dependence with other psychiatric disorders in the national co-morbidity survey. *Archives of General Psychiatry, 54*, 313–321.

Lakoff, G. (2004). *Don't think of an elephant!: Know your values and frame the debate*. White River Junction, VT: Chelsea Green.

Lambert, M. J., Burlingame, G. M., Umphress, V., Hansen, N. B., Yancher, S. C., Vermeersch, D., et al. (1996). The reliability and validity of a new psychotherapy outcome questionnaire. *Clinical Psychology and Psychotherapy, 3*(4), 249–258.

Lichter, D. T., & Campbell, L. A. (2005). *Changing patterns of poverty and spatial inequality in Appalachia*. Washington, DC: Population Reference Bureau and Appalachian Regional Commission.

Macmillan, R. (2001). Violence and the life course: The consequences of victimization for personal and social development. *Annual Review of Sociology, 27*, 1–22.

Martin, L. (2009). Cultural considerations for the provision of substance abuse treatment for Appalachian clients. Retrieved from *www.heiselandassoc.com/mydocs/martin%20%20Rigley%20APPALACHIAN%20TX.pdf*.

Martin, L., & Ripley, B. (2011). Cultural considerations for the provision of substance abuse treatment for Appalachian clients. Available at *https://heiselandassoc.com/home-studies/24/cultural-considerations-in-the-provision-of-substance-abuse-treatment-to-appalachian-clients*.

McLaughlin, D. K. (1999). Economic restructuring and changing prevalence of female-headed families in America. *Rural Sociology, 64*, 394–416.

Najavits, L. M. (1997). "Seeking Safety": Outcome of a new cognitive-behavioral psychotherapy for women with posttraumatic stress disorder and substance dependence. *Journal of Traumatic Stress, 11*, 437–456.

Pillow, W. S. (2002). Gender matters: Feminist research in educational evaluation. In D. Seigart & S. Brisolara (Eds.), Feminist evaluation: Explorations and experiences. *New Directions for Evaluation, 2002*(96), 9–26.

Rosenberg, S. D., Mueser, K. T., Friedman, M. J., Gorman, P. G., Drake, R. E., Vidaver, R. M., et al. (2001). Developing effective treatments for posttraumatic disorders among people with severe mental illness. *Psychiatric Services, 52*, 1453–1461.

Shannon, L. M., Havens, J. R., Mateyoke-Scrivner, A., & Walker, R. (2009). Contextual differences in substance use for rural Appalachian treatment-seeking women. *American Journal of Drug and Alcohol Abuse, 35*, 59–62.

Sheikh, K., Gilson, L., Agyepong, I. A., Hanson, K., Ssengooba, F., & Bennett, S. (2011). Building the field of health policy and systems research: Framing the questions. *PLoS Medicine, 8*(8), e1001073.

Sielbeck-Bowen, K. A., Brisolara, S., Seigart, D., Tischler, C., & Whitmore, E. (2002). Exploring feminist evaluation: The ground from which we rise. In D. Seigart & S. Brisolara (Eds.), Feminist evaluation: Explorations and experiences. *New Direction for Evaluation, 2002*(96), 3–8.

Smith, B. V. (1998). Rethinking prison sex: Self-expression and safety. *Columbia Journal of Gender and Law, 15,* 185–234. Available at *http://ssrn.com/abstract=982427.*

Ward, K. J. (2002). Reflections on a job done: Well? In D. Seigart & S. Brisolara (Eds.), Feminist evaluation: Explorations and experiences. *New Directions for Evaluation, 2006*(96), 41–56.

Ware, J. E., Jr., Kosinksi, M., Turner-Bowker, D. M., & Gandek, B. (2007). *Studies of SF-12v2 Health Survey. User's Manual for the SF12-v2 Health Survey.* Lincoln, RI: QualityMetric.

CHAPTER 7

Measuring Gender Inequality in Angola

A Feminist–Ecological Model for Evaluation

Tristi Nichols

Introduction

This chapter combines the use of ecological and feminist lenses to formulate an adaptable conceptual framework that measures gender inequality within an evaluation process. Practitioners and academicians, operating as part of the international development community, should benefit from a feminist–ecological framework that includes constructs developed for the following evaluation stages: (1) design, (2) implementation, and (3) interpretation of findings.

The framework presented in this chapter is intended to provide academicians and practitioners with guiding questions to measure the degree to which an intervention designed to promote democracy actually furthers female empowerment and/or minimizes gender inequity within an international context. In essence, the purpose of this chapter is to address the following pertinent questions:

1. How does an evaluator ensure that gender inequality is adequately measured?
2. What does reporting genuine progress on gender inequality entail?

As a consequence of addressing these questions, the perspectives on how a feminist–ecological lens views evaluation methodology and whose values are included in findings presented to the client(s) are also offered within this chapter.

Current Practices for Measuring Gender Inequity in International Development Contexts

Two commonly used theoretical feminist approaches for assessing the extent to which women's equality is brought into greater balance are the following:

1. The examination of the intended effects/benefits of increased access to educational opportunities and/or greater support in the workplace. Specifically, measuring changes in women's inequality is focused on determining the extent to which women's productivity has increased based on income and consumption levels.
2. Similarly, disparate measures of concepts such as self-worth reinforcement, empowerment, and strength of family support are outcomes typically reviewed to underscore changes in women's equality or ease of access to judicial or health services. Changes in self-reported confidence levels and departures from the (stereotypical) perceptions of the family role(s) are indicative of self-expression and greater freedom.

Figure 7.1 provides an illustration of the interlinkages between the two theoretical approaches.

Feminist theory has heavily influenced both of these theoretical areas in terms of providing the critical perspective related to epistemology to challenge economic, social, or psychological inequities between men and women. As a result, through the use of these two theoretical approaches, researchers, academicians, and practitioners have been able to use research methodologies to draw attention to existing forms of oppression, injustices, and inequalities experienced by women.

Limitations of the Theories

While the feminization of poverty does not lack public attention, few evaluations purposefully investigate in depth the origins of the social problem and the extent to which financial and human resources allocated through social programs have effectively changed women's beliefs, attitudes,

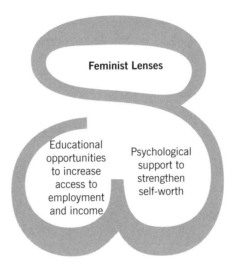

Feminist Lenses

Educational opportunities to increase access to employment and income

Psychological support to strengthen self-worth

FIGURE 7.1. Interlinkages between two theoretical approaches through which to measure changes in women's equality.

perceptions, and behavior(s). Though feminist theoretical tenets share the commonality of addressing women's inequities, there are challenges when attempting to tease out relevant (and measurable) constructs to ascertain changes/differences in women's economic, political, and social positions for evaluative purposes. This constraint is particularly prevalent within the international development context, where the practice of evaluating women's political power and participation is obstructed due to the paucity of reliable data and is therefore conceptually limited (United Nations Economic Commission for Africa, 2001). Indeed, the premise under which Bamberger, Rugh, and Mabry conceived the real-world evaluation (RWE) approach was to address budget, time, data, and political constraints, primarily experienced by evaluation practitioners in the developing world at the time of publication (Bamberger, Rugh, & Mabry, 2006, p. 18). Even within the academic setting, however, a feminist perspective has difficulty being incorporated into the mainstream and "standard," Western textbooks. In fact, "many issues addressed by the women's movement have received little coverage in community psychology literature and practice" (Campbell & Wasco, 2000, p. 777; Mulvey, 1988, p. 78).

A review of the literature revealed a gap of evaluations, guidelines, technical resources, and organizational research. Explanations for the paucity of resources in this domain are only speculative. The body of literature uncovered lacks clarity in constructs measurement (or substantive innovation/creativity) and rigor in measuring and reporting on the status of gender inequality. For instance, a community-level measure ought to reflect the nature and status of gender inequality over a period of time (decreased, increased, or remaining the same), and the extent of observed change in gender inequality should be compiled from multiple evidence sources. Based on the review, it appears that there is consistent use of advocacy for (additional) organizational support through staff capacity (i.e., sensitization training) to collect disaggregated data and thereby adhere to gender mainstreaming. The notion of gender mainstreaming is a ubiquitous strategy for considering and promoting gender equality throughout all levels, including program implementation, research, legislation, and monitoring results. A "standard measurement," addressing how (and when) women's beliefs, perceptions, attitudes, and behavior *change* over time is, however, absent. The ultimate consequence of this lack of and poorly formulated documentation is that evaluation practitioners have limited resources upon which to draw and conclude how, or if, gender inequalities have intensified or diminished over time.

Theoretical Intersectionalities

There is an intersectionality between feminist and ecological concerns that examine women's lives while they actively pursue personal needs and individual aspirations, the values within which are defined by their environment. Feminist concerns include (1) a belief that women are exploited and oppressed as subordinates in a hierarchical system that affords privilege to more valued groups, particularly the dominant racial group in a given cultural setting; (2) a commitment to empower women and change the conditions of their lives; and (3) an acknowledgment of women's experiences, values, and activities as meaningful and important (Baber & Allen, 1992, p. 9; Ryerson Espino & Trickett, 2008).

Ecological concerns, defined through Bronfenbrenner's theoretical perspectives for research (including evaluation) in human development, explain that a landscape or environment of human ecologic influences are linked (indirectly) to a person's personal development, relationships, and ability to achieve self-sufficiency. Environmental influences are presented as a nested arrangement of interrelated systems, and they are known as the micro-, meso-, exo-, macro-, and chrono-levels (Bronfenbrenner, 1986, p. 723).

The microlevel attributes changes in self as a result of interacting with others and places. While the microlevel is measured through knowledge, beliefs, values, and choices, the next level, the meso-/exolevel, refers to interrelations with other people, organizations, or/and places. It is noted that the levels are interdependent. The macrolevel, commonly used for an assessment framework, is the level that embodies changes in the social or political environment and is frequently documented through qualitative and quantitative changes in laws, regulations, and rules; social services delivered; networks established; and other democratic activities. Chronolevel measurement considers the passage of time and changes within a person; this paradigm would consider changes in women's ideology and would anticipate a marked change from a previous oppressive state. Figure 7.2 presents an illustration of the micro-, meso-/exo-, macro-, and chrono-system levels described. Through these systems, it is possible to analyze and discern program results as well as ascertain environmental influences (Bronfenbrenner, 1986, pp. 723–724).

Feminists articulate how the feminism and ecological concerns intersect by defining model components:

> The feminist ecological model considers power and power dynamics in their many forms individually and systematically, in individual, relational–social, and social–structural contexts. The objectives are to reduce power asymmetries and redistribute power. The model requires us to insert various identity markers at the personal, interpersonal, and systemic levels. . . . The Feminist ecological theory posits that

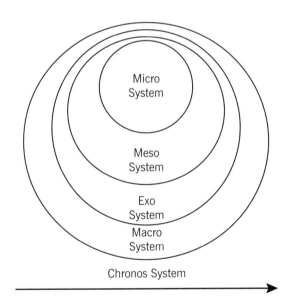

FIGURE 7.2. Illustration of Bronfenbrenner's hierarchy of the social ecology. Reprinted from Little (2013). Copyright 2013 by Todd D. Little. Reprinted with permission from The Guilford Press.

interventions should address not only the individual level, but also the socio-structural level. (Grasswick, 2008, p. 141)

While feminist scholars have published discussions regarding this inter-section in research (Ballou, Matsumoto, & Wagner, 2002; Campbell & Wasco, 2000, p. 778; Code, 2006; Gentile, Ballou, Roffman, & Ritchie, 2010; McLaren & Hawe, 2005, p. 11), the volume of research is mod-est. The connections among gender "as intertwined with other axes of oppression and social stratification are only one aspect of the deeply rela-tional nature of ecological thinking that Code recommends" (Grasswick, 2008, p. 151). Within the subject area of democracy and governance, used as an example in this chapter, the dearth of research and scholarly resources is particularly evident even though this subject area provides a clear basis to discuss women's power, including their participation in gov-ernance processes. This chapter highlights the importance of women's personal development and their understanding of democracy through decision making (within the life course) to interact within the local gov-ernance setting.

Democracy Promotion Programing in International Development

Global trends in programing designed to promote democracy and gov-ernance processes are categorized into (1) rule of law, (2) elections and democratic processes, (3) civil society, and (4) governance.[1] Given limited resources, development agencies strategically prioritize investments and target support to judicial and legal institutions, civil society organizations (CSOs), and the media.

The theory utilized for these development programs generally includes some type of service delivery to a specific target group (such as involvement in a democratic participatory process), during which an internal transformation or human development is expected to occur. The transformation is a process where a change(s) ought to take place as a result of repeated exposure to development program services/informa-tion. Similarly, within Bronfenbrenner's framework, transitions (within human development) occur throughout the lifespan, and they often serve as a direct impetus for developmental change (Bronfenbrenner, 1986, p. 724).

Further, program services provided may take on the following forms: furnishing of assets, advisory services, technical assistance (e.g., policy development, electoral planning, and proposal formulation for integrating information into an electronic-governance website), training for capacity strengthening, workshops to build consensus, and other forms of financial support. The stakeholders selected as recipients of assistance and benefits include elected/appointed officers from senior (ministry) to municipal levels, civil society organizations (CSOs) working with or focusing efforts on specific target groups within communities (including women and other vulnerable/disadvantaged groups), and media.

The transformations expected of beneficiaries include "exposure to information/training," "absorption of arguments," "change in behavior or attitude," and "internal reform." Education and information comes from capacity building, "training," "information campaigns," material support (e.g., "financial contribution," "material provisions"), and pressure (e.g., "advocacy," "lobbying," and "litigation").

Though assistance may be invested in legislative and regulatory mechanisms specifically promoting women's political leadership and representation in developing countries, it represents a minor portion of overall investment.[2] In spite of this budget reality, however, key evaluation questions for internationally funded programs frequently propose the review of women's program participation, female recipients of program services and benefits, and overall program effects on women.

Formulating the Evaluation Framework

Evaluation designs within the arena of international democracy and governance should ensure that gender inequality and ecological concerns are fully considered. In this context, measurement using a feminist–ecological lens includes the assessment of program effects on women within the following three systems of environmental influences: (1) micro-, (2) meso-/exo-, and (3) macrosystems. Table 7.1 provides definitions for each system and the corresponding key evaluative questions reflecting a combination of the feminist–ecological lenses. To facilitate the use of the systems, the names of Bronfenbrenner's three broad systems have been replaced with slightly different labels, where the microsystems have been renamed the "*individual level*," the meso-/exosystems are referred to as the "*composite–community level*," and the macrosystems are assigned the term of the "*collective level*."

The review of evaluation policy documents from international bilateral and multilateral organizations suggests that funds are generally invested to produce results that inform "the choice of methods, approaches, or instruments that are used to promote and defend democracy abroad" (International Institute for Democracy and Electoral

TABLE 7.1. Definitions for the Individual, Composite–Community, and Collective Levels and Corresponding Key Evaluative Questions Considered within a Feminist–Ecological Lens

The individual level

Definition

The *individual level* is the complex of relations between the developing person (woman) and the environment in an immediate setting *containing* that person (e.g., home, school, and workplace). A setting is defined as a place with particular physical features in which the participants engage in *particular activities in particular roles* (e.g., daughter, mother, teacher, and employee) for particular periods of time. Interrelations with places directly determine a woman's knowledge, beliefs, values, intent, and choices.

Guiding or overarching questions

1. What do women know, believe, and value about current democratic processes (or power structures)?
2. What is needed from them for democracy to work effectively?

Knowledge

What technical knowledge, provided by the development program, resonates most with female participants? What is *their* learned expertise? Based on the evidence *women* consider, the facts *they* gather, what is *their* understanding? What are the theories of knowledge about democratic processes and political power structures that *they have chosen/adopted*?

Beliefs

What specific political processes (e.g., access to justice, participation in elections, or freedom of association) are questioned and accepted? Where are their assumptions in order for political processes to effectively function? What do women believe? What points of view do women adopt and value in terms of what is needed from them to engage in the political process? What factors within the individual-level system (or immediate setting) determine how women are setting *their* priorities?

Values

What are the foci of women's attention? What is regarded as important and as unimportant? What is priority?

The composite–community level

Definition

The *composite–community level* comprises the interrelations among major settings *containing* the developing person *at a particular point in her life* and typically encompasses interaction among family, workplace, and peer group. Interrelations with other people/organizations or places are driven by cognition, learned responses, personality (intrinsic differences), and human nature (intrinsic similarities). The settings in which that person is found and thereby influence, delimit, or even determine what goes on there include community-based

(continued)

TABLE 7.1. *(continued)*

organizations, the health care system, and the educational system. Other major institutions of the society that are relevant include the world of work, neighborhood, mass media, agencies of government, the delivery of goods and services, communication and transportation facilities, and informal social networks.

Guiding or overarching questions

1. How do women respond to services, institutions, and others in support of engaging in democratic processes?
2. What is the nature of the interrelationships?
3. What is women's behavior in relation to communicating, expressing, or supporting their emotional, mental, and physical self?

Responding to services, institutions, and others

How do women apply their learned skills and knowledge from the development intervention? What are the formal and informal governance institutions within the society (structured and evolving) that support women's ability to proactively engage in political/democratic processes (voting) or with authorities?

What are the formal and informal governance institutions within the society that influence women's attitudes about and confidence in the legal/penal systems or any other system (within their community) to which they may have access?

What are the formal and informal governance institutions within the society (structured and evolving) that shape women's attitudes about accessing legal assistance (perceived equality of court system) or services to which they are entitled?

How do women communicate what they have learned to others, including what they say, how they say it, and when they say it?

Asserting political power

What interrelations within the composite–community level determine how (and when) women assert their power and engage in political processes? When do women decide/desire to influence others? How do they gain power over others? What do they write, say, and/or share? Who do they include and exclude? What is the (a) symmetry of the power (including deference, respect, leadership, or disrespect) ?

Supporting relationships related to democratic processes

What are the interrelationships that strengthen women's ability to engage in political/democratic processes? Who do women spend time with and how is the time spent?

Supporting emotional, mental, and physical self

What are women willing to tolerate and what will women take a stand on? When do women obey, submit, rebel, protest, and let go? What is the level of women's self-awareness including the responsibility taken for actions? What mental strengths do women choose to acquire, develop, and apply? What is the level of nutrition and fitness, dress, and personal hygiene?

(continued)

TABLE 7.1. *(continued)*

The collective level

Definition

The collective level is a culture/subculture that sets the pattern for the structures and activities occurring at the concrete level. This system represent laws, regulations, and rules but most are informal and implicit, carried often in the minds of the members of society as ideologies, customs, and cultural practices in everyday life (e.g., beliefs and values). Collective-level systems are also conceived and assessed within the context of social networks, roles, activities, and/or a combination of their interrelations.

Guiding or overarching questions

1. How has the broader society changed as a result of (a) women's efforts and (b) the program?
2. What are women's new ideologies?

Intent

After the postoppressive state reflecting the culture, what is the focus of women's attention? What is regarded as important and unimportant, the priorities? How do women balance inquiry and advocacy?

Choices and aspirations

What are the alternatives generated and considered? What are women's hopes and aspirations?

Assistance and Swedish International Development Cooperation Agency, 2007, p. 24). Evaluative efforts are mainly intended to enhance an organization's ability to make strategic decisions and monitor progress in achieving planned results; as a result, the scope of evaluations is limited to measuring and assessing changes in the social or political environment (in other words, primarily at the collective level) (Committee on Evaluation of USAID Democracy Assistance Programs, 2008, p. 10).

The individual and composite community levels reflect the substantive areas on which individual researchers could focus rather than those of a systematic institutional review. The combined feminist–ecological lens could be an effective tool for determining critical factors for program effectiveness and/or failure, particularly as it relates to women's involvement in politics. However, should institutions continue specifically dedicating resources to evaluative efforts wherein feminist–ecological concerns are absent, the relevant questions concerning the extent to which funded interventions *support female empowerment and/or minimize gender inequity within a country will continue* to be unaddressed.

Evaluation Methodology

This section offers evaluators a course of action, described through a case example that ought to be implemented in the event that resources are made available for the collection and interpretation of data in support of evaluations. Epistemology is a theory of knowledge (Campbell & Schram, 1995, p. 88). Feminist researchers look to women as the "knowers" in research and their experiences as knowledge. The evaluation methodology is the overall framework of methods or techniques used to collect information in response to the evaluation questions. Therefore, in applying a combined feminist–ecological lens within an international evaluation, the procedures used ought to easily elicit the perspectives, ideas, experiences, and constructions of women (Campbell & Schram, 1995, p. 89).

Since "few feminist methodologies take a strong either/or position" on quantitative and qualitative methods, a mixed-methods approach is recommended (in this chapter) to address the evaluation questions presented in the feminist–ecological framework (Campbell & Schram, 1995, p. 89) (see Table 7.1). The advantages of using mixed methods include a *"better understanding"* of social phenomena (Greene, 2007, pp. 8, 14). Through the use of multiple approaches, the evaluator effectively ensures that gender inequality and ecological concerns are fully considered. Information is collected on women's knowledge about and experiences engaging in political power structures within the three levels of environmental influences (individual, composite–community, and collective levels). This information comes from multiple resources, using an array of data-collection techniques. While analyzing and interpreting evaluation findings, the mixed-methods approach strengthens the accuracy and validity of the overall evaluative effort.

For example, the sampling process for focus groups, interviews, or/and surveys could be undertaken in clusters or in different stages, thereby ensuring an adequate level of attention to females within the sampling frame. Data sources should include literature and documents, administrative data, interviews with multiple stakeholders, focus groups, and observations. In addition, data gathering should take into account the complexities of the social context, including women's influences and roles within their families, communities, and societies. For example, in ascertaining factors that influence political behavior, the use of focus groups, as opposed to individual interviews, could effectively shape the authenticity of data collected, depending upon the comfort levels of females with male interviewers. Such factors should therefore guide how data is actually collected. Once the data is collected, checking for accuracy from informant responses and drawing from verbatim statements during the coding process are conventional practices that are essential parts of any evaluative effort.

Interpreting Evaluating Findings

The use of feminist evaluation methods not only provides evaluators with the ability to examine women's oppression, but also highlights the evaluator's commitment to empowering women and to challenging gender-related limitations and stereotypes. Interpreting evaluation findings requires an acknowledgment of culture. An evaluator who employs a combined feminist–ecological lens is also culturally competent. Such evaluators "seek to understand how the constructs are defined by cultures," including the use of that culture's language (American Evaluation Association, 2011, p. 8). The many ways in which data may be interpreted and analyzed dictates that the participant's culture be considered to determine (1) what the female subjects' views are; (2) what is valued (and what is not); (3) what is considered effective/helpful; and therefore (4) what is deemed to have impact.

Case Example[3]:
Engaging in Democratic Processes in Angola

As Angola struggled for independence from Portugal—achieved in 1975—it found itself immersed in a violent 27-year civil war fought between two opposing groups: the Movement for the Liberation of the People of Angola (MPLA) and the National Union for the Total Independence of Angola (UNITA). On two different occasions during the civil war, negotiations between the MPLA and UNITA resulted in peace agreements, first in 1991 (the Bicesse Accord) and then again in 1994 (the Lusaka Protocol), yet neither agreement enabled lasting peace. Shortly after the death of UNITA's leader, Jonas Savimbi, in 2002, the war finally ended, providing the impetus for the negotiation of a third agreement (the Luena Accord). Given a history of long civil war, the country's political and social institutions had been and continued to be challenged by a reduced prevalence of engaging in democratic practices and exercising the right of holding governance structures accountable for regular or/and effective public services.

Key Stakeholders

The Office of Transition Initiatives (OTI), part of USAID's Bureau for Democracy, Conflict, and Humanitarian Assistance, has been engaged in long-term development, fostering peace and democracy through innovative programing since 1994. In 2004, OTI had two major programs—or interventions—in Angola to help the country make a successful transition to a peaceful and democratic society, and the evaluation, upon which this case example is based, focused on one of these major programs. The Support to Angola's Democratic Transition (SADT) Program was designed to support a wide range of activities to strengthen participatory democratic practices through a small-grants mechanism. While this program was administered by OTI, Creative Associates International, Inc. (CAII—known as CREA in Angola) was the implementing partner. The purpose of the evaluation was to understand the broader lessons that OTI could learn and apply to other postconflict contexts. The evaluation scope also included exploring the impact that specific grant activities may have had.

Evaluation Design and Methods

Mixed methods were employed to respond to the principal question guiding the evaluation effort: To what extent did OTI/Angola's program meet its stated goal and objectives? This question focused on two of the OTI/Angola Strategic Plan objectives: (1) strengthening the capacity of civil society organizations (CSOs)/nongovernmental organizations (NGOs) to advocate for key issues; and (2) increasing engagement between citizens and local authorities to address community problems. Though the evaluation scope covered many areas, the second part of the strategic plan objectives—increasing engagement between citizens and local authorities to address community problems—is addressed in this chapter to demonstrate effectively how to design, measure, and interpret evaluation findings in the area of gender inequality using feminist–ecological concerns.

OTI's program theory emphasized the importance of "engagement," defined as a "process that includes identifying community needs in a participatory and inclusive fashion, negotiating and compromising to determine priorities, collaborating to acquire financial, material and human resources, and implement[ing] projects in a transparent and participatory fashion" (USAID, OTI/Angola Program Strategy, August 2003, p. 11). To satisfy this objective, OTI supported CSOs/NGOs and their activities that promoted involvement with local authorities. Specifically, most activities observed within this strategic plan objective focused on giving CSOs/NGOs assistance to promote community participation and to engage local authorities (at communal and municipal levels) around relevant community topics.

The evaluation design drew from mixed methods, including (1) a review of organizational documents, (2) a review of database information[4] on all grantees (CSOs/NGOs), (3) stakeholder interviews,[5] and (4) a survey administered to program grantees.[6] Grantee database results showed that 40% of grants were approved for (and funds obligated to) civil engagement in problem solving.[7]

The Framework and the SADT Program Evaluation: The Collective Level

The overall question is to what extent have the broader economic, social, educational, legal, and political systems shaped the CSO/NGO's ability to engage women/female citizens with local authorities to address community problems? Mixed methods were the most appropriate approach to review and analyze the broader structures that may have shaped or influenced a grantee's ability to support civic, including women's, engagement. The conceptual areas explored, falling under the collective level, concentrated on factors influencing the CSOs/NGOs' ability to support engagement with local authorities, as such elements would presumably influence women's engagement. Notably, this preliminary analysis uncovered the following areas: (1) the geographic region in which the grantee was working (and its history of exposure to the war); (2) political tension levels of the region; (3) presence of democracy and governance activities taking place in the community; (4) the size of the civil society organization; (5) demographic factors (e.g., ethnicity, experience, education levels) of those managing the CSO/NGO; and (6) other relevant elements that may have shaped the effectiveness of grantees' initiatives to engage civic engagement.

It should be noted that further analysis was undertaken to interpret findings at the collective level. However, this chapter focuses on the composite community and individual levels of the feminist–ecological framework to effectively demonstrate how the measurement and data interpretation of gender inequity may appear. Thus, while the collective level of the framework is presented in terms of overarching evaluation questions and design, and to some extent, measurement, only at the composite-community and individual levels will the interpretation of evaluation findings be fully presented in this chapter.

The Framework and the SADT Program Evaluation: The Composite Community Level

The composite community level questions are comparably more focused, examining the interrelations within the evaluand, including, but not limited to, the extent to which participants, including women, responded to NGO interventions, formal and informal governance institutions, and other major settings in support of engaging with local authorities.

Additional areas to explore could include the nature of those interrelationships that could affect (1) women's attitudes about, and therefore their confidence in, the legal/penal systems; and (2) their behavior in terms of expressing or communicating their emotional, mental, and physical selves.

Within the OTI evaluation, CSOs/NGOs used advocacy methods ranging from workshops to lectures, radio and newspaper reports, forums, theater, and one rally to raise awareness about issues and educate citizens about their rights. Survey results of program participants from CSOs/NGOs[8] revealed that women were the audience most targeted. Additional survey results from the CSOs/NGOs grantees operating in four regions (Benguela, Huambo, Huila, and Luanda) indicated that the advocacy "areas in which their organization is presently doing advocacy"[9] varied widely, with the most popular topic, land rights at 23%, followed by women's rights in the markets and elections at 19.6%, and free (of cost) education and human rights at 12%.

CSO/NGO advocacy focused on raising awareness of rights, including holding community and governance structures accountable for service delivery (e.g., education, public safety, and public sanitation). Data from in-depth interviews indicated that grantees appeared to have a solid understanding of community problems/issues, how to address them, and how to increase participation from the citizens and governing structures equally. Indeed, while survey results were mixed, all grantees clearly self-reported that community participation was "good," "high," and "participatory." Similarly, grantee reports indicated that target audience(s) were not aware of their legal rights (e.g., to free primary education, to own land, to work in the market free of harassment), suggesting that the selected projects were both warranted and suitable to the program's objectives.

As a consequence of CSO/NGO advocacy, grantees recalled that attitudinal shifts among participants, including women, had occurred. A grantee activist cited an example where he told a parent (a mother), "You have the right as a parent to send your child to school without paying." According to the interviewee, parents did not know that paying a bribe or unsystematic payment (*cobrança* in Portuguese) was not mandatory, and they were not aware that a law even existed that protected their children.

Another example, provided by a grantee, highlights the fact that women did not realize that they were entitled to work in the marketplace free of police harassment. In this case, the grantee reached audiences of women through formal lectures and "political theater" in the marketplace to educate them about their rights. The grantee reported that the women now openly discuss their rights with others in the markets. The interviewee recalled women saying that "the police have no right to harass us."

The Framework and the SADT Program Evaluation:
The Individual Level

The individual-level questions analyzed the complex relations between the woman and her environment (e.g., home, school, marketplace, and workplace). To recall, a *setting* is defined as the physical place in which the program participants engage in particular activities in particular roles (e.g., daughter, mother, teacher, and employee) for particular periods of time. Examining women's interrelations with places directly would expose and, in turn, shed more insights on their knowledge, beliefs, values, intent, and choices.

Evaluation design questions could cover all or just one of the multiple areas encapsulating knowledge, beliefs, and values: (1) the technical knowledge, provided through the CSO/NGO advocacy that resonates most with female participants; (2) what women believe in terms of their points of view adopted and their values of what is needed from them to engage with authorities; and (3) what is prioritized or regarded as important and as unimportant. In uncovering all three key areas, the remaining domains of intent and choices, as noted in Table 7.1, ought to emerge.

In addition to the mixed-methods evaluation design, it may also be helpful in a case such as this to refer to theories of adult learning processes within the rubric of raising awareness to influence attitudinal and behavioral changes concerning holding local government institutions/systems accountable. For a war-inflicted country such as Angola, it was observed that the transition to democracy required people at many levels, not only program beneficiaries, but also CSOs/NGOs, local authorities, and community leaders (some of whom were also women) to change their attitudes and beliefs. Hence, the scope of the individual-level analysis, in applying the reasoning of the feminist-ecological framework, does not have to be limited to the complex relationships and adaptations of the beneficiaries only, or in this case, the recipients of grantee advocacy messages. Indeed, evaluators should be flexible, and if possible, broaden the data interpretation to other levels where women may be making contributions.

In the case of this evaluation, it was observed that program participants experienced a process, characterized as a "journey," oscillating from lack of interest to awareness, from inaction to empowerment, and from "fear" to commitment. Transitions within women's journeys were observed based on descriptions (from CSO/NGO representatives) of their perception of women's new forms of action. For example, before participation in the CSO/NGO activities and exposure to advocacy, many women lacked awareness of their basic rights and had attitudes that were not conducive to advocating change or to engaging with others to solve community problems. One grantee described this state of mind as "very calm" (*muito calmo* in Portuguese). The following interview quotes illustrate this outlook:

> [Before the grantee's advocacy efforts], "Parents asked "How much is the bribe [*cobrança*] this year?"
> "When a woman saw a crime in the market, she would look the other way."
> "Women were scared of the police."
> "The laws don't get executed in the provinces, this is Angola."
> "The leader in the village is the LEADER."
> "People think that 'to vote means war.'"

Further examples of shifts in awareness and attitudes resulting from program participation can be seen in the following interview quotes:

> "The women would not hesitate to report a crime when observed which is different from the past. In the past, they would look the other way and going to the police was not even part of their thinking."
> [After the community meetings] " . . . the beneficiaries were more informed and showed that they had learned something; there was a new sense of consciousness to engage with authorities, saying 'let's continue this.'"
> "Now, a parent will . . . say you did not cover this or that topic well [specifying what is important for the child] or "I thought that one area was too complicated for my child in this class." Before, holding teachers accountable for their instruction was not even considered."

In spite of the observed changes of women's interrelations with authorities and shifting attitudes, beliefs, and values, however, interview data also revealed that discouragement and "fear" were other relevant factors inhibiting people's openness to new ideas and new actions. Thus, while the data were encouraging, the qualitative theme of "fear," raised through grantee interviews, was a persistent element of Angola's political culture and remained a key obstacle that limited people's willingness to explore openly civic engagement. For example, one grantee described how "their audience's [women in the markets] heads have changed, but there is still the need to eat. . . . They do not have the money to take the action." Another grantee recounted that some parents spoke out against the grantee's advocacy work, stating that they were against corruption, but they wanted their children to receive instruction.

Conclusions

This chapter covered the use of ecological and feminist lenses and pre-sented an adaptable conceptual framework to support measuring gen-der inequality within the evaluation context of interventions that support democracy and governance. Multiple approaches ensure that gender inequality and ecological concerns are fully considered at three levels of environmental influences (collective, composite community, and individ-ual levels). The following section reviews potential sampling processes, data-gathering techniques with multiple stakeholders, use of verbatim statements during the coding, and data interpretation. To elucidate these concepts and with special permission, a case example evaluating the Sup-port to Angola's Democratic Transition (SADT) Program supported by the Office of Transition Initiatives (OTI) is presented.

Concurrent to using a combined ecological–feminist lens within the evaluation process, evaluators should frame evaluation results in a fashion such that stakeholder values are presented in an accessible and nonchallenging manner. One practical strategy that evaluators could use to ensure that gender inequality and ecological concerns are fully con-sidered includes proactive approaches in guiding a temperate discussion with all relevant stakeholders (those implementing and/or financing the program). This has achieved transformative results.

Questions concerning the extent to which funded interventions sup-port female empowerment and minimize gender inequity within a coun-try will continue to be unaddressed if concerted efforts are not dedicated to honing the practice of seeking women as knowers, broadening data col-lection practices in this area, interpreting findings, and creating a stan-dard for their inclusion.

NOTES

1. Definitions are adopted from the Center for Democracy and Governance Bureau for Global Programs, Field Support, and Research, United States Agency for International Development (USAID), *Democracy and Governance: A Conceptual Framework* (Technical Publication Series), November 1998.
2. Budget estimates in this thematic area represent approximately 15% of United Nations Development Assistance Frameworks (UNDAF) reviewed. See "UNI-FEM. What Women Want: Planning and Financing for Gender-Responsive Peacebuilding," by Cueva-Beteta and Rodriguez, with contributions from Jen-kins, Goetz, Anwar, and Dore-Weeks (2010, p. 6).
3. This case example is derived from an evaluation I undertook in 2004 under Contract No. HAD-I-13-03-00124-00 with Social Impact. The Office of

Transition Initiatives (OTI) has granted me permission to use this evaluation in this chapter.

4. According to the database, a total of 55 grants had been approved for 37 NGOs throughout the program cycle.

5. The qualitative interview sample included all those who worked on the OTI/ Angola program in Washington, DC, and Angola. For grantee interviews, however, the arrangement was slightly different, where with the aid of the database, 10 to 15 projects were purposefully sampled initially. After field work, 17 projects and 14 grantees comprised the entire sample. It should be noted that some grantees were funded multiple times, and so it is for this reason that the number of grantees and projects were not identical.

6. The survey sample consisted of 35 persons, all of whom were grantees. The procedure may be characterized as convenient, based on the stratified, non-random sample. All those available for grantee interviews were surveyed, and such persons ranged from support staff to project coordinators to directors. The survey implemented included attitudinal statements, using a 4-point Likert scale ranging from "strongly agree" to "strongly disagree."

7. Figures were drawn from the program database.

8. $N = 35$.

9. Question 18 on the survey was: "Name all the areas in which your organization is presently doing advocacy (mark all that apply): (1) Land rights; (2) Rights to a free education; (3) Rights of women in the market place; (4) Labor rights for farmers and other groups; (5) Formulation of a new government; (6) Human rights; (7) Other."

REFERENCES

American Evaluation Association. (2011). *Statement on cultural competency*. Washington, DC: Author.

Baber, K. M., & Allen, K. R. (1992). *Women and families: Feminist reconstructions*. New York: Guilford Press.

Ballou, M., Matsumoto, A., & Wagner, M. (2002). Toward a feminist ecological theory of human nature: Theory building in response to real-world dynamics. In M. Ballou & L. Brown (Eds.), *Rethinking mental health and disorder: Feminist perspectives* (pp. 99–141). New York: Guilford Press.

Bamberger, M., Rugh, J., & Mabry, L. (2006). *Real-world evaluation: Working under budget, time, data, and political constraints*. Thousand Oaks, CA: Sage.

Bronfenbrenner, U. (1986). Ecology of the family as a context for human development: Research perspectives. *Developmental Psychology, 22,* 723–742.

Bronfenbrenner, U. (1995). Developmental ecology through space and time: A future perspective. In P. Moen, G. H. Elder Jr., & K. Luscher (Eds.), *Examining lives in context: Perspectives on the ecology of human development* (pp. 619–647). Washington, DC: APA Books.

Campbell, R., & Schram, P. (1995). Feminist research methods: A content analysis of psychology and social science textbooks. *Psychology of Women Quarterly, 19,* 85–106.

Campbell, R., & Wasco, S. M. (2000). Feminist approaches to social science: Epistemological and methodological tenets. *American Journal of Community Psychology, 28*(6), 773–790.

Center for Democracy and Governance Bureau for Global Programs, Field Support, and Research, United States Agency for International Development (USAID). (1998, November). *Democracy and governance: A conceptual framework* (Technical Publication Series, PN-ACD-395). Accessed at *http:// transition.usaid.gov/our_work/democracy_and_governance/publications/pdfs/ pnacd395.pdf.*

Code, L. (2006). *Ecological thinking: The politics of epistemic location.* Oxford, UK: Oxford University Press.

Committee on Evaluation of United States Agency for International Development (USAID) Democracy Assistance Programs and National Research Council. (2008). *Improving democracy assistance: Building knowledge through evaluations and research.* Washington, DC: National Academy of Sciences.

Cueva-Beteta, H., & Rodriguez, L. (2010). *What women want planning and financing for gender-responsive peacebuilding.* UNIFEM.

Fearon, J., Humphreys, M., & Weinstein, J. M. (2009). Development assistance, institution building, and social cohesion after civil war: Evidence from a field experiment in Liberia (Working Paper 194). Accessed at *www.cgdev.org/ content/publications/detail/1423322.*

Finnoff, K., & Ramamurthy, B. (2010). *Financing gender equality: Review of modalities for post conflict financing.* UNFEM.

Gentile, L., Ballou, M., Roffman, E., & Ritchie, J. (2010). Supervision for social change: A feminist ecological perspective. *Women and Therapy, 33*(1), 140–151.

Grasswick, H. E. (2008). From feminist thinking to ecological thinking: Determining the bounds of community. *Hypatia, 23*(1), 150–160.

Greene, J. (2007). *Mixed methods in social inquiry.* San Francisco: Jossey-Bass.

International Fund for Agricultural Development (IFAD). (2010). *Performance with regard to gender equality and women's empowerment: Corporate-level evaluation* (Report No. 2324). Accessed at *www.ifad.org/evaluation/public_html/ eksyst/doc/corporate/gender.pdf.*

International Institute for Democracy and Electoral Assistance and Swedish International Development Cooperation Agency. (2007). *Evaluation democracy support: Methods and experiences, joint evaluation.* Available at *www.idea. int/publications/evaluating_democracy_support/index.cfm.*

Little, T. D. (2013). *Longitudinal structural equation modeling.* New York: Guilford Press.

McLaren, L., & Hawe, P. (2005). Ecological perspectives in health research. *Journal of Epidemiology and Community Health, 59,* 6–14.

Mulvey, A. (1988). Community psychology and feminism: Tensions and commonalities. *Journal of Community Psychology, 16,* 70–83.

Organization for Economic Co-Operation and Development. (2008). Development co-operation (OECD/DAC). *Guidance on evaluating conflict prevention and peacebuilding activities working draft for application period.* Accessed at *www.oecd.org/ secure/pdfDocument/0,2834,en_21571361_34047972_39774574_1_1_1_1,00.pdf.*

Organization for Economic Co-Operation and Development. (2008). Development co-operation (OECD/DAC). *Guiding principles for aid effectiveness, gender equality and women's empowerment. Accessed at www.oecd.org/document/62/0 ,3746,en_2649_34541_42288382_1_1_1_1,00.html.*

Ryerson Espino, S., & Trickett, E. (2008). The spirit of ecological inquiry: An analysis of research relationships within published community psychology intervention research. *American Journal of Community Psychology, 42*(1), 60–78.

Social Indicator Centre for Policy Alternatives in Partnership with Academy for Educational Development (AED). (2003). Knowledge, attitudes, practices survey on the Sri Lankan peace process. Washington, DC: USAID Development Experience Clearinghouse (DEC).

United Nations Economic Commission for Africa (UNECA). (2001). *Assessing the political empowerment of women. Accessed at www.uneca.org/eca_programmes/ acgd/Publications/en_0109_political.pdf.*

United States Agency for International Development (USAID). (1998, November). *Democracy and governance: A conceptual framework.* Washington, DC: USAID Development Experience Clearinghouse.

United States Agency for International Development (USAID). (1999). *Lessons in implementation: The NGO story building civil society in central eastern Europe and the new independent states.* Washington, DC: USAID Development Experience Clearinghouse.

United States Agency for International Development (USAID). (2003, August). *Office of Transition Initiatives (OTI) in Angola program strategy/draft version.* Washington, DC: Bureau for Democracy, Conflict, and Humanitarian Assistance and Office of Transition Initiatives.

CHAPTER 8

Feminist Evaluation in South Asia

Building Bridges of Theory and Practice

Katherine Hay

Introduction

The last few years have seen renewed enthusiasm and interest in international development evaluation (Hay, 2010). The practice of evaluating women's empowerment programs or the "gender" component of development has also expanded. However, how much has this work challenged dominant ideas and approaches to development and the ways ideas of gender become rooted in interventions? What questions are evaluations raising, and what methods and approaches are being used to answer them? Is there a space to bring feminist perspectives into mainstream development through evaluation?

Feminist research has made deep and important contributions to development theory and practice. What similar or different contributions does feminist analysis bring to development evaluation? This chapter explores:

1. The contributions of feminist research (and analysis) to international development theory.
2. The value of feminist evaluation for evaluating development discourse, programs, and projects.
3. How to engage in, and use, feminist evaluation in international development.

Key Concepts and Terms

Gender bias is manifest and systematic in social institutions, and feminist analysis is a way of understanding how gender and other intersecting social cleavages (such as race, class, sexuality, caste, and religion) define and shape the experience and exercise of power in different contexts. There is no "one" feminist theory in international development but several overlapping ideas and approaches that coexist and inform each other.

Recent work by Podems (2010) illuminates the definitional confusion between feminist evaluation and gender approaches, and describes feminist evaluation as flexible and as being a way of thinking about evaluation. Podems's (2010) comparison of feminist evaluation and gender approaches gives examples of practical differences between feminist and gender evaluations. For example, Podems notes that gender approaches might identify or record the differences between men and women while feminist evaluation would explore why these differences exist and "challenges women's subordinate position" (2010, p. 8).

"Feminist evaluation" can thus be a way of describing evaluations that embody certain tenets (Podems, 2010; Seigart & Brisolara, 2003), including a central focus on gender inequities and recognition that:

- Discrimination based on gender is systemic and structural.
- Evaluation is political.
- Knowledge has power.
- Knowledge should be a resource of and for the people who create, hold, and share it.
- There are multiple ways of knowing and some are privileged over others.

I have argued that applying feminist principles to different stages in the evaluation process is what constitutes feminist evaluation in practice (Hay, 2012).

International Development: Paradigms and Trends in Development Evaluation

Development interventions such as health programs, infrastructure development, educational policies, or electoral reform schemes are informed by ideas on development and gender that are at times explicit, more often implicit, and often competing. These are the "big ideas," or the discourse, that shape our understanding of how the world works. These ideas consist of language and images, narratives, stories, and myths. At times they are unquestioned and unexplored, while at other times they are hotly contested. It may only be when one encounters an alternate discourse, or when discourse changes, that the ideas rooted in much of our policies and programs become explicit.

For example, policy responses to HIV were based on dominant discourses on HIV that evolved over time. These discourses included a gay plague discourse, a "contaminated other" discourse, an innocent victim discourse, a heterosexual-risk discourse, and most recently a development discourse (Hill, 1995). In looking back at discourses or dominant ideas around HIV, we can see quite easily how they changed over time. We can also see how these discourses shaped the ways that society responded to HIV, the kinds of programs and interventions that were developed, and how they were assessed. However, while discourses can sometimes be unpacked fairly easily in hindsight, they are often obscure (and often intentionally so) as they are lived.

Cornwall, Harrison, and Whitehead (2007) note that the creation and evolution of development policies can "be understood as a terrain of contestation in which particular framings of the problem and the solution . . . come to gain purchase" (pp. 3–4). Discourse matters because it underpins and legitimizes these framings and thus the interventions built upon them. Public spending, policies, and programs are all connected to discourse, to what society sees as important and how we understand and think change will happen. Some examples of how development theory is gendered are presented below to illustrate how evaluation can offer opportunities to critique and analyze that discourse or those paradigms.

Taking one example, Chattopadhyay and Duflo (2004) evaluated the differences in spending in a set of villages in India with female leaders and male leaders. Many development theorists had argued that if women leaders were in power they would focus spending on care, education, and health-related services, which would lead to better educated children and other positive social outcomes. However, there was little actual evidence to demonstrate whether there was a causal relationship between women's representation and policy decisions, and in what situations.

Chattopadhyay and Duflo studied the policy consequences of a 1993 amendment to the constitution of India that required states to reserve one-third of all positions of village chief to women. They surveyed investments in local public goods in a sample of villages in two districts in West Bengal and Rajasthan and compared investments made in villages that had a reserved seat for a woman leader and those that did not have a reserved seat. As village councils getting reserved seats had been randomly selected by the government of India, differences in investment decisions could be confidently attributed to the reserved status of those village councils. What Chattopadhyay and Duflo found was that in West Bengal, women complained more often than men about drinking water and roads, and that village councils reserved for women made more investments in drinking water and roads. In Rajasthan, women complained more often than men about drinking water but less often about roads, and village councils reserved for women made more investments in water and less investment in roads. Women's and men's preferences were based on the formal requests by men and women coming into the councils. Chattopadhyay and Duflo explored and did not find any evidence that these investments were driven by features other than the gender of the village chief. Their results indicate that a politician's gender influenced policy decisions in these districts, and in ways that seem to better reflect women's preferences.

However, both positive and negative gendered ideas and values find their way into development paradigms, often in simplified or uncritical ways. A good example of this is in the way that ideas of "women" appear in development discourse—often as both "victims" and "heroines" (Cornwall et al., 2007). Goetz (2007), for example, has written on the ways in which ideas on gender are included in anticorruption policies and programs. Reflecting on empirical evidence showing that women less frequently take bribes and explanations suggesting that this discrepancy is somehow intrinsic to women's nature, Goetz (2007) points out that this discourse is "based on assumptions about the way in which gender shapes people's reactions to corruption" but does not consider also the ways in which gender relations also "condition the opportunities for corrupt behavior" (p. 95). Put another way, we want to think that women are more virtuous (and design our programs accordingly), but the reality may be that they simply have less opportunity to engage in corruption. Evaluation needs to explore and be open to both explanations.

What a feminist lens brings to evaluation is not an essentialist view of women (as more virtuous, less corrupt, etc.) or a view of women as being more deserving of benefiting from development. A feminist lens brings an emphasis on power relations, the structural elements of inequities, justice, and politics. Through these foci, feminist research has made important contributions to development. For example, examining the field of economics, a feminist lens has brought extensive and important contributions to such diverse topics as women's work and the double work burden, social cleavages and overlapping sites of discrimination, the "black box" of the household, and understandings of rights that are less abstract and more lived. Researchers have both used mainstream economic tools to examine wage gaps between men and women and critiqued these tools for their limited ability to shed light on the underlying inequities behind such gaps (Figart, Mutari, & Power, 2002). Studies of unpaid work within households (the black box) have brought attention to women's unpaid work (Waring, 1988) and highlighted inequities in distribution within households (Agarwal, 1997). Tools developed by McElroy and Horney (1981) have become commonly used for understanding decision making and agency within households. A feminist lens has also led to innovations in the analysis of government budgets according to their effects on gender equity and to understanding the effects of macroeconomic policies of structural adjustment and liberalization (Grown, Elson, & Cagatay, 2000). Feminist economists have also analyzed how factors such as race and caste (Brewer & King, 2002) interact with gender and affect economic outcomes. Looking at even this very curated list of how feminist insights and analysis have strengthened the economic analysis of development suggests the extent to which feminist insights across disciplines can bring new developments, approaches, and insights to evaluation.

Like research, evaluation offers opportunities to critique dominant and evolving discourses and hold them up for scrutiny. Feminist contributions to research and deconstructive analysis (Dietz, 2003; Nash, 2002) are useful tools for such efforts. Evaluations can test whether policies and programs work on the ground (and for whom), but can also raise questions about mainstream development discourse and the way this discourse is articulated in policies and programs. As Jain and Elson (2011) note, "the very approach being taken to understanding and measuring progress, and planning for and evaluating development, needs rethinking" (p. xxxiii). Instead of only asking if a particular program is working or whether it is meeting its' objectives, for example, evaluation can also explore and examine the theory underpinning the program—or "what working" is meant to look like. That is a space where development paradigms are embedded; critiquing such paradigms thus also brings possibilities to challenge or change these paradigms. Evaluators applying a feminist lens can examine policies and programs to also ask "Who has constructed this discourse and whose experiences are not reflected?"

Ramachandran (2012) illustrates how changing discourse around education in India over the last 50 years (among educationalists, policymakers, and development agencies) has influenced programs. She maps education's conceptualization as a universal good from the point of independence, to an instrument for population control and other development goals in the 1960s, to a right by the 1980s, and to a cornerstone of women's empowerment agendas by the 1990s. In doing so she connects these paradigms to education programs on the ground, demonstrating how the programs are embedded in understandings of equity (and inequity). It is apparent that until paradigms shift there can be little space to integrate new evidence that runs counter to the dominant discourse. By examining both design and implementation, research and evaluation has strengthened and informed program and policy implementation in part by holding a mirror to the dominant development paradigms and discourses informing those policies (De, Khera, Samon, & Shiva Kumar, 2011; PROBE Team, 1999; Ramachandran, 2012).

Moving beyond domains such as education, an overwhelming feature of current international development discourse that shapes all domains is the emphasis on economic growth. While growth has been the biggest driver of decreasing global inequality in at least the past decade, many, including Amartya Sen (2011), warn that the current obsession with growth rates is misplaced given that "the lives that people are able to lead—what ultimately interest people most—are only indirectly and partially influenced by the rates of overall economic growth." Lourdes Beneria (2011) adds a feminist lens to such critiques, noting:

> The paradigm tied to global capitalism and rational Economic Man, with its conceptual frameworks and economic policies, has failed us not only because it has brought some "development" while neglecting "human development" for all, but also because, despite progress towards gender quality at many levels, it has done so within a paradigm of social inequality that feminists need to question. (p. 70)

The Consequences or Limits of Mainstream Development Evaluation

Dominant development discourse matters. It shapes what we think is important, our understanding of "how things work," and thus our views on how things might change. Elson (2011) notes that a feminist lens can challenge the idea of "rational economic man" and can help us to "rethink the criteria we can use to evaluate economic and social policies and to construct better ones that are more likely to realize the dreams of social justice and women's rights" (p. 3).

Implicit (or explicit) theoretical underpinnings of programs will vary among actors and can change and shift over time. Evaluation can serve to embed, challenge, or formally reflect those underpinnings. There is an opportunity for feminist evaluators to identify and test various dimensions of theories underpinning policies and programs—including examining sets of programs. Such evaluations could interrogate not only the outcomes of the program but also the underpinning theory of the programs. To give an example, India has a set of programs that have some parallels with Depression-era works programs of the United States, including a $9 billion program designed to create jobs through building infrastructure in rural areas called the Mahatma Gandhi National Rural Employment

Guarantee Scheme (MGNREGS). Analysis of this program illustrates that the design of that program was gender-sensitive in a range of ways (equal wages for men and women, participation of women in committees, and provision of a daycare center on work sites, etc.). However, evaluations with a feminist lens have demonstrated that daycare centers are often not set up (an implementation failure) and also that women workers are more comfortable leaving infants with other older children, whether at home or on the site (a program theory failure) (Sudarshan & Sharma, 2012). The second finding speaks to the design itself and the ideas and discourse informing that design (specifically, that women would prefer to leave their children with workers at crèches rather than with family members). By getting the design and the implementation wrong, older girl children began missing school to provide child care to allow mothers to work. The program design failed to account for gender norms and preferences around child care that did not change, despite adding a new opportunity for earning into the context. In this case assumptions about gender roles, child care, and women's labor unintentionally moved domestic burdens onto girl children by further engaging women in development work. A mainstream evaluation might simply probe whether crèches were in place in the locations where the program intended them to be. A feminist evaluation might push further and question the nature of the program design itself, the assumptions behind the design, and the dominant and gendered ideas around child care implicit in the design. In doing so evaluation can both test whether a program is "working" but also critique "what working looks like," and who benefits, does not benefit, or is harmed, by the program. Building from this example, one can question the extent to which programs targeting "the household" ignore the lived realities of stakeholders who may be very unequal within that household. This type of questioning opens a rich space where feminist analysis, research, and evaluation theory can come together. For example, realist synthesis (Pawson, 2006) builds on the principles of realist evaluation (Pawson & Tilley, 1997) to develop and test theories about how, for whom, and in what contexts policies and programs work. A feminist realist synthesis could be developed to unpack theories and discourse on ideas of the household that inform policies and programs but are often themselves untested (or known to be false). Such efforts could demonstrate how understandings of the household are embedded in policies and help develop and test theories about how, for whom, and in what contexts programs targeting households might and do work.

Feminist critique and analysis can examine the ways in which dominant discourses become lodged in policies, programs, and projects, and evaluate whether the implicit assumptions behind these discourses resonate with women's actual lived experiences. In doing so, a feminist lens in evaluation offers opportunities to generate findings that strengthen program and policy implementation but also critique the dominant discourse informing those policies, and bring greater diversity of views and values into that discourse.

Why Questioning Paradigms Matter: The Case of India and Bangladesh

Of what value is feminist evaluation for evaluating development discourse, programs, and projects? Beginning with a case study of India and Bangladesh, this question is illustrated with some examples from theory and practice.

India and Bangladesh are neighboring countries with many cultural and historical connections. If one focuses on growth rates to examine the development of the two countries, India comes out far ahead. India's gross national product (GNP) per capita is over double that of Bangladesh. However, a feminist lens might suggest looking at other dimensions. For example, what if one were to look at sex ratios (the ratio of males to females in a population)? The natural sex ratio at birth is estimated to be 106 boys to 100 girls (Grech, Savona-Ventura, & Vassallo-Agius, 2002). Cultural preference for one sex, typically males, is significantly skewing the naturally occurring ratio in some populations, particularly since the introduction of ultrasound scans in the 1980s.

Bangladesh's sex ratio is 978 females per 1,000 males. India's sex ratio, among children ages 0–6 years, declined to 914 girls per 1,000 boys in 2011. The sex ratio is declining because families are choosing sex-selective abortion (aborting female fetuses), and because girls that are born have a lower chance of surviving than boys because of inequitable distribution of resources within families (such as food or medical treatment). India has enacted laws targeting sex selection. It is illegal for ultrasound technicians to reveal the sex of the fetus or to abort based on the sex of the fetus. However, the sex ratio continues to worsen. Preliminary data from the 2011 census recorded districts with sex ratios less than 850. It is the range and depth of discriminations against women and girls that supports the decline.

In another comparison, one can look at maternal mortality (the annual number of deaths of women from pregnancy-related causes per 100,000 live births). In Canada, seven of every 100,000 pregnant women die during pregnancy and childbirth each year (Hogan et al., 2010). India reported 250 deaths per 100,000 live births in 2005–2009 (UNICEF, 2011), while Bangladesh reported 194 deaths for 100,000 live births in 2010. Particularly impressive in Bangladesh is the decline achieved from 1989 when 574 of every 100,000 pregnant women died (Bangladesh Maternal Mortality and Health Care Survey, 2010). While the numbers are still unacceptably high, this progress in one of the poorest countries in the world is important to understand. How did Bangladesh achieve this decline? While more research is needed, Glassman (2011) suggests that the decline is based on a combination of investments in family planning, delayed age at marriage (possibly in part due to investments in girls' education), increased awareness, and increased availability of obstetric care.

In examining the cases of sex ratio and maternal mortality, if policymakers focused on development paradigms that emphasized these indicators rather than growth, how might this influence the questions being asked? Perhaps evaluators would be asked to examine the relative success in Bangladesh of such measures and how these successes are connected to different development efforts and their intersections over time. While researchers and policymakers may speculate on the links between strategies, policies, and results, evaluation could help capture more evidence on what is working and not working for women and girls in India and Bangladesh. Why would such evaluation matter? Even with no systematic evaluation of why laws and policies are not working and which programs show the most (or least) promise, cash incentive-based programs are increasingly used to target son preference in India. Examples of cash incentives include cash grants and saving bonds redeemable on the daughter's 18th birthday if she meets certain targets such as being unmarried or achieving certain educational levels. On the positive side, these policies recognize the value of changing attitudes, rather than trying to legislate against the practice of son preference (through sex-selective abortions), which has not changed behaviors. However, studies show that sex ratios are not positively impacted by increases in income (Jha, 2011).

The dominant discourse or paradigm of economic rationality underpins development understandings and thus economic rationality underpins the solutions (policies and programs) designed to change these behaviors. This is despite evidence that economic rationality is not the primary driver of son preference. Paradigms are powerful. Because we are convinced by our discourse that economic growth is the answer, and economic rationality is its manifestation at the individual level, we seek out solutions that reinforce and support our assumptions and continue with them despite all evidence to the contrary. As Jain and Elson (2011) write, "It is not enough to call for . . . the empowerment of women within existing paradigms of development . . . [it is the paradigms] themselves that need questioning and transforming" (pp. xxxiii–xxxiv).

If equity were the dominant international development model rather than growth, or in addition to growth, we might begin to question why India's growth success does not seem to have translated into success in gender equity. If we were to begin to ask, "What would promote success?," we would be asking an important question. The next section explores how feminist evaluation at the policy, program, and project level can help to do this.

Using Feminist Evaluation to Examine International Development Policies, Programs, and Projects

Evaluation theories and theorists and the evaluation approaches they espouse are sometimes associated with particular methods. Such evaluation approaches are prescriptive in nature; that is to say, following such approaches also entails following a prescribed set of methodological steps. For example, doing experimental impact evaluations will always include randomizing a treatment across a control group and a treatment group. However, there are many other evaluation theories and approaches that take a stance on particular evaluation issues, but that do not prescribe a specific or required set of methods. Such evaluation approaches may, for example, lay out principles and/or develop and include frameworks, while not prescribing a specific set of methods for evaluations guided by these principles. As I have argued elsewhere (Hay, 2012), applying feminist principles to different stages in the evaluation process is what constitutes feminist evaluation in practice. Feminist evaluation, therefore, it is argued here, is among this latter category of nonmethodologically prescriptive evaluation theories and approaches. What this looks like in practice is that at each stage in the evaluation process the evaluator asks a series of questions to explore and ensure the integration of feminist approaches in their evaluation work. Different evaluation theorists and practitioners would categorize this process into different stages, but, in general, there is a start or a *planning phase* that includes deciding what to evaluate and what questions to ask; this is followed by a *design phase* of determining what methodologies and methods will best generate the kind of knowledge and evidence needed; there is also an *implementation phase* where data is gathered and analyzed; and finally, a *phase of use* where the evaluation findings are shared, taken up, and used. These phases usually overlap in different ways depending on the nature of the evaluation (Hay, 2012).

Figure 8.1 demonstrates a set of stages in conducting evaluations. Applying the feminist principles at each of these stages is how one does feminist evaluation (Hay, 2012). What this means for the practitioner is that applying the principles of feminist evaluation will determine the nature of the evaluation design and methods for that particular evaluation. The process is reflexive and adaptive and one in which the evaluator

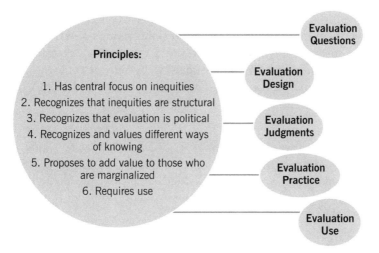

FIGURE 8.1. Feminist principles and the stages of evaluation.

must weigh and balance decisions (on design, method, process, and use) along the way. What is offered is thus not a prescriptive design, but rather a set of principles and values that shape and guide practice and decision making.

For example:

1. At the questioning stage, as described earlier in the case of the rural employment scheme, a feminist critique can identify gaps in program theory that weaken opportunities to address gender inequities. Feminist evaluators can raise and explore new or different questions by negotiating with evaluation commissioners to integrate such questions into the evaluation terms of reference.

2. At the design stage, while a rigorous feminist evaluation would be one that used the range of methods that best matched the questions, some designs do not address (indeed they attempt to factor out) the perspectives and experiences of marginalized groups in the evaluation process. Feminist evaluation designs would start with the principle of including those voices.

3. Making a judgment about what works and what does not work is a fundamental purpose of evaluation. At the judgment stage, feminist evaluations would recognize that in any program there are different or competing definitions and criteria of success. Feminist analysis would bring those criteria to the surface for debate and critique.

4. Feminist evaluation practice is characterized by what I have termed a "healthy discomfort" (Hay, 2012) that comes with trying to negotiate and insert feminist principles into a time-bound, resource-bound, judgment-oriented exercise. It is "healthy" because it comes with reflection, analysis, and adjustment that moves evaluation closer to feminist principles. This reflexivity also comes with

> a groundedness or situatedness of the evaluator within the evaluation process . . . and, this situatedness relates to questions of evaluation work that is sought, considered, or rejected, what is negotiable and nonnegotiable, how they see themselves in the evaluation process and, how this relates to the way they see themselves in the broader contexts in which they operate. (Hay, 2012, p. 333)

5. Feminist evaluation brings with it the evaluator's responsibility to take action on findings. Particular pathways may be risky (for the program or the women's movement more broadly), others blocked, and some strategic—but all are understood as negotiated and constructed (Hay, 2012).

The opportunity for practitioners, particularly given the relative newness of feminist evaluation thinking and writing, is that it will be the documenting of practice that further deepens and informs the body of work and practice that constitutes "feminist evaluation." Given that evaluation theory has arguably had few major theoretical leaps in over a decade, this is new, important, and exciting terrain.

However, in attempting feminist evaluation, factors in the international development environment that evaluators need to understand and respond to include:

- Positions on methodological choices.
- Debates (and their disciplinary roots) on rigor.
- Calls for accountability and what that means and to whom.
- Competing and dominant ideas on how change happens.
- Challenges to acting on findings.

These factors are flagged because they are the spaces where mainstream development discourse is often embedded and articulated, particularly in terms of challenges to alternatives (whether development alternatives or evaluation alternatives). As such, the kinds of alternative conceptualizations or approaches that a feminist evaluation approach may offer is likely to be contested along one or more of these lines. They are thus flagged in the following section as areas that evaluators using feminist approaches should pay particular attention to as spaces for potential tensions or conflict with dominant development understandings.

Methodological Choices

Evaluations with a feminist lens can be situated within different approaches to evaluation and draw upon differing traditions in design, methodology, and approaches to rigor and validity found in those approaches. However, the questions feminist analyses pose are often different from mainstream development questions. Mainstream development, and by extension mainstream evaluation, grapples with mainstream questions. This has resulted in designs, approaches, and tools that may be more or less suited to addressing those questions, but may not be particularly well suited to addressing questions arising from feminist critiques of development policies and programs.

Methodological choices are also situated within, and reflect broader trends in, evaluation and development. While international development evaluation is diverse and heterogeneous, there are broad trends or patterns that characterize some aspects of that field. For example, the centrality of economics in development, and increasingly development evaluation, is one dimension of the current landscape. Jackson (2007) argues that both separate and shared interests are central to understanding household dynamics, but they remain largely silenced in the research of large agencies, in part because of the dominance of economists as researchers "for whom gender disaggregation and comparison is methodologically more tractable than researching the relational significance of gender" (p. 109).

The influence of economic approaches is also seen in growing debates on experimental (randomized) and quasi-experimental designs. Critics of randomized approaches argue that these approaches do not address (indeed they attempt to factor out) context and the complexity of overlapping development processes. Other criticisms include technical critiques that they do not have external validity and "have no special ability to produce more credible knowledge than other methods, and . . . are frequently subject to practical problems that undermine any claims to statistical or epistemic superiority" (Deaton, 2010, p. 424).

Some of the impetus for randomization comes from a logical desire to start small, test what works, and then scale up. However, as Woolcock (2009) notes, the assumption that scaling will work, or that bigger will be better, is questionable for projects where success is reliant on a range of changing contextual factors and where implementation can look very different in different sites. For example, in a health program she evaluated in

India, Khanna (2012) found partners in different sites implementing very different efforts; one partner was only looking at antenatal care and institutional delivery, another was focusing on safe abortion as an entry point on sexual and reproductive rights, while a third let the community lead programing and in this case the project emphasized getting identity cards (as a way to help women access government benefits and programs). A randomized design might require getting rid of the "noise" created by this variation. Alternative designs could start by understanding the ways in which community health workers understand and adjust programs based on different contexts and their own different visions and skill sets. This can create space to dialogue and engage on different theories of change, as Khanna (2012) did, and to use this dialogue for transformation.

On the surface, none of this is problematic, as the proponents of randomized designs are not arguing that such designs should be used in all cases. However, trends in evaluation, which themselves are shaped by trends in dominant development paradigms, encourage some designs over others and potentially influence program managers to implement programs in ways that suit the evaluation design, rather than vice versa. The tail in such cases, can begin to wag the dog, particularly when evaluation users may be largely unfamiliar with the range of different evaluation designs. They may be prone to calling for randomized designs, even when such designs are not particularly well suited to answering their evaluation questions or those of other stakeholders in the evaluation process.

Evaluators working with a feminist lens do and must continue to draw on a range of approaches including those focused on measuring attribution and others emphasizing process, context, engagement, transformation, and stakeholder's perspectives. For the latter set, there are rich traditions in evaluation to draw from. Robert Stake (1995), for example, argued for "thick description" and case-based approaches; Lincoln and Guba (1986) took a constructivist stance and argued that an evaluator's duty is to present the values of differing stakeholders; and House (1990) argued that evaluation should give voice to the underrepresented or those whose voices are excluded. The transformative evaluation paradigm (Mertens, 2009), theory and work from Fetterman (1996) on empowerment, and Cousins and Whitmore (1998) and King (1998) on participatory evaluation also offer insights. This volume, of course, also provides a rich body of theory and practice from which to draw.

Rigor

Discussions of rigor can be found in the work of many bodies of research, including feminist research. To convincingly argue for the use of evidence and findings, evaluators need to respond to questions of quality and rigor. The question here is "What counts as valid evidence?" Feminist evaluation does not consist of one design or one set of methods, but of a lens or standpoint that influences choices made in design and methods. A rigorous feminist evaluation is one that uses a range of methods that best match the questions and the types of change the policy or program is addressing. Individual methods per se are not feminist or nonfeminist; their suitability (and rigor) in any given evaluation is a function of their ability to generate valid and reliable data that speaks to the nature of the inequity and the change the program is attempting to promote.

When drawing on different evaluation designs and methods, evaluators must recognize that different types of knowledge, expressed through different methodological traditions, have different power in decision-making structures. Evaluators also recognize the credibility of some designs (and of quantification more generally) among some intended users of evaluation. They thus may also weigh concerns for including voice, drawing out difference, and highlighting lived experiences, with the practical value of drawing on such designs. For example, Sudarshan and Sharma (2012) note:

> [In our experience,] qualitative methods have been more conducive to exploring the "why" and "how" and in revealing any relevant unanticipated changes that may have come up as a result of the intervention. . . . However, figures are often more effective in advocacy . . . and [respond to] the demand for quantification . . . from the implementer/donor [or both]. . . . (p. 309)

Noting that grass-roots women's organizations in India avoid quantitative and macrodata, Khanna (2012) integrates quantitative methods in her evaluations to increase the capacity of such groups in quantitative analysis. This is a practical strategy. The feminist lens brings recognition of the power of quantitative data and the transformative potential of empowering women's organizations with the capacity to use both quantitative and qualitative data through the evaluation process itself.

Cornwall et al. (2007) write that the "power relations within development ensure that feminist thought remains marginal" and "it is seen as perfectly respectable . . . to regard it as the responsibility of gender experts to convince the mainstream of its relevance" (p. 16). This would certainly be equally applicable to feminist evaluation. Thus, alternative designs need to recognize and respond to dominant discourses, including those within evaluation. While arguably more energy has been applied to developing quality standards for assessing randomized controlled trials, a number of researchers have developed quality criteria for qualitative research and evaluation (Boaz & Ashby, 2003; Lincoln & Guba, 1986). Such standards do not draw rigor from sample size or addressing attribution questions, but rather from other factors. For example, the Medical Sociology Group criteria for quality include, among other questions: Are the research methods appropriate to the question being asked? Is the relationship between the researchers and researched considered, and have the latter been fully informed? Are researchers clear about their own position in relation to the research topic? (cited in Boaz & Ashby, 2003).

As noted earlier, feminist evaluation may draw on more naturalistic approaches that seek to understand phenomena in context-specific settings as well as more positivist approaches that use experimental methods and quantitative measures to test hypothetical generalizations. What is important to note is that these different approaches are drawn from fundamentally different paradigms of inquiry. Where positivist approaches seek causal determination, validity, and generalization of findings, naturalistic approaches seek understanding and extrapolation to similar situations. The knowledge they seek is different, and what constitutes rigor or quality is also different for both. However, it is not necessary to pit these paradigms against each other.

Patton (1990) advocates paradigm choices and seeking "methodological appropriateness" as the primary criterion for judging methodological quality. I argue the same should apply to feminist evaluation. Such choices allow evaluators to respond appropriately to the evaluation questions and context they find themselves in in ways that strictly following one paradigm or another will not. In international development evaluation conceptualizations of rigor are used to inform both evaluation design and the use of findings and their credibility in policy and program spaces. This can be particularly challenging given that questions of rigor are usually framed within the dominant discourse, which may privilege some designs over others. A deeper understanding of rigor is not an academic exercise; evaluators attempting to use alternative designs require language, frameworks, and strategies to inform the rigor question.

Lincoln and Guba (1985, p. 300) developed alternative criteria corresponding to those typically employed to judge quantitative work (see Table 8.1). Lincoln and Guba's approach includes the rigor that comes from the groundedness or situatedness of the evaluator within the process. Feminist standpoint theory (Harding, 2004; Hartsock, 1983) has informed feminist research for over two decades and it can also inform the approaches that evaluators use in their practice. Standpoint theory offers conceptualization of rigor and validity that are rooted in principles of situated and constructed knowledges that acknowledge positionality, and begin from "lived experiences." This has some parallels with Patton's

TABLE 8.1. Comparison of Criteria for Judging the Quality of Quantitative versus Qualitative Research

Conventional terms	Naturalistic terms
Internal validity	Credibility
External validity	Transferability
Reliability	Dependability
Objectivity	Confirmability

(1990) stance on "empathy," but it also calls for an examination of the stance and position of the evaluator in the evaluation process.

Ultimately bad evaluation, whether positivist or naturalistic, feminist or not, is to be equally condemned, and good evaluation is always going to be incremental at best in terms of providing society better understandings of what is working or changing, for whom, and how. The good work in both cases will be open to critique and examination and be able to withstand scrutiny and refutation. However, contexts privilege certain methods and approaches over others, so evaluators applying feminist analysis to their work need stronger language and evidence for demonstrating and speaking to the strengths, rigor, validity (and limitations) of the approaches they are using. In contexts where other evaluation approaches dominate evaluation discourse and top the lists of what donors and national governments consider credible, such work is both essential and contested.

Accountability

Many countries have gone through phases of development evaluation that correspond with the major development paradigms of planned development and liberalization.

> In the liberalization period, the influence of international donor agencies became particularly important. The origins of this push for more and better quality evaluation during this period was largely a push for upward and external accountability to donors. The push itself was in part a response to growing demands within donor countries for greater accountability and demonstration of impact [of tax spending] from public sector audit bodies and parliaments in the case of some bilateral donors and from individuals and boards in foundations. With a few exceptions, this . . . phase of evaluation has been dominated by

northern-based organizations and individuals, particularly funding
agencies. This created and reinforced inequalities in the global evaluation field by overemphasizing the values, perspectives, and priorities
from the north and underemphasizing those from the south. . . . (Hay,
2010, p. 224)

New calls for impact are being overlaid on a landscape that has
been historically shaped by a dominant focus on external accountability.
Increasingly in international development, even for small-scale projects,
funders demand demonstration of impact or "value for money," at times
with little recognition of what they mean and what they are asking for. By
"impact," do they mean statistically proving the intervention caused a set
of changes on the ground? That is often (but certainly not always) impossible to do with statistical certainty in the absence of large sample sizes. In
asking for "value for money," is there clarity on value for whom and what
value they ascribe to things that can be difficult to value such as gender
justice or increased rights?

Again, though not particular to evaluation with a feminist lens, evaluators should demand a more thoughtful discussion on who evaluation is
intended to serve, on appropriate measures when measuring impact is not
possible or central, when abstract actuarial attempts to ascribe monetary
value to complex social changes may not be the most important issue,
or when there is no clarity on what values are being measured. Making
a judgment about what works and what does not work is a fundamental
purpose of evaluation (Mark, Henry, & Julnes, 2000); however, figuring
out whether something works entails articulating what "working" actually
might look like. In any program, and certainly in large-scale programs,
there are often different or competing definitions and criteria of success
held by groups of stakeholders with more and less power.

A feminist lens sees programs as a political space where competing discourses informing program theory can be examined. Jandhyala's
(2012) account of a large program in India for women's education and
empowerment describes how an external donor made funding for the
program contingent on targets that reflected a fundamentally different
theory of change than that of the implementing organization. The funder
wanted to show progress toward achieving the Millennium Development
Goals (MDGs), a product of a particular development discourse. Through
the MDG lens, women's mobilization through the program can be seen as
a way to reach goals around elementary education. Millennium development Goal 3 is to promote gender equality and empower women, but the
indicator and thus the target of this goal is to eliminate gender disparity
in education. One (implicit) theory is that more educated and informed

women are more likely to send their daughters to school. In this view the education of the women is a means to another end: the education of their daughters. This instrumentalist approach is quite different from the theory held by program implementers who saw the empowerment of women as the end in itself. The monitoring and evaluation framework became the space where theories on the nature of structural inequities and empowerment resided and were articulated. It was in monitoring and evaluation discussions that these competing views of the world, the program, and of women's place within both became manifest. A feminist lens can ask, "To whom, and for what, is the program accountable?" In doing so, feminist evaluation can focus attention on variables that may not be deemed central based on the dominant program theory and use these variables to assess the success of the program. One area where this has occurred is in examinations of women's time and women's drudgery in evaluations of development programs, particularly income-generating projects (Murthy, 2012; Sudarshan & Sharma, 2012). Jain and Elson (2011) note that "the kind of reasoning that has dominated policy in the last 40 years ignores the issue of equality of outcomes" (p. xxxviii); they suggest new investments first be assessed by equity-focused criteria—such as whether they are likely to reduce or increase time spent on unpaid work. Such questions can be included in evaluations even when time use was not considered in the original program design (reflecting the undervaluing of women's labor in dominant development discourse), questions on unpaid work can be included in evaluations.

How Change Happens

Closely linked to the idea of success and measures of success is the idea of trajectories and linear results chains. Development has been quite taken by methods that use chains or logical frameworks to represent complex processes more simply. They are often referred to as performance- or results-based management, and performance- or results-based measurement. Performance (or results-based) management has been defined as "a broad management strategy aimed at achieving important changes in the way government agencies operate, with improving performance (achieving better results) as the central orientation" (OECD, 2000, p. 6). Performance measurement is "concerned more narrowly with the production or supply of performance information, and is focused on technical aspects of clarifying objectives, developing indicators, collecting and analyzing data on results" (OECD, 2000, p. 6). The proposed benefits of this reductionist approach are that it is methodical, intuitive, and facilitates planning and control. It is increasingly being criticized, however, for not working. An evaluation of results-based management (RBM) approaches among United Nations agencies (Office of Internal Oversight Services, 2008) identifies a range of concerns with the approach at both conceptual and practical levels. Among other findings, it noted that "the formalistic approach to codifying how to achieve outcomes . . . can stifle the innovation and flexibility required to achieve those outcomes" (p. 20) and concluded damningly that "RBM in the United Nations has been an administrative chore of little value to accountability and decision-making" (p. 21).

Results chains may be useful planning tools, but they can become dangerous when the proxies for change (indicators) become confused with the intended change. For example, many programs targeting violence against women look for change in indicators such as incidence in violence. In order to understand whether the incidence is increasing or decreasing, they may use reporting on violence as a proxy. However, reporting of violence is not the same thing as the occurrence of violence. Studies in India have shown that an increase in women's representation in local government actually leads to a significant rise in documented cases of crimes against women. Evidence suggests that this rise is actually positive because it reflects increased reporting of crime rather than increasing incidence of crimes (Iyer, Mani, & Topalova, 2011). With this evidence in hand, the change in documented cases makes sense; as women become more empowered, they are more likely to report violence in the household. Empowerment is not increasing violence—it is increasing reporting (Iyer et al., 2011). However, given the limited available rigorous evaluation on issues of empowerment, we have little material to draw from on what indicators to use and what change actually looks like; thus we need to plan ambitiously but measure cautiously. A feminist lens could both attempt to capture change as it unfolds and make sense of that change (including by developing new indicators) around the nature of change the program expects to see (and why that is the case) and exploring whether change is actually happening (or is likely to happen) in those ways.

Even if one does have good measures, expectations that violence, for example, should be reduced in expected ways over an expected trajectory if the intervention is the right one and is done well are problematic. For many areas of inequities we often do not understand well the problem, we do not know what interventions work, and we need research and development to help us understand what trajectories may be. Development is increasingly critiqued for being informed by a view that change is linear and upward (Woolcock, 2009); this in turn lends itself to measurement that assumes that this linear change comes in regular installments and can be tracked in that way. We actually know very little about the actual trajectories of change in different sectors. Our implicit and false assumptions of those trajectories limit our opportunities to better understand how and what makes societies change. For example, drawing on their work in evaluating women's development programs in India, Sudarshan and Sharma (2012) argue that this view of development (as positive and linear) creates an implicit assumption that the emergence of conflict represents failure. Feminist analysis can create space to understand and indeed, to expect that efforts to change power relations may lead to resistance, and in the short term increase conflict between different groups. Things can become worse before they get better.

A view of development as being only positive and linear has little space for expecting, tracking, and learning from setbacks, by influencing development programs to only find and demonstrate positive and upward change. Sudarshan and Sharma (2012) consider part of their role in the evaluation process (which they describe as being one of responsible feminism) as validating an alternate discourse—where change is not always linear and the way that challenges are faced is an important part of the change story. Evaluation becomes an opportunity to make explicit a view of development that is more consistent with lived realities—a reality where change and empowerment is often met with resistance, and where things can get worse before they get better.

Evaluation with a feminist lens may include valuing and generating knowledge on process results and unintended outcomes. This is not specific to feminist evaluation, of course. Several evaluation theorists (Mertens, 2009; Morell, 2005) have made secondary effects and unintended consequences a focus of their work. However, it is particularly important in evaluations relating to structural inequities, as interventions may further reinforce inequities in ways that were not anticipated or attempting to shift those inequities may create conflict or reinforce other divisions. Feminist evaluations should attempt to retain space to reframe, adjust, or raise new questions as the evaluation unfolds.

Many feminist analysis frameworks are rooted in ontologies and epistemologies that validate connectedness to change processes on the ground and create space for co-construction of understanding how change happens with those whose lives are changing. Thus evaluators applying a feminist lens may be quite uniquely poised to begin to find ways to identify changes that may "appear small and insignificant," but "are actually enormously significant as having ushered in a new direction of thought and movement" (Sudarshan & Sharma, 2012, p. 311). They are also well positioned to develop and explore theories of change and change trajectories that are rooted in the lived experiences of organizations and groups trying to engage in social change on the ground, and the experiences of people whose lives are being changed.

Acting on and Recognizing Results

A challenge with all evaluation is use, whether to modify a small project being rolled out on the ground or using findings from multiple evaluations to change thinking on an issue (and everything in between). Resources (of time and money) to generate evidence are always limited; the women's movement and other development and equity movements need to increasingly see feminist and gendered evaluations as a body of evidence that needs to be tapped. Given the amount of evaluation happening, opportunities are lost for synthesizing and generating deeper understandings on how the development process is affecting change (positive or negative). Knowledge being generated through evaluations is generally not broadly shared, made available, or used (with other evidence) to explore questions beyond the particular evaluations. The vast majority of policy-relevant evaluation simply does not enter the public domain; this limits the opportunities to triangulate, challenge, or reinforce other bodies of knowledge around issues of social change and equity.

Multiple pathways are being and should be sought to use feminist evaluations. However, research and evaluation does not happen in a political vacuum (Weiss, 1976). There is a rich branch of evaluation theory centered around utilization, most notably the work of Patton (2008). Recent insights from research and evaluation theory can inform development discourse, but as Gita Sen (2005) has noted, powerful institutions control discourse. González de la Rocha's (2007) examination of how her own work on urban poverty in Mexico has been used offers interesting insights on that process. González de la Rocha's work in the 1980s covered a period of economic crisis in Mexico when the urban poor suffered a dramatic decrease in purchasing power. Her work illustrated poor people's strategies for survival and the ways that poor urban households responded through social networks, household restructuring, and turning to the informal sector. González de la Rocha argues that her work and other studies led to the creation of the "myth of survival" or the idea that the poor have an unlimited capacity to withstand shocks, but her later research following the 1994 Mexico financial crisis brought this "myth" into question. She argues that her work has since then been selectively used by key development institutions such as the World Bank, with her early work highlighting the strategies and agency of the poor being picked up, and her later work showing the limitations of those strategies being ignored. This example illustrates how the work of researchers and by extension evaluators can be co-opted and used to reinforce broader discourses such as economic liberalization, even as they attempt to critique and offer alternate conceptualizations of development.

As Sudarshan and Sharma (2012) write, "Responsible feminism requires recognition of the contextual constraints and the feasibility of recommended courses of action and choices . . . pointing out specific changes and actions that in our analysis would empower women . . . [while reflecting] what is possible or desirable, given any particular context and capacities" (p. 317). Feminist evaluators recognize that the underlying structures and systems that create inequities cannot be programed away within contexts that perpetrate and reinforce those systems. Embedding this political lens on utilization-focused approaches to evaluation appears to be a promising space theoretically for engendering policies and programs on the ground.

Conclusion and Lessons Learned

A feminist lens and feminist analysis could be further used to critique and call for transformation of mainstream development discourse and the ways in which it manifests in programs and projects. Bringing feminist analysis into evaluation at all levels creates opportunities to generate new and different knowledge and to suggest new and different development approaches and possibilities. Linking critiques of dominant paradigms to practical evaluation of policies and programs has promise for shifting norms and inequities in the field, and strengthens and reinforces both evaluation theory and practice. With the deep connections between feminist theory and practice, this work may make important contributions to understanding which paradigms, policies, and programs have promise of supporting more equitable societies. Given the persistence of inequities and the failure of dominant models of development to deliver equity, this is a promising and needed space for new work, effort, and energy.

REFERENCES

Ackerly, B., & True, J. (2009). Reflexivity in practice: Power and ethics in feminist research on international relations. *International Studies Review, 10,* 693–707.

Agarwal, B. (1997). "Bargaining" and fender relations: Within and beyond the household. *Feminist Economics, 3*(1), 1–5.

Banerjee, A., & Duflo, E. (2011). *Poor economics: A radical rethinking of the way to fight global poverty.* New York: PublicAffairs.

Bangladesh Maternal Mortality and Health Care Survey. (2010). Retrieved from *www. dghs.gov.bd/dmdocuments/BMMS_2010.pdf.*

Beneria, L. (2011). Globalization, labor, and women's work: Critical challenges for a post-neoliberal world. In D. Jain & D. Elson (Eds.), *Harvesting feminist knowledge for public policy* (pp. 70–92). New Delhi: Sage.

Boaz, A., & Ashby, D. (2003). *Fit for purpose? Assessing research quality for evidence based policy and practice.* Retrieved from *www.kcl.ac.uk/content/1/c6/03/46/04/wp11.pdf.*

Brewer, R. C., & King, M. (2002). The complexities and potential of theorizing gender, caste, race, and class. *Feminist Economics, 8*(2), 3–18.

Chattopadhyay, R., & Duflo, E. (2004). Women as policy makers: Examples from randomized policy experiment in India. *Econometrica, 72*(5), 1409–1443.

Cornwall, A. (2003). Whose voices? Whose choices? Reflections on gender and participatory development. *World Development, 31*(8), 1325–1342.

Cornwall, A., Harrison, E., & Whitehead, A. (2007). Gender myths and feminist fables: The struggle for interpretive power in gender and development. *Development and Change, 38*(1), 1–20.

Cousins, J. B., & Whitmore, E. (1998). Framing participatory evaluation. In E. Whitmore (Ed.), Understanding and practicing participatory evaluation. *New Directions for Evaluation, 1999*(80), 3–23.

De, A., Khera, R., Samon, M., & Shiva Kumar, A. (2011). *PROBE revisited.* New Delhi, India: Oxford University Press.

Deaton, A. (2010). Instruments, randomization, and learning about development. *Journal of Economic Literature, 48*(2), 424–455.

Desai, M. (2007). The messy relationship between feminisms and globalizations. *Gender Society, 21,* 797–803.

Dietz, M. (2003). Current controversies in feminist theory. *Annual Review of Political Science, 6,* 300–431.

Elson, D. (2011). Economics for a post-crisis world: Putting social justice first. In D. Jain & D. Elson (Eds.), *Harvesting feminist knowledge for public policy* (pp. 1–20). New Delhi, India: Sage.

Fetterman, D. (1996). Empowerment evaluation: An introduction to theory and practice. In D. Fetterman, S. J. Kaftarian, & A. Wandersman (Eds.), *Empowerment evaluation: Knowledge and tools for self assessment and evaluation.* Thousand Oaks, CA: Sage.

Figart, D., Mutari, E., & Power, M. (2002). *Living wages, equal wages: Gender and labor market policies in the United States.* New York: Routledge.

Glassman, A. (2011, March). *Maternal deaths are rare in Bangladesh.* Retrieved from blog post on Global Health Policy: *blogs.cgdev.org/globalhealth/2011/03/maternal-death-now-rare-in-bangladesh.php?utm_source=nl_weekly&utm_medium=email&utm_campaign=nl_weekly_03082011.*

Goetz, A. (2007). Political cleaners: Are women the new agents of anti-corruption? *Development and Change, 38*(1), 87–105.

González de la Rocha, M. (2007). The construction of the myth of survival. *Development and Change, 38*(1), 45–66.

Grech, V., Savona-Ventura, C., & Vassallo-Agius, P. (2002). Unexplained differences in sex ratios at birth in Europe and North America. *British Medical Journal* (Clinical Research Ed.), 1010–1011.

Grown, C., Elson, D., & Cagatay, N. (2000). Introduction. *World Development, 28*(7), 1145–1156.

Harding, S. (2004). Rethinking standpoint epistemology. In S. Harding, *The feminist standpoint theory reader* (pp. 49–82). New York: Routledge.

Hartsock, N. (1983). The feminist standpoint: Developing the ground for a specifically feminist historical materialism. In H. S. Harding & M. Hintikka, *Discovering reality: Feminist perspectives in epistemology, metaphysics* (pp. 283–310). New York: Springer.

Hay, K. (2010). Evaluation field building in South Asia: Reflections, anecdotes, and questions. *American Journal of Evaluation, 31*, 222–231.

Hay, K. (2012). Engendering policies and programmes through feminist evaluation: Opportunities and insights. *Indian Journal of Gender Studies, 19*(2), 321–340.

Hay, K., & Sudarshan, R. (2010, January 16). Making research matter in South Asia. *Economics and Political Weekly*.

Hill, R. (1995). Gay discourse in adult education: A critical review. *Adult Education Quarterly, 45*(3), 142–158.

Hogan, M., Foreman, J., Naghavi, M., Ahn, S., Wang, M., Makela, S., et al. (2010). Maternal mortality for 181 countries, 1980–2008: A systematic analysis of progress towards Millennium Development Goal 5. *The Lancet, 375*(9726), 1609–1623.

House, E. (1990). Methodology and justice. *New Directions in Program Evaluation, 1990*(45), 23–36.

House, E. (1993). *Professional evaluation: Social impact and political consequences.* Newbury Park, CA: Sage.

Iyer, L., Mani, I. M., & Topalova, P. (2011). *The power of political voice: Women's political representation and crime in India* (Working Paper, Harvard Business School). Cambridge, MA: Harvard University Press.

Jackson, C. (2007). Resolving risk?: Marriage and creative conjugality. *Development and Change, 38*(1), 107–129.

Jain, D., & Elson, D. (2011). Introduction. In D. Jain & D. Elson (Eds.), *Harvesting feminist knowledge for public policy* (pp. xxxiii–xivi). New Delhi, India: Sage.

Jandhyala, K. (2012). Ruminations on evaluation in the Mahlia Samakya Programme. *Indian Journal of Gender Studies, 19*(2), 211–232.

Jha, P. E. (2011). Trends in selective abortions of girls in India: Analysis of nationally representative birth histories from 1990 to 2005 and census data from 1991 to 2011. *Lancet, 377*(9781), 1921–1928.

Khanna, R. (2012). A feminist, gender and rights perspective for evaluation of women's health programmes. *Indian Journal of Gender Studies, 19*(2), 259–278.

King, J. (1998). Making sense of participatory evaluation practice. In E. Whitmore (Ed.), Understanding and practicing participatory evaluation. *New Directions for Evaluation, 1999*(80), 57–67.

Lincoln, Y. S., & Guba, E. G. (1985). *Naturalistic inquiry.* Beverly Hills, CA: Sage.

Lincoln, Y. S., & Guba, E. G. (1986). But is it rigorous?: Trustworthiness and authenticity in naturalistic evaluation. In D. D. Williams (Ed.), Naturalistic evaluation. *New Directions for Evaluation, 1986*(30), 73–84.

MacKinnon, C. (2006). *Are women human?: And other international dialogues.* Cambridge, MA: Belknap Press of Harvard University Press.

Mark, M., Henry, G., & Julnes, G. (2000). *Evaluation: An integrated framework for understanding, guiding, and improving policies and programs.* San Francisco: Jossey-Bass.

McElroy, M., & Horney, M. (1981). Nash-bargained household decisions: Toward a generalization of the theory of demand. *International Economic Review, 22*(2), 333–347.

Mertens, D. M. (2009). *Transformative research and evaluation.* New York: Guilford Press.

Mohanty, C. (2003). *Feminism without borders: Decolonizing theory, practicing solidarity.* Durham, NC: Due University Press.

Morell, J. (2005). Why are there unintended consequences of program action, and what are the implications for doing evaluation? *American Journal of Evaluation, 26*(4), 444–463.

Murthy, R. K. (2012). Reflections on a decade of micro-finance and livelihood projects from a gender and equity lens. *Indian Journal of Gender Studies, 19*(2), 279–302.

Narayn, U. (1997). *Dislocating culture: Identities, traditions, and third-world feminism.* New York: Routledge.

Nash, K. (2002). Human rights for women: An argument for "deconstructive equality." *Economy and Society, 31*(3), 414–433.

OECD. (2000). Results-based management in the development co-operation agencies: A review of experience. Accessed at *www.oecd.org/dataoecd/17/1/1886527.pdf.*

Office of Census Commissioner. (2011). *Government of India Ministry of Home Affairs.* Retrieved from size, growth rate and distribution of child population India 2011: *www.censusindia.gov.in/2011-prov-results/data_files/india/Final%20PPT%202011_chapter4.pdf.*

Office of Internal Oversight Services. (2008, Sept. 22). *Review of results-based management at the United Nations.* Retrieved from *www.un.org/ga/search/view_doc.asp?symbol=A/63/268.*

Patton, M. Q. (1990). *Qualitative evaluation and research methods* (2nd ed.). Newbury Park, CA: Sage.

Patton, M. (2008). *Utilization-focused evaluation.* Los Angeles: Sage.

Patton, M. Q. (2010). *Developmental evaluation: Applying complexity concepts to enhance innovation and use.* New York: Guilford Press.

Pawson, R. (2006). *Evidence-based policy: A realist perspective.* London: Sage.

Pawson, R., & Tilley, N. (1997). *Realistic evaluation.* London: Sage.

Podems, D. (2010). Feminist evaluation and gender approaches: There's a difference? *Journal of Multi-Disciplinary Evaluation, 6*(14), 1–17.

PROBE Team. (1999). *Public report on basic evaluation in India.* New Delhi, India: Oxford University Press.

Ramachandran, V. (2012). Evaluating gender and equity in elementary education; Reflections on methodologies, processes and outcomes. *Indian Journal of Gender Studies, 19*(2), 233–258.

Seigart, D., & Brisolara, S. (Eds.). (2003). Feminist evaluation: Explorations and experiences. *New Directions for Evaluation, 2002*(96), 1–114.

Sen, A. (2011, Feb. 28). *Growth and other concerns.* Retrieved from The Hindu at *www.thehindu.com/opinion/op-ed/article1451973.ece.*

Sen, G. (2005, Sept. 1). *Neolibs, neocons and gender justice: Lessons from global negotiations.* Retrieved from United Nations Research Institute for Social Development at *www.unrisd.org/publications/opgp9.*

Shiva Kumar, A. (2010). A comment on "evaluation field building in South Asia: Reflections, anecdotes and questions." *American Journal of Evaluation, 31,* 238–240.

Stake, R. (1995). *The art of case study research.* Thousand Oaks, CA: Sage.

Sudarshan, R., & Sharma, D. (2012). Gendering evaluations: Reflections on the role of the evaluator in enabling a participatory process. *Indian Journal of Gender Studies, 19*(2), 303–320.

UNICEF. (2011, Nov. 1). *UNICEF.* Retrieved from *www.unicef.org/infobycountry/indian_statistics.html.*

Waring, M. (1988). *If women counted: A new feminist economics.* San Francisco: HarperCollins.

Weick, K. (1995). *Sensemaking in organizations.* London: Sage.

Weiss, C. (1976). Using research in the policy process: Potential and constraints. *Policy Studies Journal, 4,* 224–228.

Woolcock, M. (2009). Toward a plurality of methods in project evaluation: A contextualized approach to understanding impact trajectories and efficacy. *Journal of Development Effectiveness, 1*(1), 1–14.

Latin American Feminist Perspectives on Gender Power Issues in Evaluation

Silvia Salinas Mulder
Fabiola Amariles

Introduction

In Latin America, where conceptual and methodological approaches for gender, human rights, and feminist evaluations are still under construction, undertaking a feminist evaluation[1] can be particularly challenging for several reasons. While the political environment of the region favors the creation of a culture of evaluation based on equity, mainly because of the strengthening of mechanisms for social control in different countries, understanding and accepting gender-responsive approaches as mainstream as an international mandate for governments and development programs is still slow and even decreasing in some political and cultural contexts. National agendas and other internal and geopolitical issues are gaining prominence; within countries with strong sovereignty discourses, feminist issues are usually stigmatized, women's subordination is linked to colonization, and gender claims are commonly perceived as trends imposed by development corporations.

While this juncture has evidenced the importance of attending to the complex power relations and articulations between gender, class and ethnicity, which Westernized Latin American feminist approaches may have promoted, it has also led to an overall weakening of the gender-inclusion agenda. This is true even in countries with advanced constitutional and legal frameworks for women's rights, but weak enforcement mechanisms. Ethnocentric evaluation processes reinforce such stands and resistance, and evidence the importance of articulating gender responsiveness in evaluation with culturally sensitive though reflexive and critical approaches.

In our opinion, complicating the implementation of a feminist evaluation approach, the weak evaluation culture that prevails in the Latin American region, or a limited understanding of its fundamental purposes and potential, does not facilitate the collection of evidence from evaluations to enhance programatic effectiveness and support feminist activism and advocacy. Thus, implementing a feminist evaluation is political per se and transgresses conventional patterns not only in terms of addressing gender and its relation to human rights, social justice, poverty reduction, and development, but also with respect to this weak evaluation culture.

The purpose of this chapter is to share with readers our Latin American experiences, reflections, and practical recommendations about applying principles and practices of human rights and feminist evaluation theories (mostly created in the "North," as are many other evaluation approaches) to real development evaluations. We also propose, based on discussions held in recent regional feminist forums, that efforts invested in technical assistance, methodological training, and institutional advancements in the region have often missed the political essence of feminist/gender-responsive valuations,[2] and thus lost focus on the key issue of unequal power relations,[3] with few encouraging and solid results.

From our perspective, feminist evaluation must center its attention on power relations in three dimensions: (1) the context, (2) the evaluation object (the program or project), and (3) the evaluation process. The feminist evaluator thus has the mission to analyze the context from the perspective of power, evaluate changes in unequal (gender) power relations related to the intervention, and finally discover, make visible, and whenever possible disentangle unequal power relations intrinsic to the evaluation process. The evaluation task, where the evaluator is a subjective, interpretative, and powerful actor (not an objective spectator) is thus simultaneously technical, strategic, and ultimately political.

Within this framework we consider the evaluative process as a knowledge-building and -sharing process permeated by power and subjectivity, and thus it can be either empowering or disempowering, according to the way it is designed and implemented. By challenging conventional rules and hierarchical structures, yet applying rigorous ethics, evaluations may best contribute to gender equity and equality in developing countries. We also emphasize the relevance of context analysis—national, subnational, etc.—and how it is translated into practical elements and situations at the microlevel. In the following sections the reader will find a combination of concepts, experiences, analytical perspectives, and tips and practical recommendations from our work as evaluation practitioners, which aim to contribute to global discussions and increased capacities to implement feminist principles in development evaluations. As Latin American feminists, we consider this chapter an opportunity to share our experience-based views and reflections "from the South to the North," to enrich the global discussions around power issues in feminist evaluation, and to move beyond good intentions and formal commitments toward concrete actions to operationalize the feminist agenda in evaluation practice in the region and further.

The Latin American Context: Opportunities and Challenges

Program evaluations do not take place in a vacuum. This is particularly true for feminist evaluation that faces political, cultural, economic, and technological factors, among others, that may inhibit or facilitate the fulfillment of its objective of contributing to greater social justice. These factors may be found at the regional, national, or local level, and evaluation practitioners must be aware of their existence in order to anticipate scenarios and creatively develop context-specific strategies to succeed in the implementation of feminist evaluations, challenging the status quo and changing paradigms.

Faúndez and Abarca (2011) analyzed trends of several evaluations conducted on programs and projects of the United Nations and governments of the Latin American region during the period 2005–2010, and found five key contextual elements that (from their perspective) define opportunities and shape the "state of the art" of gender-responsive and human rights-oriented evaluations in the region. In Table 9.1, we summarize these key elements outlined by Faúndez and Abarca and complement the analysis by identifying related limitations and threats based on our recent experiences assessing the status of gender-responsive evaluation mainstreaming in development corporations (international donors), civil society, and government organizations.[4]

Based on their analysis, Faúndez and Abarca (2011) conclude that though incipient, the region presents a progressive and enabling environment for evaluations that have a focus on gender equality and human rights. We basically agree with this general contextual analysis and balance, but still highlight that the challenges to mainstream a feminist or gender-responsive perspective in development evaluations remain large, and tackling gender inequities that lead to social injustice in realities that are diverse, complex, and under permanent change is still difficult. From our perspective, three key success factors are missing to take advantage of

TABLE 9.1. Our Experience in Comparison with Five Previous Key Contextual Findings by Faúndez and Abarca (2011)

Key contextual elements and opportunities detected by Faúndez and Abarca (2011) for gender-responsive and human rights-oriented evaluations in Latin America	Our perceptions on limitations and threats based on our recent practical experiences
The implications of the change of emphasis from women in development (WID) to gender and development (GAD) approaches has caused a shift toward incorporating gender mainstreaming language in evaluations, and a progressive mainstreaming of gender issues in public policies in the region.	These *changes are not of a general nature* and not always progressive, and the *belief that gender refers exclusively to women and women's programs prevails* in many contexts.
There has been a reemergence of issues related to citizen participation in Latin America, linked to a greater capacity of social movements—including women's movements—to influence public policy through evaluation and social control.	"The other side of the coin" is that the *emergence of social movements*—including women's movements—as increasingly influential actors in the public arena *is highly politicized*; thus the gender agenda is frequently undermined as one that weakens the collective and structural social, indigenous, and Afro-descendant claims.
There is an increased positioning of a human rights approach in the region, linked to particular inequality and diversity groups and issues.	This is also *tainted with political confrontations* that frequently bring up historical injustices to legitimate acts that can be questioned from a rights perspective. *Tensions between individual and collective rights* also illustrate the complexity of the actual Latin American panorama regarding a human rights' approach.
There is an increased availability, over the last two decades, of conceptual and methodological tools, standards, and rules for program and country gender- and human rights-responsive evaluations.[a] Several international conferences, the creation of evaluation networks and organizations, as well as national evaluation associations in countries of the region, have contributed to create greater awareness and opportunities for gender- and human rights-responsive evaluations.	Different barriers *limit the wide and sustainable use* of these *resources available*, even in organizations where gender-responsiveness mainstreaming is a mandate. Furthermore, *gender and human rights capacities tend to be too generic* to respond to specific contexts, themes, and issues—for example, gender and climate change, gender and economic crisis, and gender in a specific rural setting.

(continued)

TABLE 9.1. *(continued)*

Key contextual elements and opportunities detected by Faúndez and Abarca (2011) for gender-responsive and human rights-oriented evaluations in Latin America	Our perceptions on limitations and threats based on our recent practical experiences
A growing process of institutionalization of evaluation practice is taking place: for example, the creation of United Nations Evaluation Group (UNEG) and the evaluation unit in UNIFEM in 2008 (more recently under the newly created UN Women), as well as the presence of new specific evaluation agencies in the public sector in several countries.	The *use of evaluation findings and evidence* to guide and support decision-making processes *remains weak*.

[a]Since the creation of international evaluative norms and standards by the Organization for Economic Cooperation and Development (OECD)/Development Assistance Committee (DAC) in 1991, several evaluative frameworks have been developed to incorporate the principles of gender equality and human rights into development policies and programs. For example, DAC guidelines and concepts on equality between women and men (1998); the United Nations "Gender Score Card" for accountability on gender equality, created after the Resolution of the 59th Session of the UN General Assembly on Gender Mainstreaming (2004); and the establishment of the Evaluation Policy of UNIFEM (now UN Women) in 2009, among others.

existing opportunities and effectively tackle gender inequalities: political will, evidence-based decision making, and specialized strategic and implementing practices to mainstream gender-responsive approaches.

Participatory Is Not Always So Participatory

As is discussed in several sections of this book, and as presented by Salinas-Mulder and Amariles (2011) at the American Evaluation Association annual meeting, multistakeholder participation, inclusion, and ownership of the evaluation process is critical to achieving one of the goals of feminist evaluation. It is important to influence policymakers, public opinion, and other key stakeholders by providing evidence that incorporates considerations of equity and gender equality. This can support the development of public policies toward a broader systemic change of societies and their cultural values.

Participation of stakeholders in all phases of the evaluation is also important and contributes to the empowerment[5] of actors, a success factor for most development programs or projects. However, participation is not always understood as a process that should involve not only methods to gather data and information from target groups and other stakeholders of the program or project, but also strategies to ensure that the voices of those most excluded are valued and heard.

In our experience, participation in evaluations often gets reduced to including the privileged voices of program managers and evaluators who then issue conclusions and recommendations. Most of the time there is only a quick interaction with community representatives, usually male, and a selected group of the most accessible—and thus typically most privileged—"beneficiaries," often chosen by the implementing organization and strongly expected to participate.

In development discourse it is common to keep calling the target population of a program "beneficiaries." This expression has been questioned by the Latin American feminist movement, as it represents the old trend of development programs three decades ago (the women in development [WID] era) where *assistance to women* was the predominant trend without questioning unequal gender roles. The subsequent gender and development (GAD) approach seeks to eliminate gaps in gender power relations. We agree with this feminist position and add that it is the evaluation that can provide evidence of whether women or other target groups in fact benefited from the intervention. Addressing target groups as "beneficiaries" from the beginning thus reflects the assumption that people are so disempowered, poor, and vulnerable that they will benefit from *any* external action. It may also ignore women's self-determination and critical capacities.

The restricted interactions with excluded groups, and particularly women, reproduce hierarchical power relations between the evaluator and the interviewed people, which may shape participation patterns, as well as affect the honesty and reliability of responses. As Rance (2002) emphasizes, "dialogue is an ideal, maybe a utopia. It belongs to a dream world where we could sit face to face with a person or group of people listening and recognizing each other as equals."[6]

Some common attitudes of evaluators tend to limit the scope of participation of excluded groups, particularly women; for example, by focusing on their own questions and interests, they narrow the evaluation to a search for arguments that support their explicit and implicit assumptions. Salinas-Mulder, Rance, Serrate Suárez, and Castro Condori (2000) *describe* this practice as a "fact-seeking drive," interpreting what we hear and see just on the basis of our limited knowledge, background, and biased interpretations, disregarding context and culturally meaningful expressions and meanings, including resistance to participate; for example, "We arrived at R's house and asked for her. Her children told us she was not at home. A few minutes later, when we were at a distance, we saw her leaving her house." It became evident that R did not want to be interviewed.

> **Tip:** Interviews should be dealt with as dialogues where people have the opportunity to express their priorities and points of view.
>
> Do not limit your interactions to a question–answer dynamic. Let people speak freely and "listen actively" to discover what is essential to them. Respect and interpret the silences and do not insist on answers to your questions; rather, focus on trying to understand the underlying meaning and reason for each reaction. This will allow an eventual reconstruction of how change is occurring (theory of change) for the specific intervention and context, even if it has not been explicitly stated in the program/project design. Also, as evaluators, we tend to focus on verbal communication, ignoring the importance of tone and gestures. Make sure you are alert to less explicit but key messages, and register them. Be aware that this requires specific competences; capacity-building programs for evaluators should consider the importance of building these communication abilities. Also remember that for marginalized women, frequently these are unique opportunities for socialization, exchange, and learning, which enhance their self-esteem and contribute to their empowerment.
>
> _____
>
> *Note.* The theory of change is defined as "a thinking–action approach that helps us to identify milestones and conditions that have to occur on the path towards the change that we want to contribute to happen" (Retolaza, 2011). Applied to planning and evaluation, it means making explicit assumptions about how a program is supposed to work and create social change. It focuses on the causal relationships between resources, activities, short-term and long-term outcomes, and the context of the intervention, including its unintended consequences. This way the approach helps to identify what should be evaluated, when, and how.

The "Real" Cultural Context: Overcoming Paternalism and Unconditional Respect

In Latin America, where a diversity of cultures converge and are often permeated by very hierarchical power structures,[7] evaluation practitioners must be aware that building ample participation and ownership of the evaluation process is often a challenge. A thorough knowledge and understanding of the local culture, actors, and power dynamics is required to define the appropriate communication strategies and channels to ensure an effective though inclusive, respectful, and participatory process.

For example, as evaluators, we may tend to consider rural communities as homogenous entities and pay little attention to internal diversity, inequality, and power dynamics. Also, "cultural sensitivity" is often interpreted as following the established social, political, and cultural organization and representation patterns, and thus frequently limiting the participation to those most powerful, recognized as legitimate, formal

> *Tip:* **Combine context-relevant approaches with strategies to neutralize power relations that inhibit the free and voluntary participation of most excluded groups like women.**
>
> For example, pay attention and listen to formal leaders and representatives, but also search actively for the marginalized and most excluded people, enabling secure and confidential environments for them to speak. Ask them about themselves and their views, but also allow them to give their worldviews and more general perspectives. The role of cultural brokers or members of the evaluation team knowledgeable of the local culture is key to achieve an inclusive, context-sensitive approach to the evaluation.

representatives, who are mainly adult men. Rural authorities, especially indigenous ones, are usually considered to represent the only valid collective perspective. "Common people," particularly women, are not expected to dissent. Frequently this fact implicitly authorizes male leaders to be present and to "supervise" women's meetings or interviews, illustrating Hofstede's (2001) hypothesis that less powerful members of organizations and institutions often accept and expect the reality that power is distributed unequally. This is usually an accepted practice at the community level, one that inhibits the evaluator from obtaining the full and sincere perspectives of women and other most marginalized people.

Frequently, as evaluators, we unconsciously assume paternalistic attitudes toward marginalized people, and women in particular. Thus we do not enable or facilitate their participation but rather reproduce exclusionary communication patterns: "Vulnerability and protection are sociocultural constructions, often based on a paternalistic underestimation of others' capacity to resist, and overestimation of one's own ability to take care and provide" (Salinas-Mulder et al., 2000, p. 107). It is important to consider the truths that power is relational and that no one is completely powerless. For example, during an action-research project with women farmers in the Bolivian highlands, one of the researchers—a white, urban, and young psychologist—was perceived by local people as a "vulnerable outsider" requiring special attention and care (and control), which were ultimately intended to keep her in a subordinate and marginal position.

Participation: Right or Obligation?

Under normal circumstances, in evaluations of development programs and projects, especially those in rural areas, members of the target population are usually treated as information resources but not as key

> *Tip:* **Everyone should have the real opportunity to participate and also to decline from participating (e.g., informed consent), and should not fear any implications of such a decision (e.g., formal or informal exclusion from future program activities).**
>
> Emphasize with the program/project-implementing actors that having people decide about their own participation is a good indicator of ethical observance in the process.

audiences, owners, and users of the findings and recommendations of the evaluation. This very functional approach contradicts our reciprocity perspective: in one way or the other, participants—and mainly marginalized people—should directly benefit from the evaluation process and results with symbolic or material resources, knowledge, and other assets. In any case, they should not leave with less capital than when they arrived, and this oftentimes also includes attending to material issues.

For example, it is usually expected that "beneficiaries" obtain their own transportation to the interview and collaborate with the evaluation as a form of gratitude to the program or project. In our opinion, this reproduces unequal power relations and adds to other restrictions like gender, age, and geography, limiting the opportunity—not the obligation—of participation for many women. Furthermore, participation is usually circumscribed to a quick, functional interaction with no further communication or feedback. Thus, the notion of participation must imply symbolic recognition and valuing of participants' contributions, and sometimes even monetary reimbursements, especially for those women who make sacrifices to have their voices heard, such as traveling by horseback for hours to come to a focus group of a program evaluation, or spending their own money for transportation and food.

From "Defensive" Spectators to Key Actors: Program Staff Participation

Goetz (1992) and other authors (MacDonald, Sprenger, & Dubel, 1997; Rao & Kelleher, 2005) confirm that organizations tend to reproduce societal gender inequalities and even women's organizations normally operate within patriarchal institutional and macropolitical contexts. At the same time, in contexts where other issues like indigenous rights and inclusion are prioritized, program managers are often directly confronted with serious external obstacles to move the gender and women's rights agendas forward.

For example, as already mentioned, in several Latin American countries, despite the existence of equity-favorable norms and public institutions formally established to mainstream gender responsiveness and guarantee women's rights, these frequently lack the minimum technical and financial capacities to fulfill these mandates, as resources are often applied to other interests. In these cases, staff involved in the implementation of the program or project are probably the best resources to

---

Tip: **Organize a reference group that includes staff members from different levels of the organization/program and from diverse perspectives.**

The group will be the voice of staff in matters related to evaluation design and development. External actors may sometimes be invited to participate. The reference group is also a vehicle to share information with relevant decision makers beyond the implementing and/or financing institution, in order to facilitate ownership and responsibility for the process. Build a strong relationship with the group as a source of feedback for the evaluation team, but also to reflect on how the mission of the program is being followed by its members, and how human rights and equity issues are being dealt with internally. Be prepared to account for power imbalances among its members; ensure that everyone feels able to speak and contribute to the evaluation, by interacting with subgroups with similar characteristics (administration staff, programatic staff, etc.), or making one-to-one meetings as required. Make feedback from staff appear visible (though anonymous) in draft reports so that everybody knows the positions and perspectives of other subgroups. If possible, include an attachment with the responses/actions of the evaluation team with regard to comments and other considerations from the reference group. Also, write and test the recommendations in a consultative way with the reference group. Communicate with them frankly and openly, get and give feedback, and explicitly value their participation and inputs. Also, act as an evidence-based feminist activist and use strong arguments to position the evaluation exercise in the agenda and hearts of the different key stakeholders, and win them over as change agents who will promote women's rights and gender equality at different levels, including national and/or subnational policymaking.

Note. The creation of a reference group is a technique broadly applied in development evaluations, to help external evaluation teams to identify data sources and to access them. "They validate the evaluation questions, and discuss conclusions and recommendations. The reference group allows a variety of points of view on the evaluated intervention to be expressed" (European Commission—EuropeAid Cooperation Office; retrieved January 3, 2013, from *http://ec.europa.eu/europeaid/evaluation/methodology/methods/mth_stg_en.htm*).

illuminate the essential aspects of an evaluation linked to a deep understanding, not only of the context opportunities and challenges, but also about how equity issues are being addressed within the implementing institution.

However, participation of program managers and technicians in evaluations is often addressed in a questioning–defending pattern, with little room for reflection, self-evaluation, and learning. Changing the philosophical starting point and main purpose of an evaluation may open enormous opportunities to make use of valuable "secret knowledge" usually hidden in the bookshelves and minds of the implementing program staff.

Approaching program/project staff as "participant allies" may also allow for identifying and analyzing hidden innovative ideas, proposals, and best practices, which are not part of the "official" history. Tools like "Appreciative Inquiry"[8] and "MDF Organizational Assessment with Gender Perspective"[9] have been especially useful to us in performing organizational analysis with gender responsiveness as a self-assessment within the evaluation process. The application of these tools is part of the negotiations for the evaluation design at the beginning of the process, and the results have proved valuable to the analysis of efficiency and efficacy of the program or project, in addition to the gains in commitment and ownership of the process by staff members. External evaluations and internal self-evaluations thus are not necessarily different, incompatible processes. On the contrary, tools for organizational assessment with a gender and human rights perspective will help evaluators to identify, through the self-reflections and feedback of implementing staff, those internal and external issues that may be hindering or facilitating impact, as well as limiting the complete unfolding of the organizational and individual potential to contribute to women's rights and opportunities.

(Hidden) Politics in Feminist Evaluation

Donna R. Podems (2010), citing Sielbeck-Bowen, Brisolara, Seigart, Tischler, and Whitmore (2002), ratified the political essence of evaluation in one of the six tenets of feminist evaluation that several authors have defined: "Evaluation is a political activity; the contexts in which evaluation operates are politicized; and the personal experiences, perspectives, and characteristics evaluators bring to evaluations (and with which we interact) lead to a particular political stance" (p. 4). Rance (1999) emphasizes that politics belongs to the arena of struggle, confrontation, and trying to get advantage of a partially conflictive situation: "When we are defending a stand in relation to a—real or imagined—opposition of some force that we estimate as potentially superior, we recourse to politics to make ours prevail" (p. 1).[10]

Actors . . . Act

The dynamics and decisions involved in an evaluation create a particular micropolitical atmosphere, which depends on each specific circumstance and interaction that takes place. Based on her research and evaluation experience, Gracia Violeta Ross (2003), a Bolivian activist for the rights of people living with HIV and AIDS, and particularly women, emphasizes that in each interaction the political characteristics and connotations are defined by the role the researcher/evaluator assumes (e.g., researcher, woman with HIV, activist leader), who the informant is (e.g., doctor, person living with HIV, activist leader), and the particular situation where the data is generated (e.g., interview, public forum, medical consultation). Figure 9.1 is a graphic example of a "relationships map" prepared by Ross (2003) to illustrate the different roles and power relations she envisioned in her research with women living with HIV. The central circle describes

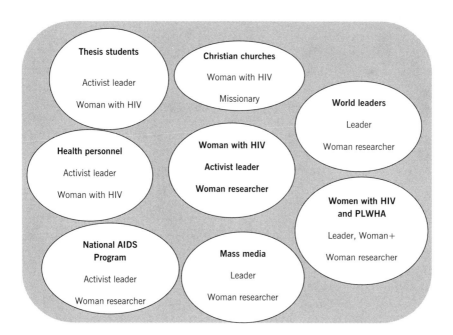

FIGURE 9.1. Relationships map. From Ross (2003). Copyright 2003 by Gracia Violeta Ross. Translated from Spanish by the authors. Reprinted by permission.

> *Tip:* **Mapping stakeholders, roles, interests, and power relations, including our own position as feminist evaluators with multiple identities and interests, facilitates a better understanding and interpretation of the data we gather.**
>
> While it is true that recognizing intrinsic and inevitable power relations is not sufficient, it enables us to contextualize and analyze the responses and reactions of different actors within each specific circumstance and its determinants. It is important to remember that identities and roles are not only what or who we say we are, but also (and mainly) how others perceive and interpret us. This is usually not explicit but should be part of our understanding of the context. Construct your map with community actors, identify and analyze similarities and differences in their perceptions, discuss and reach consensus about power factors that may affect the results, including the contributions of every actor (and evaluators) to the process, and strive to respect the others' knowledge and points of view.

the three main identities that, from her own perspective, she displayed during the research: woman with HIV, activist leader, and woman researcher. The circles around the center represent each type of actor (in bold on the first line)—for example, PLWHA (people living with HIV/AIDS)—and, below the actor, how the researcher was perceived, which simultaneously shaped each relationship.

Not Everything That Shines Is Gold: The Politics of "Success"

"Success"—to prove it or to disregard it—is, beyond a technical issue, a central political battle in development evaluations, exacerbated by the reduced availability and thus increased competition for financial resources in the Latin American region. On the one hand, the approach of success as an objective and logically derived conclusion of "neutral" analysis usually omits its power essence and intrinsic political and subjective dimensions. On the other hand, evaluation cultures that privilege limited funder-driven definitions of success reproduce ethnocentric perspectives, distorting experiences and findings, and diminishing their relevance and usefulness.

In fact, the analysis made by Batliwala and Pittman (2010) of more than 50 monitoring and evaluation (M & E) frameworks and tools used by women's organizations found that M & E is more likely to be undertaken because (1) donors require it, (2) it helps to make the case for obtaining funding, and (3) it supports advocacy work. They confirm that this donor-driven approach to evaluation "distorts the purpose and potential value of our M & E work" (p. 5). In our experience, the design and evaluability of "gender responsiveness" in program design is often very weak, with technical shortcomings and indicators that do not reflect context-relevant representations of a particular gender phenomenon, and are thus inadequate to determine social change and "success." Thus, as evaluators, one of our first challenges and decisions has to do with how to deal with deficient gender equality indicators. While usually technical limitations regarding indicators can be detected from the beginning, context-relevance and cultural responsiveness require a more complex analysis, particularly when we are acting in unfamiliar arenas.

Another key issue has to do with the capacity of a selected set of indicators to represent advancement (or lack of advancement) regarding social change, frequently in non-Western contexts. In extreme though not infrequent situations, we have encountered programs that have "successfully" complied with their "standard" gender equality indicators and targets, but have contributed little in terms of transforming gender power relations and the conditions for women's empowerment.

Even more, we have experienced cases where the pressure to achieve the established "gender targets" (e.g., in credit allocation) has resulted in violation of women's rights (e.g., exercising pressure on women and/or husbands to accept credit) and has led to negative consequences over women's position, self-determination, and even economic situation, contradicting the essence of the program's objectives.

Also, in some women-only rural agricultural programs, it was discovered that though women signed on as formal "beneficiaries," it was actually men who were controlling them, having their wives as "vehicles" to access and benefit from the program resources. An evaluation concluded that the women-focused strategy had been inadequate for the sociocultural and economic context, and recommended an "indirect strategy" to effectively privilege women's access and benefit from program resources, including identifying female roles and targeting needs related to women's productive activities. This approach proved to be culturally sensitive and much more effective in terms of gender transformations.

Finally, the pernicious combination between a weak evaluation culture, the low priority attributed to gender responsiveness, cultural and anticolonialist stands, and approaches that privilege validation of success over learning usually implies very inflexible and nonrigorous gender evaluation standards that can lead to erroneous conclusions in development evaluations. Beyond ethical and political implications, these evaluations set precedents that have prejudicial multiplier effects over the future commitment to and quality of the gender responsiveness of programs,

Tip: **Openly discussing the client's and donor's ideas about "success" and their expectations regarding a "good evaluation" beyond the terms of reference diminishes resistance to rigorous analysis and constructive criticism.**

Based on our evaluation experiences (e.g., an evaluation of a complex multiactor and governmentally led HIV prevention and attention program) we have learned that communication is key. So, it is important to include strategies such as communication and negotiation to permanently reinforce trust and a shared commitment and the benefits of an evaluation linked to legitimacy, transparency, accountability, and future vision.

Tip: **In the field, listen carefully and adhere to the principles of grounded theory: discovering theory through the analysis of data.**

Regarding evaluability, cultural appropriateness, and the relevance of the gender equality indicators, time spent in the field to gather evidence on the quality and usefulness of the indicators to account for social change is valuable. Do not focus on the indicators but search for mainstreamed perceptions among different groups of actors and systematically analyze your data to provide evidence of any changes. Analyze afterward whether or not, and to which extent, these transformations are (or are not) captured and reflected by the indicators. You may also uncover gender equality indicators, which are context-relevant and culturally meaningful to nourish feminist knowledge and evaluation, e.g., gendered responses and differentiated impacts of climate change, rural development, migration, infrastructure, etc. linked to the specific intervention being evaluated.

Note. In international development language, the "terms of reference" is the document that sets out a road map for a project, committee, meeting, or any activity for which people work together to accomplish a shared goal. In an evaluative process, the terms of reference describe the objectives, context, criteria, scope, evaluation questions, deliverables and timeframe for the evaluation, as a common understanding among participants. In the case of external evaluations, it describes the task assigned to the consulting team selected. The terms of reference are usually incorporated in the consulting contract signed with the evaluator(s).

implementing institutions, donors, and future similar initiatives. Thus, while we recognize the importance of being sensitive by highlighting and valuing processes and changes considering context realities beyond abstract ideals, we also emphasize that gender requires the same committed, professional, and rigorous assessment as any other evaluation criteria such as effectiveness, efficiency, or sustainability.

The P-Art of Policy Influence

Another political dimension of feminist evaluation is based on the expectation that the evaluation findings contribute with evidence to *incidencia política*, or advocacy,[11] and to public policy change in a particular context. Feminist evaluations not only bring the tools to find evidence and data to demonstrate gender gaps and inequities as an integral part of the evaluation process, but their findings, validated models, recommendations, and lessons learned may contribute to additional advocacy efforts for public policies to overcome gender inequities and reduce poverty. Also the evaluation should build capacity for the construction of an ex-post advocacy strategy by the program staff and feminist groups—tools, information, results, and also for building a theory of change for the program or project.

One of the main obstacles to achieve these objectives is that often evaluation-based advocacy remains an afterthought, since concrete products, methods, actions, and resources to influence policy design and implementation are not planned or anticipated to follow the evaluation process. A second important limitation is the belief that decision making in the public realm is mainly an information issue and not a complex, oftentimes "irrational," process that involves multiple dimensions within a context of male-dominated paradigms, power relations, and interests. In addition, highly unstable and continuously evolving dynamics among public program staff frequently aggravate this situation (Bronfman, Langer, & Trostle, 2000). Finally, a third inhibiting factor refers to the legitimacy of the process and findings, which is directly related to the participatory quality and ownership of the evaluation.

Tip: **Carefully inform all participants and target groups from the beginning about the purpose of the evaluation, the process and methodology, and the background of the evaluators, to build their interest, foster "buy-in," and to promote potential use of the findings to improve their advocacy capabilities.**

Create and transmit a positive vision of the potential of the evaluation to contribute to policy changes, program effectiveness, and reduction of gender inequities, in an environment of shared commitment by all parties. Take into account that publication and/or dissemination of the evaluation report—findings, conclusions, lessons learned, and recommendations—is effective for information and accountability purposes, but does not automatically strengthen advocacy competencies, promote decisions based on evaluation findings, or instigate policy changes.

Practical Recommendations
for Disentangling Power Relations

The design and implementation of an inclusive and participatory feminist evaluation often faces resistance as well as power and political obstacles that need to be overcome in order to produce useful results. Evaluators need to consciously and consistently apply feminist principles and practices throughout all phases of the evaluation process, convincing and attracting as many "change agents" as possible, so as to ensure ownership of the evaluation results and their broad application as evidence for policy design and implementation toward social change.

Based on our experience in Latin America, we provide some recommendations/practical ideas for different phases of evaluation of development interventions, with examples whenever possible. At the end of this section we offer an illustrative case based on a real evaluation.

Demarcating the Agenda, Defining the Field of Play, and Gaining Allies

The initial planning is one of the key phases of the evaluation to introduce some actions, methodologies, and principles that address changes in the lives of women and the reduction of gender inequality. The following tips elaborate on the guidelines prepared by the United Nations Evaluation Group (UNEG, 2011) on integrating human rights and gender equality in evaluation:

Terms of Reference

These are not engraved in stone; ensure that they comply with the following characteristics, among others: to be participatory, reflexive, and evaluation criteria that go beyond the traditional ones of relevance, effectiveness, or efficiency. It is important to explore other aspects of gender and to allow cultural appropriateness.

Work Plan

Use this to specify, fix, and clarify any relevant issues regarding gender responsiveness in the evaluation—and be sure to check for consistency and feasibility. Take into account accessibility and other factors that will facilitate and/or inhibit your fieldwork, particularly in rural, indigenous areas. Consider that within communities, marginalized groups (e.g., women) can be more difficult to reach; allow enough time for each interview, anticipating communication and language challenges that you may face. Also, allow ample time to examine not only the immediate results of the program/project but also its intended and unintended effects on women and on other special disadvantaged groups (e.g., young and elderly people).

Evaluation Questions

Go beyond the traditional questions, reframe them to be gender-responsive, and add new ones to ensure that evidence of change (or no change) in women's lives is gathered. Add questions about transformations in gender power relations and specific female concerns and interests, but also include questions that unearth women's contributions to "general development issues" (e.g., effective climate change strategies) and promote gender analysis in topics frequently perceived as "gender-neutral" (e.g., productivity). In rural contexts, where the family is considered the basic unit of analysis, include provocative questions to identify possible inequalities in how individual family members access, control, and benefit from available (program) resources.[12] Also include questions to capture self-reflections on how the program managers and staff are dealing with issues of human rights and gender equity within the program and organization.

Rapport and Common Language

Strive to build rapport with project managers, participants, and donors. In Latin America, like in other places, the word *feminist* has been stigmatized and sometimes produces resistance; you do not need to use the word, but the use of the concepts, principles, and arguments associated with feminist approaches promotes gender responsiveness and social justice and improves the quality and effectiveness of any development intervention. Be provocative, but not hostile, and use available facts and resources to build consensus and common language. For example, at the beginning of a diagnostic assessment of a health program, we used secondary information about access and use of contraceptive methods by men and women in the region (El Salvador, Central America). The information revealed that in the case of men an important obstacle was their cultural resistance to visit "women's hospitals" where free male sterilization was offered; the procedure made them feel like they were losing their masculinity. The discussion about this finding at the beginning of the assessment not only demystified gender issues but allowed the evaluators to build rapport with program staff by talking about gender equity and equality "in their own language," thus facilitating further interaction and construction of an appropriate framework for the study using a gender-responsive approach.

Ethics

Explicit consideration of the ethics of the study is required; propose concrete context-specific measures in your work plan to guarantee the implementation of ethical principles in the process; for example, to safeguard confidentiality you need to ensure certain conditions and infrastructure for the interviews and carefully safeguard your records; to protect particularly vulnerable key informants—such as women victims of violence—from any possible reprisals, you need to anticipate risks and apply secure strategies to access their testimonies; to ensure that beyond systematic application, the substance and purpose of informed consent are transmitted, you need to be aware of evaluator–informant unequal power relations and consciously give potential participants "real" opportunities and confidence to withdraw from participating. Furthermore, some experiences have shown that in some contexts complying with Western-defined ethical norms like informed consent can lead to unethical practice—for example, during a research project in rural Bolivia illiterate women offered to "sign a blank sheet of paper" (Salinas-Mulder et al., 2000).

Selection of Participants

Select a stakeholder mix and ensure that all relevant, directly and indirectly involved, and affected actors are included in the evaluation process, from the most powerful to those frequently excluded for "practical reasons," such as and especially marginalized women, rural women, victims of violence, adolescent and young women, girls, transsexuals, sex workers, women with HIV, etc. Disaggregate them by age, ethnicity, class, language, education level, and so on to be able to capture and analyze usually ignored internal group diversity and disparities. Suggest the inclusion of other strategic actors and potential users of the evaluation results, for example, members of the international development cooperation (donors), representatives of the national mechanism for the advancement of women in each country, and other NGO staff.

Confronting "Reality" in the Field

Always remember that despite all planning and anticipation, fieldwork will always challenge your flexibility and creativity, offering unexpected opportunities to make key findings regarding gender issues and add empowering and redistributive[13] potential to the evaluation through participation.

Be Creative

Evaluation techniques are the means not the end, and can thus be created, re-created, and adapted to each situation and context. For example, use *"conversatorios"* (rather flexible and informal round-table discussions with key actors and informants, as opposed to the more structured and strict technique of focus groups) to gather people with diverse backgrounds and perspectives to discuss a particular aspect of the evaluation. In addition to the innovation that these less-structured methods may bring to the evaluation, they allow evaluators to react to situations of uncertainty, generating "methodological answers" adapted to specific cultural contexts and situations. They may also counteract imbalances in power relations. Participants usually appreciate these reflective spaces and feel motivated to speak "outside the box," while evaluators obtain a holistic overview of the topic and the setting. In meetings with marginalized women, use drawings, charts, storytelling, and other creative methods as means to capture their sense of change and success. Nature-related analogies may also be useful in rural settings to search for meaningful male–female representations and analyze power relations. Also, build with participants the "desired future," which can help program managers to compare it with their own theory of change and build recommendations around that.

Expand Your Sources and Understanding

Analyze who came for the meeting and who did not and why. Whenever possible, visit the families and make gender-sensitive participant observations in community meetings, health services, schools, and the like. Identify women's and men's difficulties but also their capacities and abilities, trying to understand within this context the contribution and rationale of the intervention, with particular attention to gender transformations.

Capture Diversity

Identify relevant differences and inequalities between and within genders. Even within apparently "homogenous" groups, remember that women do not necessarily or always privilege their "gender identity" over other identities like class and age, and do not undervalue dissent in your analysis.

"Listen" for the Meanings

Include actors as co-analysts, not only as "informants," by asking them for explanations and interpretations. Gather and surface gender-relevant issues and problems from a feminist perspective. Visualize and chart cause–effect relations to understand why and how changes were set in motion, and then analyze the role and specific contributions of the program, involving the stakeholders' diverse perspectives whenever possible.

Evaluation Report, Recommendations, and Dissemination of Results

The evaluation report with its recommendations is an important vehicle for feminist evaluation to create and disseminate knowledge and contribute to the reduction of gender inequality.

Diverse Evaluation Products

While products for target populations need to focus on key findings and arguments to comply with ethically expected feedback and to strengthen their negotiation agenda, for decision makers the findings need to be specifically translated into evidence-based public policy recommendations. What this advice brings up is not only an issue of contents but also of the types of products, the language, and the vocabulary used for each audience. Prepare—whenever possible—specific evaluation communication products (e.g., videos, executive reports, and public policies recommendations) for different audiences and uses.

Validation and Ownership

Promote ownership and use of the evaluation findings among participants—particularly women and other most marginalized groups—for advocacy purposes. The report should be the result of a close interaction between the evaluation team, the participants, the reference group, and other involved actors who need to ensure that the recommendations will be followed. Also plan specific communication activities and products to ensure that the results and findings (produced knowledge) are shared with each stakeholder group in a understandable, relevant, pertinent, and useful manner, thus increasing the participants' capacities to understand their situation, strengthen their position, propose, negotiate, make decisions, and find solutions.

Form and Style Matter

Be creative in how you structure and write the report to reduce barriers. It must be friendly and attractive to enhance access and use. Include quotes extracted from interviews extensively throughout the document and in presentations and workshops, to support the findings and reflect the voices of those not normally heard. Be positive in your appreciation of findings: apply methods like "appreciative inquiry" or "most significant change" (Davies & Dart, 2005) that are being widely used to identify what is functioning well and why this is changing the lives of women. In general, start with the positive findings: remember that change processes are usually slow and it is necessary to highlight "small victories" that could serve as an example for other programs and motivate further progress toward gender equality. Emphasize the findings as learning opportunities, which the program staff will be able to utilize to make evidence-based improvements.

Change Orientation

Ensure that the recommendations include concrete steps and advice on follow-up actions. Being strategic and creative: Emphasizing the promising orientation of an evaluation on HIV prevention in Bolivia, we wrote an "inverted" evaluation report that presented the challenges and recommendations first, followed by the evaluation findings that support and explained the recommendations. The Bolivian Ministry of Health has decided to publish it. Focus on practical recommendations. Present them in a strategic and creative way and highlight the general benefits and multiplier effects of favorable gender-responsive measures. Ask for a management response that ensures follow-up and future actions.

Targeting Decision Makers

When planning dissemination, pay particular attention to decision makers in terms of their limited time availability, particular language, and specific interests regarding information and recommendations. Inform yourself and frame your presentation within prevailing development paradigms and current policies. Sensitize politicians, decision makers, and society about prevailing human rights and gender injustices and their negative impact on poverty reduction and development. Provide decision makers with evidence, arguments, and concrete ideas for gender responsiveness in culturally sensitive policy design and implementation. Promote replication and scaling-up of successful models and strategies to address gender inequalities within diverse sociocultural contexts.

Promising Perspectives?

The following example illustrates how we confronted key political aspects referred to above when introducing a feminist approach in an already planned "neutral" evaluation of a regional project for agricultural technical assistance in Central America that did not have women as a specific target population.

One Inspiring Case: Transforming a Gender-Neutral Evaluation into a Feminist Evaluation

Description of the Intervention[14]

This evaluation examined a regional rural development program of agricultural technical assistance that covers seven countries in Central America and has been funded by seven international agencies. The program is based on agricultural demands within each country, with the objectives of creating conditions for agricultural activities to become more productive, competitive, with more appropriate management of the environment, and to contribute to rural poverty alleviation. The intervention is advocacy-focused, with two of its four objectives explicitly directed toward creating capacities to formulate policies and move agricultural agendas toward sustainable rural development. However, the participation of women's groups, particularly rural women, in its conception and execution was not evident.

Challenging the Terms of Reference of the Evaluation

An external evaluation team had been selected through an international competition process, with predefined terms of reference prepared internally to guide the evaluation. During the design and inception phase, ample discussions were held between the evaluation team and project managers (mostly men) about modifying the terms of reference. Given the high potential of the results of the program to contribute to change, the evaluation team highlighted the importance of introducing a feminist perspective (naming it "gender-responsive analysis") within the evaluation to collect more evidence on the situation of rural women and how the project could make contributions to changes in public policies for gender equality in the rural sector. The main argument was to evaluate the extent to which the needs of rural women had been taken into account by the intervention, and to analyze the factors, including power relations, that may be restricting rural women's empowerment as elements to be considered in policies for rural development. Getting another perspective and involving more marginalized rural women in the evaluation process would contribute to advancing the feminist agenda to fight poverty and gender inequity.

The Strategy to Make the Most of the Evaluation Results in Political Terms

Starting from the design phase of the evaluation, interactions between the evaluation team and project managers were very active, with at least four stages to gain political legitimacy throughout the process: (1) Convincing stakeholders that the evaluation process by itself would support advocacy on issues of interest for the project, especially with regard to gender equality and poverty reduction; the argument being the potential of the project to influence changes in public policies through the evaluation results; (2) gaining legitimacy and ownership by stakeholders through the inclusion of key actors (authorities, opinion leaders) as active participants in the evaluation, with a methodology oriented to reflection and analysis; (3) strengthening the implementing organization by means of an analysis of its performance with a gender-responsive approach; and (4) valuing evaluation findings and recommendations as evidence for public policies, through the utilization of results by the organization and its stakeholders.

Operationalizing the Gender Approach

With advice from the gender expert on the evaluation team, the evaluation questions were reviewed to include gender issues for each evaluation criteria; gender was also dealt with as a separate thematic analysis. An online survey was conducted with program staff using the SurveyMonkey tool to reach more people and groups. Differentiated analyses were applied to responses from men and women surveyed; focus groups as well as individual and group interviews were also conducted using a gender-responsive approach in their design; and the team also sought actively to include remote rural women. In short, gender issues were handled as an integral part of the evaluation, including the implementation of the gender checklist of one of the donor partners, the International Fund for Agricultural Development (IFAD), for interviews and analyses.

There was an explicit intention to involve the most marginalized women in the assessment process, to capture their needs, interests and opinions, so as to correlate gender analysis with rural poverty and provide the opportunity for women to influence public policymaking.

Concrete Actions to Enhance the Results of the Evaluation

To maximize the contribution of the evaluation to create knowledge and promote learning to support rural policies and programs from a gender-responsive perspective, there were some specific actions:

1. During the design phase there was an ample interaction between the evaluation team, the director of the organization, and the representatives of partner agencies. A reference group was formed to gain legitimacy throughout the process. Data collection tools (interviews, focus groups, surveys) were designed with a gender-responsive perspective, that is, including questions to gather information as to how/where gender equity was present in the activities, objectives, and strategies of the program. Throughout the evaluation process there were self-reflexive sessions with staff of the program at different hierarchical levels about the organizational capacities, strengths, and weaknesses to institutionalize gender-responsive practices.

2. The potential of the program to influence public policy through the evaluation results was highlighted by the evaluation team, especially in regard to gender equality and poverty reduction. There were specific commitments to use the evaluation results to emphasize the role of women in social development and to recognize that social change requires engaging women. Although the program had developed some gender equity projects before, the evaluation served as a reminder that gender equality needed more attention.

3. Key stakeholders (authorities, opinion leaders) were included as active participants in the evaluation process, with a methodology oriented to reflection and analysis. Most important, after the evaluation, there was a follow-up process during which results were shared with different actors, including workshops with civil society to internalize the results and recommendations.

4. A rapid institutional analysis with a gender-responsive perspective supported the formulation of conclusions and recommendations to promote gender mainstreaming in the routine activities of the program,

with specific instructions on strengths and weaknesses regarding gender-responsive institutional capacity.

5. Results of the evaluation and its recommendations were recognized as evidence for public policy change, through their appropriation and use by the organization and its stakeholders. Further actions included establishing links between women's organizations and decision makers through the intervention of the program. In rural development, the focus was on improving relationships between the local communities and policy decision makers.

Enabling Factors

One of the most important factors that we found was the openness shown by the representatives of the contracting agency to adjust the terms of the evaluation to include a gender-responsive perspective. This was facilitated by the priority given to gender issues by some partner agencies, and also by the coherence between the objectives of the institution and gender equality as a key factor for sustainable development and poverty reduction.

The broad scope of the project allowed the development of a participatory process, demonstrating a trend regarding the examination of gender issues in the country. Thus, the evaluation process itself served as a means of increasing awareness of gender issues among many people involved with rural development in Central America and who are responsible for the development and implementation of policies.

The presence of a gender expert on the evaluation team gave legitimacy to the analysis and recommendations and facilitated the development of tools with gender-responsive components.

Limiting Factors

The paradigm that "gender" refers only to equal participation of men and women in project activities, or that development activities are gender-neutral, had prevailed at the organization, with only a few projects that addressed specific needs of women among the group of "vulnerable populations." Given that previous evaluation exercises had not addressed gender issues in depth, no actions had been taken before to introduce formal gender analysis or to detect the existing differential needs of women and men in rural development, except for specific projects for women. Similarly, the organization had not developed a mapping exercise to visualize actors, including rural women, to analyze and understand their needs, and to put them in connection with rural development plans and policies.

The evaluation team also faced the limitation that partner agencies gave different levels of priority to gender issues. While for some agencies gender equity was a mandate, for others the inclusion of a gender approach in their work was not an issue.

Conclusions

The described experience presents a strategy that was key to gaining trust and credibility, which are important issues for the success of an evaluative process. Through a proactive attitude from the evaluation team, and using negotiation skills to reach agreements and consensus with project managers and key stakeholders, the evaluators could achieve two objectives: one, linking results and recommendations to sustainable gender equity and equality; and two, sensitizing program staff and other actors about the importance of addressing gender equity issues in order to advance social change and development. In this process it was important to challenge power relations and make clear that the evaluator and the "evaluated" need to respect the knowledge of each other and understand that both are part of a change process and share objectives that contribute to a better society.

The case illustrates how, from the perspective of a Latin America reality and evaluation practice, the central political objectives of a feminist evaluation were accomplished. Based on evidence, the evaluation process challenged the paradigms of intracommunity homogeneity and equality. The process and its results also served to sensitize politicians, decision makers, and local communities on prevailing human rights and gender injustices and their negative impact on poverty reduction and development. Similarly, the evaluation provided evidence and arguments that can contribute to policymaking toward broader objectives of inclusion, equity, and equality.

To conclude, in our opinion, although there is advancement in the promulgation of feminist principles and implementation of feminist practices and rights-based evaluations in the region, there is still a long way to go to position and institutionalize the political, strategic, and practical gender-responsive dimensions of inquiry into most program evaluations. There is, however, hope that despite complex and often disempowering environments, evidence and new waves of transformation and social control in the region will consolidate innovative perspectives to allow feminist evaluation principles to nourish the commitment toward equitable, inclusive, and nondiscriminatory societies.

NOTES

1. Globally we have perceived persistent conceptual discussions and lack of clarity or even overlapping between, for example, "feminist evaluation," "gender-responsive/sensitive evaluation," and "rights-based evaluation." In the Latin American context the concept of feminist evaluation and its focus on uneven power relations and social change; that is, "questioning authority, examining gender issues, examining the lives of women and promoting social change" (Seigart, 2005) is not widely used and practiced as such. There is, however, a trend in applying gender and human rights approaches to evaluation, which is evolving in a complex and often ambiguous and contradictory context, which we try to portray in the following section of this chapter.

2. A virtual forum sponsored by the United Nations Development Program (UNDP) in September 2011 analyzed the strategic validity and effectiveness of training to mainstream gender. Among other issues assessed, the forum discussed whether training efforts were actually developing the required capacities to transform gender disparities in personal and institutional practices. Among the conclusions, the depoliticization of training contents and a weakening of the transformative spirit of the trainings were highlighted as a key limitation. This report was retrieved on January 3, 2013, from *http://mainstreaming.americalatinagenera.org/wp-content/uploads/2011/09/ S%C3%ADntesis-Foro-capacitacion.pdf,* pages 2 and 4.

3. Rance (cited in Tellería & Rance 2002) graphically represents and analyzes the interpretations of different authors on the issue of power. From the ideas represented in this graphic, we basically adhere to Focault's relational approach to power as a network of relationships that sustain a dominant model. However, we also recognize situations in our practice that are in line with Jane Flax's arguments that power is exercised by certain actors to challenge historical forces and influence the terms of daily life. Also, we find evaluation dynamics analogous to Lyotard's idea of power like a chess game, where surprising moves can distract and destabilize the challenger.

4. Our experience is based on assessments made of gender responsiveness, processes, and level of institutionalization, most of which remain as confidential reports for the use of the contracting agencies.

5. We adhere to the general World Bank "Empowerment," n.d., para (1) definition of *empowerment*: "The process of increasing the assets and capabilities of individuals or groups to make purposive choices and to transform those choices into desired actions and outcomes." Women's empowerment, though, is a more refined strategy addressed at the Fourth Beijing Women Conference (1995), which emphasized that the concept of empowerment does not refer to dominating others (men), but to the ability of women to increase their self-confidence, make decisions, and influence change.

6. Translated from Spanish by the authors.

7. Hofstede (1991) measured the degree of inequalities in society through the Power Distance Index (PDI) which has demonstrated high power distance

values for Latin countries (both Latin European, like France and Spain) and lower values for the United States, Great Britain and its former Dominions, and for the remaining non-Latin part of Europe.

8. The American Evaluation Association (AEA) dedicated special issue No. 100 of *New Directions in Evaluation* (Preskill & Coghlan, 2003) to this tool: "Using Appreciative Inquiry in Evaluation."

9. MDF Training and Consultancy, The Netherlands.

10. Translated from Spanish by the authors.

11. The word "advocacy" is used here as the translation for *incidencia política*, a Spanish expression widely used in Latin America to mean "organized community efforts to influence the formulation and implementation of public policies and programs, through persuasion and pressure on authorities or other institutions of power to decide. It is one of the mechanisms by which different sectors of civil society can advance their agendas and have an impact on public policy" (BioAndes, 2008; translated from Spanish by the authors).

12. The UNICEF Women's Equality and Empowerment Framework (WEEF), designed by S. Longwe (1991) is a good resource to help frame evaluation questions that guide on matters related to women's access, awareness of causes of inequality, capacity to direct one's own interests, and taking control and action to overcome obstacles to reducing structural inequality.

13. From economics; it refers to measures taken to reduce inequalities.

14. By decision of the program's managers, the full evaluation report was not made public. However, results were presented to several audiences, mainly governmental counterparts, donors, and participating agencies of the organization (stakeholders).

REFERENCES

Batliwala, S., & Pittman, A. (2010). *Capturing change in women's realities. A critical overview of current monitoring and evaluation frameworks and approaches.* Association for Women's Rights in Development (AWID). Available at www.awid.org/About-AWID/AWID-News/Capturing-in-Womens-Realities.

BioAndes. (2008). Material de Sensibilización y Capacitación: Incidencia Política. Retrieved April 20, 2012, from www.agruco.org/bioandes/pdf/Peru/Revistas%20informativas/INCIDENCIA%20POLITICA%20Cajamarca.pdf.

Bronfman, M., Langer, A., & Trostle, J. (2000). *De la Investigación en Salud a la Política: La Difícil Traducción.* México D.F.: Instituto Nacional de Salud Pública, Editorial El Manual Moderno.

Davies, R., & Dart, J. (2005). *The "most significant change" (MSC) technique: A guide to its use, Version 1.00.* Available at www.mande.co.uk/docs/MCSGuide.pdf.

Empowerment. (n.d.) Retrieved August 8, 2013, from http://web.worldbank.org/WBSITE/EXTERNAL/TOPICS/EXTPOVERTY/EXTEMPOWERMENT/0,,menuPK:486417~pagePK:149018~piPK:149093~theSitePK:486411,00.html.

European Commission. Europe Aid Cooperation Office. (2006). The reference group. Retrieved January 3, 2013, from http://ec.europa.eu/europeaid/evaluation/methodology/methods/mth-stg-en.htm.

Faúndez, A., & Abarca, H. (2011). *Principales Hallazgos de la Sistematización de Evaluaciones con Enfoque de Igualdad de Género y Derechos Humanos en América Latina* (Document for discussion at the Forum on Evaluations with Gender Equality and Human Rights Approach in Latin America, RELAC, Latin American and Caribbean Evaluation Network). Available at *http://api.ning. com/files/p13aejfdq90CY5M7KldFdepod731wbss23EUuV3qpBuSVmDHRqef-skXRxfKQLUrpiQZsw/Cuq495RtskxdPhQF5tFF7hGuPu/SistematizacinPresent-acinQuitoFinal.pdf.*

Foro Virtual: Capacitación, Capacitación y más Capacitación: ¿Una estrategia agotada? Alcances y limitaciones de la capacitación como estrategia para el mainstreaming de igualdad de género. Agencia Catalana de Cooperació al Desenvolupament, UNDP. Retrieved January 3, 2013, from *http://main-streaming.americalatinagenera.org/.*

Goetz, A. M. (1992). Gender and administration. *IDS Bulletin, 23*(4), 6–17.

Hofstede, G. (1991). *Cultures and organizations: Software of the mind. Intercultural cooperation and its importance for survival.* The Netherlands: McGraw-Hill International.

Hofstede, G. (2001). *Culture's consequences: Comparing values, behaviors, institutions and organizations across nations* (2nd ed.). Thousand Oaks, CA: Sage.

Longwe, S. (1991). Gender awareness: The missing element in the third development project. In T. Wallace & C. March (Eds.), *Changing perceptions: Writings on gender and development* (pp. 149–157). Oxford, UK: Oxfam.

MacDonald, M., Sprenger, E., & Dubel, I. (1997). *Gender and organizational change: Bridging the gap between policy and practice.* Amsterdam, The Netherlands: Royal Tropical Institute.

Podems, D. R. (2010). Feminist evaluation and gender approaches: There's a difference? *Journal of MultiDisciplinary Evaluation, 6*(14). Retrieved June 12, 2010, from *http://survey.ate.wmich.edu/jmde/index.php/jmde_1/article/view/199/291.*

Preskill, H., & Coghlan, A. T. (Eds.). (2003). Using appreciative inquiry in evaluation. *New Directions for Evaluation, 2003*(100). San Francisco: Jossey-Bass.

Rance, S. (1999). *Política y Ética: Una Deslealtad Declarada.* Paper prepared for the "Subcomisión de Política y Ética." La Paz: Comité de Investigación, Evaluación y Políticas de Población y Desarrollo (CIEPP), UNFPA.

Rance, S. (2002). Diálogo de Saberes. In *Experiencias en Investigación Sociocultural* (pp. 29–39). La Paz: Comité de Investigación, Evaluación y Políticas de Población y Desarrollo (CIEPP), UNFPA.

Rao, A., & Kelleher, D. (2005). Is there life after gender mainstreaming? *Gender and Development, 13*(2), 57–69.

Retolaza, E. I. (2011). *Theory of change: A thinking and action approach to navigate in the complexity of social change processes.* Guatemala: UNDP/Hivos.

Ross, G. V. (2003, May). *Cuestiones de Ética, Política y Poder en mi Investigación Autobiográfica con las Mujeres Viviendo con VIH en la ciudad de La Paz.* Paper presented at the Regional Meeting "Sexuality, Health and Human Rights in Latin America." Lima, Peru.

Salinas-Mulder, S., & Amariles, F. (2011, November). *Challenging gender blindness in conventional evaluation.* Presentation made at the annual conference of the American Evaluation Association (AEA), Anaheim, CA.

Salinas Mulder, S., Rance, S., Serrate Suárez, M., & Castro Condori, M. (2000). Unethical ethics?: Reflections on intercultural research practices. *Reproductive Health Matters*, *8*(15), 104–112.

Seigart, D. (2005). Feminist evaluation. In S. Mathison (Ed.), *Encyclopedia of evaluation* (pp. 154–157). Thousand Oaks, CA: Sage.

Sielbeck-Bowen, K., Brisolara, S., Seigart, D., Tischler, C., & Whitmore, E. (2002). Exploring feminist evaluation: The ground from which we rise. In D. Seigart & S. Brisolara (Eds.), Feminist evaluation: Explorations and experiences. *New Directions for Evaluation*, *2002*(96), 3–8.

Tellería, J., & Rance, S. (2002). *El Antimétodo–advocacy participativo*. La Paz: MASQUE V Fondo Editorial.

United Nations Evaluation Group (UNEG). (2011). *Integrating human rights and gender equality in evaluation–Towards UNEG guidance* (UNEG/G[2011]2). Available at *www.unesco.org*.

SECOND REFLECTION

Saumitra SenGupta
Sharon Brisolara
Denise Seigart

A s we move from feminist evaluation to feminist research, we move from a relatively more programatic focus to more exploratory questions. Some of the themes we explored in the previous section continue in the research articles as well.

Before exploring the content of the chapters, let us examine some of these common threads first. As we revisit the issue of whether a study should be classified as research or evaluation, the reader will find once again that the boundaries are fluid. The chapters by Seigart (Chapter 10) and Galiè (Chapter 11) perhaps exemplify this dilemma most. Both of these authors examine specific programs or initiatives in depth and draw conclusions that are similar to evaluation report findings. Seigart utilizes an interpretive case study method in her research that has also been widely used in the program evaluation literature. However, despite the methodological commonality, Seigart examines the issue of school-based health programs cross-nationally in contexts that widely vary from each other. As a result, the study formulates its research questions and how to answer these questions in a more flexible way than a traditional evaluation would. She also notes that her funding sources were varied, unlike most evaluations, which can be tied to a specific funding stream or funder. It could be said that her work lays the foundation for future program definition in the three countries, streamlining goals and delivery systems that will lead to a more defined program evaluation study in the future. At the time of her study, there were many open and unknown issues that could only be addressed using a flexible, exploratory research framework.

255

Galiè looks at an agricultural initiative in the context of Participatory Plant Breeding (PPB) in Syria where the overarching content, aim, and methods resemble program evaluation most closely. Using a participant/stakeholder-defined model of empowerment for feminist participatory action research, she examines the differential impacts between villages where PPB was or was not used. This could very well be classified as a program evaluation chapter in the present volume. There is no crystal ball for determining such things. The length of the study, the confluence of contextual factors, the open approach to defining the study indicators, and the analysis and presentation of the findings tilted our judgment toward including this chapter in Part III. Compared to Seigart's and Galiè's chapters, we had less difficulty classifying Dietsch's (Chapter 12) study of traditional midwives in rural southern Kenya as a good example of feminist research. If we go back to Mathison's distinctions between research and evaluation, all three studies presented in Part III will likely fall within the category of applied research. Dietsch's study falls more toward the basic research end of the applied research spectrum. We can also look at her chapter from the perspective of feminist evaluator roles identified by Whitmore (Chapter 3). There is resonance with many of the evaluator roles or skills that she employed in this study such as facilitation, language, reflexivity, "soft" (people) skills, and activism/advocacy. This has been a deliberate decision on the editors' part to limit this volume to feminist evaluation and feminist applied research because there is a gap in recent literature. Texts on theory and basic feminist research have been published recently including the primer and the handbook both edited by Hesse-Biber (2012). In feminist research, we again encounter the issue of applying the "feminist" label to a study, at which stage and in what context it is applied. This is a discussion that the reader will find continued from Podems's Chapter 5 in Part I. The commonalities among the three chapters in this last section are unmistakable. All three authors clearly label their research as feminist and provide succinct reasons for doing so. However, the reader will notice a difference in how and when the studies evolved into feminist research.

Seigart and Dietsch are perhaps more similar in their approaches. Both acknowledge the difficulties or hurdles encountered in the proposal stage when studies are submitted as feminist research projects. Seigart provides a detailed discussion on gaining entry to schools and health care institutions using her school-based health care study example in three countries. She adopts a matter-of-fact approach in presenting her methodology in a way that makes clear that a feminist lens will be used without necessarily having to introduce herself as a feminist evaluator. Dietsch reflects deeply on this issue and questions why, despite never being in doubt about using a feminist research approach and ethics, she considered this study to be primarily a critical study.

Galiè takes a very different approach in setting the stage for her research on PPB. But before discussing her chapter, we must acknowledge that this research was conducted during a relatively more stable time in Syria. Since the time when this chapter was written for inclusion in this volume, times have changed and large fatalities have resulted from the Syrian uprising. We sincerely hope and pray for the safety of the women and men with whom Galiè collaborated so closely for a number of years, and whose living experiences from that period are so vividly displayed in this chapter.

Galiè introduces and frames her study more openly as feminist research. She pursues an empowerment model for what can be characterized as participatory action research in the context of female participation in Syrian agriculture. She underscores the importance of not stopping at outlining or uncovering gender inequities, but emphasizes the empowerment approach in her work to bring about social justice for women. She also documents a participatory process for defining what empowerment means for the study participants and engages them in defining suitable indicators of empowerment that were then used throughout the study period to establish any differences that PPB approach may have brought about in terms of Syrian female farmers' empowerment.

Regardless of how each of these studies was labeled, including the ones in Part II, and the very diverse ways that the authors have gone about or recommended formulating the study questions and research/evaluation approach, there is one common theme that emerges from all these chapters, that is, examining, analyzing, and discovering the underlying power structures that impact different demographic or cultural groups differently, and in particular, how women might be adversely impacted. We previously discussed this in the context of privileging of information and gender equity. Here we highlight some continuing themes from the next three chapters.

Seigart starts out with a "neutral" stance and strives to make herself almost "disappear" while opening a communicative space and raising consciousness. She uses intersectionality to define a holistic, all-encompassing vision of health care at the outset to replace the pervasive positivist, biomedical, approach to health care research. This is an important distinction to acknowledge and one that fosters active listening; allows the researcher to discover uncharted, not premeditated pathways; and, most importantly, keeps open the possibility of following unexpected leads that expose gender and cultural fissures. We can see the results of this approach in stating and questioning findings in a rather unexpected way. An example of this can be found in her discussion of the disparate impact of structural inequities borne by certain professions that are predominantly occupied by women. Sometimes the cultural or other demographic inequities stand out more prominently than gender inequity, a point made by Brisolara (Chapter 1) and

Mertens (Chapter 4) in their respective chapters in Part I. Seigart provides a very succinct example of this when she examines the issue of health disparity faced by Aborigine children.

Dietsch uses a critical framework to conduct feminist research that exposes oppression and power exerted over women. Dietsch's and Seigart's operational definitions of power are similar in that both identify withholding of resources from others as the manifestation of exertion of power. The resources can be concrete, physical in nature as well as more conceptual; perceptual; or abstract. The latter is exemplified by the recognition of privileges accorded by a professional title and how that marginalizes traditional knowledge and wisdom based on thousands of years of lived, culturally grounded experience.

There are two important issues that emerge from Dietsch's exposition of this global structure that discriminates against traditional midwives. First, it is perhaps easier to identify the oppression of women than who the oppressor is. The oppressor is not simply men. The power structure is nuanced. It consists of structural, systemic, and established layers that are not always easy to disentangle. What she eloquently captures as the power of Western hegemony through a biomedical industrial complex that permeates through this structural imbalance, is identified by Seigart and Galiè as well. In Seigart's case, it is the withholding of resources, whereas in Galiè's study it is the components of empowerment including recognition, opportunities, resources, and decision making.

Second, Dietsch also demonstrates that the oppression of women through withholding of resources is global in nature and exists across cultural, developed–developing, and North–South divides. It manifests in different forms as she compares her findings on the experiences of birthing women in Kenya to that of the closing of maternal units in rural Australia. The justifications and manifestations in each case are vastly different, yet the results are strikingly similar in terms of women experiencing the ill effects of such structural inequity.

Examining the issue of intersectionality that appears as a recurring theme throughout this volume gives us a way to analyze and interpret power structures across cultures and countries. All three chapters in Part III provide examples of discovering nuanced power structures that have polarities not as sharply divided along gender, nor are these power structures identifiable solely along any of the other possible demographic or cultural dimensions. However, using a feminist approach, we do see that the polarities are stacked rather differentially along gender lines disfavoring women.

In Part I, Whitmore (Chapter 3) articulated the importance of paying attention to the language of evaluation including cultural competence, particularly when working in a cross-cultural and/or cross-national setting. All three authors in Part III pay very close attention to this issue. Seigart acknowledges the relatively short-term visits to two countries away from her home in the United States and emphasizes the notion of cultural humility in working in other countries. Galiè ensures that the concept of empowerment, arguably a Western term and concept, is vetted and sufficiently operationalized by the participants/stakeholders in the study. Dietsch is very mindful of the pitfalls and shortcomings of language interpreters. She spends significant time and effort ensuring that the understanding of the fundamental premises of the study is shared by the interpreters, and that translation does not become value-laden or assume the language of the very power structure that one is trying to unmask.

In her reflections on this volume at the end, Jennifer Greene (Final Reflection) observes that today's social inquirers are seldom tied to a single framework. Rather, they "construct their own blend of aspects of multiple assumptive and methodological frameworks." This aptly describes the variability in methods and roles that feminist evaluators and researchers have applied to their work. It also captures the diversity of labels they have applied to their approach depending on the context. Perhaps one can draw a parallel to what Christiansen (1997) describes as *innovative disruptions* in describing the technological evolution and revolution in the past hundred years. Innovative disruptions are now being considered in health care delivery systems as well as in its nascent stage in applications to social change.

One of the ideas that Christiansen promoted in revising his earlier notion of disruptive technology is that these are not by themselves, fully disruptive. That is because, he argues, the conceptual innovation is what ultimately disrupts current thoughts and practices; new technologies only provide the tools of the trade for disruptive innovations. And yet, there are economic and social forces pushing for innovation; businesses speak of an innovation crisis and both evaluators and researchers are faced with assessing and supporting the development of the innovative strategies and projects that emerge. Patton (2011) has also recently introduced into the evaluation literature the Developmental Evaluation model, which draws on complexity concepts to further enhance innovation as well as shore up the use of evaluation processes and findings.

One can look at the change in the way applied social science researchers and evaluators have modified their thinking and practice and draw some parallels here. The whole genre of concepts and methods such as transformative research, empowerment evaluation, cultural competence or humility, and participatory action research, to name a few, together constitute an innovative disruption to a positivist-dominated social science research approach or causal pursuit in program evaluation. Such models acknowledge the complexity of existing relationships and encourage new ways of seeing. Like innovative disruptions in business and technology, these came to rely on not a single matrix of epistemological positions and methodological certainties. Rather, the diversity that we are seeing exemplified in this volume is reflective of that very disruptive innovation happening in evaluation and applied social research.

Like any disruptive innovations in business and industries, the disruptive innovation that we see in this volume will need to continue to evolve to create the opportunities for all practitioners to adopt its position, language, and palette of tools. But that change is already palpable and is unmistakably taking hold in the modern social science literature and practice. The chapters in this volume provide some ideas and tools for the applied feminist researchers and evaluators to become active participants in this change.

REFERENCES

Christiansen, C. M. (1997). *The innovator's dilemma: When new technologies cause great firms to fail.* Boston: Harvard Business School Press.

Patton, M. Q. (2011). *Developmental evaluation: Applying complexity concepts to enhance innovation and use.* New York: Guilford Press.

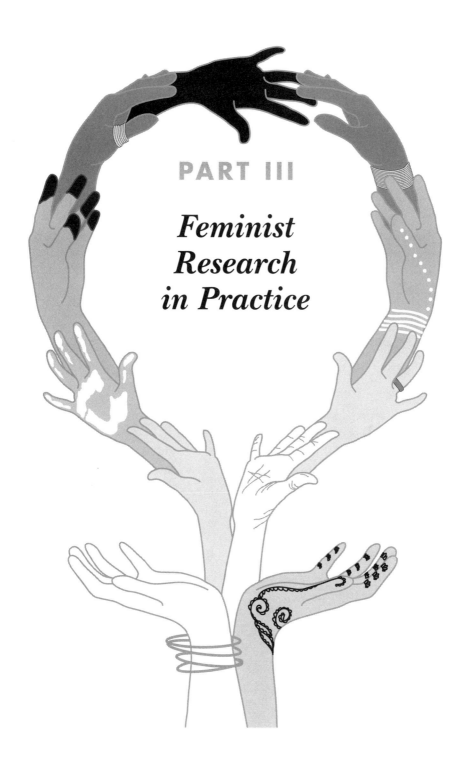

PART III

Feminist Research in Practice

CHAPTER 10

Feminist Research Approaches to Studying School-Based Health Care

A Three-Country Comparison

Denise Seigart

A great novel heightens your senses and sensitivity to the complexities
of life and of individuals, and prevents you from the self righteousness
that sees morality in fixed formulas about good and evil.
—AZAR NAFISI (2004), *Reading Lolita in Tehran*

Introduction

Like a great novel, a great evaluation or research project, in my opinion,
creates the conditions for learning and change, particularly for the benefit of women. This chapter discusses the implementation of a feminist
evaluation/research approach during the study of school-based health
care in three international settings: the United States, Canada, and Australia. In the process of implementing a qualitative study of school-based
health care, I utilized a feminist lens and feminist methods, including
reflexivity; interviews focused on active listening and the experiences of
the interviewees; collaborative examination of the data with interested
stakeholders, other feminists, and nonfeminists; and diverse dissemination of the results for the purpose of promoting dialogue, health care
reform, and social justice for children. It was my intent to create conditions for a critical feminist exploration of school health care for children
across the three countries, to share this information, and ultimately, to

promote community learning, action, and change. I do not refer to this project primarily as evaluation, because I was not evaluating one particular program, nor was I responsible to any particular funder.

What Feminist Evaluation Is

Feminist evaluation, like other evaluation approaches, is concerned with measuring the effectiveness of programs, judging merit or worth, and examining data to promote change. The difference between feminist approaches and other evaluation models generally lies in the increased attention paid to gender issues, the needs of women, and the promotion of transformative change (see Brisolara, Chapter 1, this volume, for a more extensive discussion of the differences). Feminist evaluation approaches are specifically interested in promoting social justice, particularly for women, but includes other oppressed groups as well. Attention is paid not only to gender but to race, class, sexual orientation, and abilities.

> For feminist evaluators, recognizing the ways in which discrimination is deeply imbedded within society—how key institutions (such as churches, temples, mosques, schools, and governmental programs), popular media, and culture reinforce the dominant patriarchal paradigm—is critical. (Brisolara & Seigart, 2012, p. 300)

Feminist evaluation approaches are a natural outgrowth of the influence of the feminist movement, feminist theory, and feminist research on the evaluation field, as mentioned earlier in this text. As feminist researchers have challenged the boundaries of how to do research, their ideas have influenced the way evaluators with feminist leanings approach evaluation. Feminist researchers have contributed to dramatically different views of what it means to do research, to critically examine gender issues, to explain the lives of women, and to promote social justice (see, e.g., Hesse-Biber, 2012). Feminist research has evolved over the years from feminist empiricism (utilizing traditional research methods to examine women's issues), to feminist standpoint theory (which argues that women approach research with different perspectives and therefore different abilities to examine problems than men), and finally to postmodern and postcolonial feminisms. This stream of feminist thought argues against the creation of new versions of old approaches that were implicitly sexist, racist, and classist. Postmodern and postcolonial feminists advocate for actively listening to multiple perspectives, exploring multiple realities in the process of research and/or evaluation, and avoiding the creation of grand theories that are deemed to suit all.

In the field of evaluation, collaborative and emancipatory evaluators have addressed some of the issues of concern to feminists, and have contributed much to the development of alternative approaches to evaluation. Evaluators such as Guba and Lincoln (1989), Greene (2007), Fetterman (2000), Patton (1997), and Mertens (2008) have made significant contributions to debates regarding evaluation practice, including which questions should/can be asked, how they should be asked, who should be included in the process, what methods can be used to answer critical questions, and how results should be shared. In spite of the inclusiveness of collaborative or empowerment-oriented evaluation approaches, however, they often still do not meet the guidelines generally considered critical for feminist evaluation practice (see Brisolara & Seigart, 2012). Research has demonstrated that even collaborative approaches can be co-opted by powerful parties or ingrained cultural interests, and thus may not adequately represent the voices of those with less power, frequently women. While feminist evaluation approaches tend to be collaborative in nature, more attention is paid to the power of gender expectations and relationships, the position and voice of oppressed groups, and the ethics of the study, the methods, and research processes.

Exploring Feminist Methods

Labeling evaluation models or approaches specifically as "feminist" is a fairly recent phenomenon. Within the evaluation field, there remains considerable resistance to alternative paradigms or approaches to evaluation, and often alternative methods continue to be regarded as inappropriate, biased, unreliable, and not truly "evaluation." Today, backlash against feminism and feminist work, as well as other alternative evaluation approaches, often creates a hostile environment for feminist evaluators and the possibility of exclusion from job opportunities for those who label their work as feminist in nature. For this reason, evaluators are often reluctant to label themselves as feminist (see Bheda, 2011, or Podems, Chapter 5, this volume), or their work as feminist, although their approach and methods may have a very feminist orientation. The language of feminism, the word *feminist* itself, is laden with particular meanings and stigma, and it continues to be the subject of debate among professional evaluators whether or not labeling an evaluation as "feminist" is desirable. Some authors argue for the use of different words (e.g., *transformative, gender-responsive*) in order to promote social justice-oriented research and evaluation, particularly in contexts where feminism is regarded as extremely controversial (Bamberger & Podems, 2002; Mertens, 2008; Patton, 2002). It is not my intent, however, to delve into this topic here. Whether or not they are "labeled" as such, feminist methodologies are generally reflective of the following:

> Feminist methodologies include epistemological arguments on how to apprehend the social; the evaluation of specific research questions and designs that capture the historical, intersectional, and transnational dimensions of women's lives and gender relations; attention to the ethical and policy implications of research; acknowledgement of the representational quality of research and scholarship; and attention to the outcomes of research including the development of multiple strategies for dissemination of research findings. (Chakravarty, Cook, & Fonow, 2012, p. 693)

In health care research, for example, the predominant positivist paradigm for research and evaluation is primarily focused on finding "cures" for particular diseases, whereas feminist researchers working in health care settings are more inclined to utilize an intersectional approach which is much more focused on finding "interventions designed to change broad systems of race, class, gender, and other dimensions of inequality, including those outside health (e.g., economy, jobs, education, law) that shape health" (Weber & Castellow, 2012, p. 437). The focus of feminist research in the health care arena is often not on individual problems, but on the power systems and structures that reinforce the oppressive systems that lead to poor health. Participatory or collaborative research designs are often favored by feminist researchers not only to ensure that local issues are addressed, but also to promote community learning and empowerment (which can theoretically produce more lasting action and change). Lykes and Herschberg (2012) refer to feminist participatory approaches as "an iterative set of processes and outcomes performed in one of three ways: (1) to reposition gender, race, and class; (2) to excavate indigenous cultural knowledges and generate voices; or (3) to deploy intersectionality as an analytic tool for transformation" (p. 331). The purpose is not only to help people identify problems and possible solutions, but to promote an environment of learning that will lead to transformative change.

Feminist evaluators recognize that mixed and multiple methods also provide an excellent base from which to investigate social problems, create conditions for learning, and produce results that will influence program leaders, policymakers, funders, and/or other important individuals and groups (Chakravarty et al., 2012; Greene, 2007). Feminist approaches often incorporate qualitative methods and are particularly focused on active listening, the power and status of the interviewer and the interviewee, reflexivity, relationships, language, and the ethics of the study. As noted by DeVault and Gross (2012):

Active listening means more than just physically hearing or reading; rather, it is a fully engaged practice that involves not only taking in information via speech, written words, or signs but also actively processing it. It means allowing that information to affect you, baffle you, haunt you, make you uncomfortable, and take you on unexpected detours. (p. 216)

The process of active listening can lead to detours and changes in the "design" of a study, something that may not be tolerated within a funded evaluation, particularly if the funder is looking for quick results and a particular focus. Surveys and other quantitative methods are often preferred merely because they can gather data more rapidly, and the focus is not on promoting learning among participants, but upon producing reports to validate the success of a program (or the money spent).

The Context: School-Based Health Care in the United States, Canada, and Australia

This study expanded upon my previous research, which examined the potential for fostering community learning while conducting a participatory evaluation of school-based health care in the United States (Seigart, 1999). Also based in participatory and qualitative frameworks, this international study added a feminist lens to the examination of school-based health in order to promote dialogue about the health needs of children and types of care provided, as well as the models for providing that care in various countries. Since feminist evaluators value an action orientation, it was the intent during this study to foster dialogue and community learning about various models for providing care for children, particularly with regard to the care provided for girls and young women. School-based health care is often a politically contentious approach to providing care for children. Thus utilizing a feminist approach ensured an opportunity to ask critical questions from a feminist perspective, thus "opening communicative space" as described by Kemmis (2008) to foster community learning. Often religious objections to certain types of health care (e.g., birth control education, provision of contraceptives) make school-based health care models targets of debate. This can interfere with the implementation of these models in more schools.

Feminist evaluation, as I define it, adheres to the early tradition of "consciousness raising" utilized by feminists in the 1960s, an approach that values feminist perspectives and creates opportunities for increased dialogue and learning during the evaluation/research process. As mentioned previously, traditional forms of evaluation and more participatory forms of evaluation often share aspects of feminist evaluation, but lack the feminist lens and critical questioning typically associated with a feminist approach. Emergent questions might not be asked, detours might not be taken. More recent efforts to incorporate a feminist lens during the evaluation process and facilitate community learning through evaluation are an attempt to repair this omission (Seigart & Brisolara, 2002). School-based health care and advocating for comprehensive health services in schools is increasingly accepted, but not yet widespread (Dryfoos & Maguire, 2002; Kolbe, 2005; Lear, 2007; MacDougall, 2008). Australia, Canada, and the United States have all engaged in various forms of school-based health care for children.

The United States, in particular, has focused on implementing school-based health centers, in addition to more traditional models of school-based health care. However, since the start of school-based health centers (SBHCs) in the United States in the early 1960s, their acceptability and proliferation has been steady, but inadequate (Gustafson, 2005; Kruger, Toker, Radjenovic, Comeaux, & Macha, 2009; Pheterson, 2008; Summers et al., 2003). Research indicates that the benefits of more comprehensive school health services are varied and can include increased school attendance, better maintenance of chronic health conditions, and enhanced health promotion activities (Fauteux, 2010; Guo et al., 2005; Nabors, Troillett, Nash, & Masiulis, 2005; Ricketts & Guernsey, 2006; Scudder, Papa, & Bray, 2007; Sidebottom, Birnbaum, & Nafstad, 2003; Veugelers & Fitzgerald, 2005). However, given the current global economic climate, school nursing services and SBHCs continue to be frequent targets for cutbacks. In the United States, school systems often share a school nurse. In the Canadian and Australian systems, many students do not have access to on-site comprehensive health services and the role of school nurses is poorly understood or valued (Fauteux, 2010; Moses et al., 2008; Resha, 2010). During this study, frontline professionals, parents, and community leaders identified multiple health care needs of children in schools and identified barriers to that care.

Gaining Entry

During the period of this research I encountered many issues including the occasional lack of access to a school or health care site. There can be an exclusionary habit among funders, publishers, and agencies that are the focus of research, if gender or feminist questions arise. Long periods of approval processes through multiple human subjects review committees may be required, making it nearly impossible to conduct research within a context that is hostile to feminism or transformative change.

Participatory processes can be regarded as subversive, and the power of the knowledge can be so dangerous as to prohibit the sharing of that knowledge, lest we cause something akin to an "Arab spring."

I personally do not present myself as a feminist evaluator who is coming to unearth embedded structures that promote or sustain oppression and social injustice. I presented my research plan, my interview questions (primarily dealing with school-based health care and the health care needs of children), my approval by two university ethics committees, and my resume. In my resume, it is apparent I do feminist work. This is perhaps enough to be threatening to some agencies, but it is not possible at this point to hide my interest in feminist approaches (any Google search will demonstrate my long involvement in this work), nor do I want to hide it. I do not know if the evidence that I do feminist work was the reason I was denied access to nurses/teachers at some agencies, but it may have been a factor. Completing a human subjects review process at every agency and school I was interested in was impossible time-wise, and larger scale approvals (statewide) seemed to be unavailable, so I sometimes accessed and interviewed individuals outside their agencies. Since I was working on a short timeline (2 months in Australia and 2 months in Canada), I did not have time to proceed through the multiple steps (barriers) that some agencies required in order to enter their agency and interview staff (health care agencies, schools). I had completed two human subjects reviews at two universities and the study was found not to violate any ethical principles. Therefore, I utilized snowball sampling and informed consent with each participant, whether I accessed them through an agency or outside an agency. I also informed participants if I did not have agency approval and allowed them to decide whether or not they desired to speak with me, and I guaranteed them confidentiality.

Agencies will sometimes deny researchers/evaluators access to their staff internally because they don't want to know how their program is doing, are afraid research will prove controversial, that it may lead to discontinued funding, or because they have had too much research ongoing in their facilities. I took a more investigative journalism approach, sometimes accessing individuals outside agencies through snowball sampling, as I believe that individuals have the right to decide whether or not they would like to speak with me and whether or not the research is important. This is consistent with social science and investigative journalism ethics, as discussed by Ian Richards (2010) in his article "Uneasy Bedfellows." I also conducted interviews until I felt I had reached a point of saturation (hearing the same concerns/topics over and over) and when I noted a particularly interesting or troubling theme, I followed up on these by trying to access those individuals who would have more information (e.g., when some teachers, nurses, administrators expressed the view that Aboriginal patients didn't mind sitting in an emergency room [ER] all day to get care, I sought out staff who specifically work in a clinic for Aborigines to garner their point of view on this attitude). My intent was to give voice to teachers, nurses, parents, and administrators who recognize the needs and attempt to provide health care for children every day through schools.

Methods

This study involved a series of interpretive case studies in three countries during 2008–2009, utilizing qualitative methods to compare and contrast the provision of health care for children through schools in the United States, Australia, and Canada. Since school-based health care is a complex process deeply influenced by the communities in which it takes place, a case study approach was implemented. In this study, data were gathered from in-depth interviews with key health care providers, teachers, and other stakeholders involved in school-based health care. On-site observations of various models for providing school health care were also utilized. Institutional reports and other literature were also consulted to enhance the understanding of the school health care environment. Patton (2002) has stated that "the major way in which qualitative researchers seek to understand the perceptions, feelings, and knowledge of people is through in-depth, intensive interviewing" (p. 21).

Interviews (mostly face-to-face), lasting approximately 1 hour each, were conducted with a total of 73 school nurses, teachers, administrators, parents, and community leaders in New York, Pennsylvania, New South Wales, Queensland, Victoria, Quebec, and Ontario. Snowball sampling was utilized as the method to obtain the names of key stakeholders (since I was an outsider in these settings) via the recommendations of these nurses, teachers, administrators, university faculty, parents, and other community leaders. Individuals included in the interview process were regarded as well informed about school-based health care or their children had utilized the services of a school health program, and they were frequently recommended by other interviewees as being well informed about school-based health care. The majority of the interviews were completed with school nurses or community health nurses who work in schools ($n = 40$), and these were supplemented by interviews with parents, teachers, administrators, nursing faculty, and other community leaders ($n = 33$) in order to compare differing perspectives on health care as provided through schools. Each interview utilized a strategy of "active listening," and participants often engaged with me in extensive conversations about school-based health care.

Information about school health models in other countries was often shared during these interviews, and added to the richness of the exchange. For example, school nurses in Australia were often surprised to learn that nurses in the United States were frequently based in one school only. Australian teachers were often surprised to learn that nurses could be on-site daily; in fact, one Australian principal of a school for children with special needs stated she had "never seen a nurse" at the school in the 5 years she had been principal there.

Data analysis strategies utilized were congruent with those used in grounded theory approaches. These included analysis of interview transcripts, field notes, and records of observations for emerging themes. Contextual analysis was completed by coding apparent themes from the transcripts of taped interviews and field notes of observations conducted in schools, and then categorizing these themes interpretively. While coding the data, I also attempted to reflect on how a feminist would view this data. Much like Christians who wear a WWJD (What Would Jesus Do?) bracelet, I would don my WWAFS (What Would a Feminist See?) glasses. Within each category of data that emerged, a feminist analysis of the context, structures, and processes was applied.

I asked questions of the data. For example, Why were teachers (largely female) consistently being asked to assume duties outside their scope of practice? Why were nurses (largely female) routinely spread so thin among schools? Why were childrens' health needs often ignored? Why did religious views play such an important role in the selection of available health care in schools? Although I was not able to share the transcripts with individual interviewees due to travel and time constraints, preliminary themes and data were shared with nursing faculty and community leaders during large forums held in Australia, Canada, and the United States as the themes were refined and examined for internal consistency and conceptual distinctiveness (Strauss & Corbin, 1990). The emergent themes were also shared with three other nurse scientists (including a feminist) along with the original data for independent comparison and critique. This study utilized the "trustworthiness" criteria for qualitative methods as outlined in Guba and Lincoln (1989), including credibility, transferability, dependability, confirmability, and authenticity. Credibility can be achieved through prolonged engagement and persistent observation. I spent 1 month in Canada and 2 months in Australia interviewing and observing school health care. I have spent much more time engaged in the study of school health care in the United States, and as a nurse, have a deep understanding of the functioning of school nurses and the health care needs of children. This perhaps gives me the ability to establish trust with interviewees earlier in the relationship, and

I sometimes heard the comment, "I can't believe I told you all that, it will be confidential, right?"

Transferability is achieved through "thick description" of the context and study, so that readers can assess the environment, data, and results and judge its applicability to their own settings. In other writings related to this research, I have focused on thick description of school-based health care and the needs of children. Dependability and confirmability are often achieved through external audits of the data and the process. While I did not have formal external audits, I did share the data and my analysis with stakeholders and other researchers/evaluators who were involved in the research, including feminists. Their perspectives and comments contributed to the final analysis I shared through presentations and publications. I also looked for triangulation of the data (interviews with observations and document review).

Emergent Issues

As noted previously, a feminist lens was applied to the analysis of data. Thus when I noted phenomena that impressed me as being structurally connected with sexism, racism, and classism, I paid attention to these issues, because as a feminist evaluator it is important to focus intensively on those findings that indicate the reinforcement of social injustice. Asking questions about structural inequalities is not necessarily built into research and evaluation projects, or appreciated when they are, but paying attention to emergent questions is an important part of what a qualitative researcher, and feminist evaluators, must do. In this study, for example, the plight of children with special needs in schools became an important focus as teachers, parents, and administrators discussed the struggles each face with regard to providing health care and quality educational opportunities for these children. Additional problems noted included restrictions on health care due to religious objections of certain community members, elimination of school nurses (largely women) from school systems, and the burdening of teachers (largely women) with health care responsibilities outside their scope of practice. Political influences can be so strong as to prohibit the asking of important questions or even the inclusion of important words within a study, and controversial topics are often avoided so as to prevent any disruptive questions being asked.

Since this study deals with school-based health care (which can be controversial due to sexuality issues, particularly at the high school level), schools and health care organizations may deny researchers/evaluators access to their agencies. While interviewing individuals or conducting focus groups, I worked hard to maintain a "neutral" stance in that I did not advocate for any particular type of care (feminist) or voice an opinion as to whether or not I thought the care being provided was good and/or bad. It was my intent to "disappear" in a sense, and let the participants describe what school health care is like in their settings, although the probes I utilized might be regarded by some as controversial (e.g., What type of sex education is provided for students in this school?). As per the interview protocol, I asked interviewees to describe the health care needs of the children they work with, the current health care system in their schools, and the barriers they perceived to providing health care for children through schools.

From a cultural competency perspective, as an outsider looking in, an American examining Australian and Canadian school health systems, this study required an important level of collaboration and help with interpretation, referenced by my colleague Elaine Dietsch (Chapter 12, this volume) as cultural humility (Foster, 2009; Tervalon & Murray-Garcia, 1998). In each context (Australia, United States, and Canada), I worked closely with local nurses and nurse scientists to carefully analyze the school health systems and promote learning for transformative change. These individuals helped me with the snowball sampling (suggesting key informants), as well as data interpretation and dissemination. I also attempted to access individuals who had specific knowledge about health care for underserved populations. My Canadian nurse scientist colleague is of First Nations heritage. My Australian colleague is noted for her work with Aborigine and African women. In addition, when I noted data that seemed to indicate an underlying prejudice (racism, sexism, classism), I followed up on these by asking additional questions for the rest of the study (which is consistent with attention to emerging themes in qualitative methods).

For example, it became apparent early in my study that whether or not a nurse is present in the school has a great impact on the education/inclusion of children with special needs. I added specific questions to my interviews early on regarding the health care issues of children with special needs to more fully understand this phenomenon. As mentioned previously, I also noted an apparent prejudice toward Aboriginal children and parents on the part of some teachers, nurses, and administrators. I followed up on this issue by probing deeper during interviews (e.g., What do you believe causes the health care issues you have noted in Aboriginal children?) and sought out alternative points of view (e.g., the views of staff who work directly with Aboriginal children/families in a clinic specifically designed for providing Aboriginal care). Specific results of this study are presented in the following discussion.

Results/Interview Themes Regarding School Health Care

Scope of Practice

Limited resources and physician control of nurses' practice continue to affect the quality of school-based health care provision for children (a historical/structural issue that persists in our current health care systems, reflecting the control of women by men and/or powerful groups). For example, Canada and Australia have a relative scarcity of nurse practitioners (NPs), as this model of care is only recently becoming acceptable in these countries. Much opposition from physician groups exists to the expansion of the scope of practice rights for NPs in all three countries.

> The Australian Medical Association continually claims that NPs offer a second-class service. The AMA puts out more press releases attacking the concept of NPs the more they see NPs gaining a foothold. Many NPs said they were acutely aware of the responsibility of being pioneers, and felt if they did anything wrong it would be seized on by the doctors. NPs work within clinical guidelines which have been a major area of contention. Initially, the process of developing the guidelines was laborious, partly because it involved the AMA, which is opposed to the very concept of NPs who aren't supervised by doctors. Some doctors attempt to limit NPs' practice by opposing their clinical guidelines. (New South Wales Nurses and Midwives Association, 2006)

> Nurse practitioners are an idea whose time has come—except in Quebec. . . . The problem, Desrosiers explained, has been with hospital administrators, unfamiliar with the NP role. . . . Diplomatically, she avoided suggesting that MDs might also be a little reluctant about a bigger role for NPs. Today, there are just 41 nurse practitioners in Quebec. By comparison, Ontario has 800. (Lamontagne, 2009)

In the United States NPs are more accepted; however, there is continued resistance to expansion of their scope of practice here as well (For more information on this issue, see Robert Wood Johnson Initiative at the Institute of Medicine, 2010). In New York, for example, there are approximately 9,000 practicing NPs and 900 midwives. If NPs and midwives (largely women) were allowed to practice to the full extent of their abilities, this could greatly relieve the growing burden for primary care providers, including those serving children in schools.

Increasing Stress

Educators in most schools (predominantly women, especially at the grade-school level) reported increasing stress regarding administrative expectations that they will provide health care for children, a function well outside their training and licensure. Teachers described their "duty of care" and recounted situations where children could not attend school if the teachers were not willing to administer medications or provide some other type of health care:

> "We have a line-up of children taking their meds . . . it's very busy, very difficult to deal with . . . we have more and more to do. In one school the teachers were being required to give meds, teachers are very strong here, they will not give meds. Teachers are becoming more and more resistant to taking on that kind of responsibility. The teachers have so many other things they have to do! . . . Teachers feel very overwhelmed. I have one student who had to have blood pressures every 2 hours . . . she finally left the school, no one wanted to take responsibility for the medications . . . it was after the girl had chemotherapy." (Quebec focus group with six school nurses, Spring 2009)

In Canada and Australia, there is currently little demand by parents to have a nurse present in each school (because there is limited history of this kind of service), and while there has been pressure to maintain the school health services available on-site in the U.S., economic pressures and education cutbacks are making nurses easy targets for desperate administrators.

Devaluing the Nurses' Role

A lack of understanding or valuing of nurses as the providers of school health care is common, and often contributes to the loss of nursing positions in schools. Some parents and administrators believe, "They just apply band-aids all day." Others argue that to keep a nurse will cause the loss of a teacher, and that schools really ought to be about education, not health care. In spite of international efforts to promote the health of children (e.g., antiobesity campaigns), health programs within schools are often not led by nurses. Physical education teachers or health teachers are frequently recruited to oversee "health programs," and in more and more cases nonlicensed personnel are being recruited in schools to provide health care and emergency care for children, even secretaries and janitors. The results of these trends can range from children being sent home from school more often (Pennington & Delaney, 2008) to the death of a child in the school setting (Bergren, 2010; Thomas, 2012).

Rural and Religious Communities

The influence of conservative and/or religious organizations on school health care can also be dramatic. Restrictions on certain kinds of care, or the access nurses have to schools, can be impacted by the tenor of the local community and the risks perceived by administrators. For example, in some Australian communities, access to some kinds of health care like birth control or abortion are restricted because Catholic facilities have a strong presence and physicians do not want to alienate administrators, since they have privileges in those institutions.

> "In NSW a 14-year-old can get a termination of pregnancy [TOP], but not here [in this town], public health insurance does not pay, it can cost $300–400. In Victoria you have to be 16 to get TOP without parental consent. I have had pregnant 12 year olds sometimes, this is an automatic DoCS [Department of Community Services] referral. I sometimes have to transport teens to other cities for TOP. The physicians won't support bringing in another MD (from the next city over) to do abortions or vasectomies. . . . [T]hey don't want to alienate the private Catholic hospital. . . . [T]hey also have privileges there. This is a very conservative area. We have a fairly high teen pregnancy and birth rate in comparison to other parts of Australia. I sometimes have trouble getting into the schools to do sex education. I hear such sad stories, one disabled girl told me during a sex ed class—'I don't need contraceptives, I don't have sex, I just give the guys blow jobs during lunch break for cigarettes.'" (Australian teen health community nurse, Fall 2008)

This trend can be observed in the United States as well, particularly in rural areas, with more than 60% of SBHCs in the United States being prohibited from dispensing contraception, a policy determined most often by school districts (Strozer, Juszczak, & Ammerman, 2010). This fact does not deter conservative groups and legislators, however, from portraying SBHCs as "sex clinics," as noted in the recent media attention given Rep. Bachman (Siegel & Bachmann, 2009). Notably, Canadians did not seem to have the same level of problems with conservative or religious attitudes affecting health care in schools, according to those interviewed.

Other Structurally and Culturally Embedded Issues

Many other structurally and culturally imbedded issues were noted during the period of this study. Racism, classism, sexism, and attitudes regarding the deserving versus the undeserving poor were noted. For example, it was often noted that poorer families (those without private insurance in the United States and Australia) were subjected to different levels of health care than those with insurance. Longer wait times, or lack of access to any care at all, were common problems (particularly in the United States). Selected groups were regarded by some as undeserving of care (e.g., illegal immigrants, Aboriginals). The lack of school health care was not regarded by some school administrators as a problem for schools. As stated by one Australian principal, "The Aborigines go to the ER, they're happy to sit there, at the hospital . . . it's cool and they watch the TV all day." Some parents did not believe that children with special needs should be mainstreamed, as the cost of providing care for these children in schools would take away from those children "deserving" of care and education. Some children with special needs are denied access to mainstream schools because there are no on-site nurses to provide the important health care procedures these children often need, and their parents are unable to pay for private-duty services. Rather than considering health care a right of every child, many regard it as an expensive privilege, something you should work for, and if you can't afford it, then you just won't get it. There is no "preferential option for the poor" as advocated by Paul Farmer (2005), and those without health care are regarded as somehow inferior. The structural violence of the current health care systems noted by Farmer (particularly those in the United States) often forces the uninsured to seek health care through charities, or to go without health care completely. As noted by Janet Poppendieck, a rise in "kindness" reflects a decline in justice:

> The resurgence of charity is at once a symptom and a curse of our society's failure to face up to and deal with the erosion of equality. It is a symptom in that it stems, in part at least, from an abandonment of our hopes for the elimination of poverty; it signifies a retreat from the goals as well as the means that characterized the Great Society. It is symptomatic of a pervasive despair about actually solving problems that has turned us toward ways of managing them: damage control, rather than prevention. More significantly, and more controversially, the proliferation of charity contributes to our society's failure to grapple in meaningful ways with poverty. (as quoted in Farmer, 2005, p. 154)

Current political debates in the United States and elsewhere predict a bruising battle on our journey toward justice in health care and other arenas. Recent votes in Wisconsin refusing to recall the Republican governor and reinforcing the destruction of labor unions, the current Republican effort to recall the Obama health care initiatives, and other global events foretell a period of increasing desperation and suffering for many, and yet, if we could learn to listen to one another, there might still be hope.

Creating Conditions for Learning

It is my belief, that whenever possible, feminist evaluators and researchers should set up the conditions for learning to occur during an evaluation or research study. In debates I have heard about the role of the evaluator, I often reflect on my own functioning, and have decided that my favorite role is as "catalyst." In the same way that Azar Nafisi, a professor who was banned from teaching literature and writing in Iran, continued her classes in her home and thus created the conditions for her students to learn (2004; *Reading Lolita in Tehran*), evaluators should position themselves and their studies in such a way that participants will have the opportunity to learn from each other and the data that are produced. As I strived to do in this case, the inclusion of stakeholders in studies and discussion of problems can lead to learning and transformative change, especially those regarding gender issues and programs serving women. Rani Parker (1993) suggests that gender analysis cannot be transformative unless the people being analyzed are involved in the study. Participatory and collaborative approaches to evaluation and research begin to produce these kinds of conditions, but I believe they often miss the important structural and cultural influences that restrain any true transformative change. As noted by Kemmis (2008), evaluation and research should be about promoting dialogue:

> The central purpose of evaluation is *to create opportunities for communication about themes and issues arising in social and educational programs and settings.* Beneath this overarching purpose, communicative evaluation has purposes of (1) *revelation*—helping people to understand cultural, social and interpersonal dynamics in and around programs and settings, (2) *anticipation*—helping people to orient towards the future in increasingly unsettled times, and (3) *building communication and partnership*—helping people to work together for transformation not only at local levels, but also in relation to global issues, trends and tendencies. (Unpublished paper shared with author)

ɪfortunately, feminist approaches to evaluation or research are
ɪt pursued, due to a variety of reasons. Bamberger (2009) outlines
ˀollows:

  is often not adequately addressed in program evaluation, and
  ᵛ" approaches to evaluation and research are often shunned
  ɪriety of factors including:

1. Additional costs (more personnel, more time).
2. Additional time (qualitative methods, increased sampling).
3. Qualitative methods not considered by many stakeholders as "professional research."
4. Many agencies reluctant to address questions relating to "culture."
5. Gender equated with "feminism" which has a negative image for many people.

However, if evaluators are concerned with the quality of their work, and ultimately producing conditions where transformative learning can occur (which will benefit women and all oppressed groups), I do not believe feminist approaches can be ignored. As noted by Greene:

> Evaluation can offer a space where the practices of reason and delibera-tion are engaged, where evidence of multiple kinds displaces rhetoric, and where conversation is directed toward shared goals of social better-ment and practical wisdom. Evaluation can create a space where differ-ence is accepted, respected, and viewed as an opportunity for listening and for learning, for learning to listen. Evaluation can be a space that welcomes, even celebrates values of tolerance, dialogue, integrity, and social responsibility. (*AEA Newsletter*, September 2011)

Creating opportunities for learning should be a central goal for feminist evaluators and/or researchers. Feminist evaluation, or gender-responsive evaluation, should not, however, position the needs of the eval-uator or researcher above those of the participants in the research. Active listening entails truly paying attention to the needs of the participants, changing the direction of the study as needed in any particular context, and being careful to prevent harm in the process of conducting evalu-ations and promoting learning. For example, a study observed by Paul Farmer (2005) is a good example of disrespect for the needs of the local stakeholders:

> The women of Guatemala City were conducting a "gender sensitivity" workshop. They had asked each of those present—about twenty locals, mostly young women, . . . to draw a scene from childhood. The adult pupils sat crammed into children's desks, supplied with crayons. One of the facilitators would hold aloft the drawing and ask the artist, and occasionally the audience, questions about it. The theme of the ques-tions was gender relations. . . . It seemed to us that the exercise was demeaning—the participants, having survived genocide and displace-ment, were now being treated like children. They were being asked to respond to an agenda imported from capital cities, from do-gooder organizations like ours, from U.S. universities with the "right" answers to their every question. (pp. 3–4)

Conclusion

I believe it is always important to consider the needs of women and other oppressed groups when designing evaluations and/or research projects. I do not believe that we should move forward in any project without considering ways that we may design into the project the opportunity for learning. This is not just a "nice" option, but in my opinion an imperative. If we are to make progress in the world with regard to the rights of women, if we are to promote social justice and cultural competence, we must "set up" the conditions for learning whenever we can. Involving all stakeholders in the process in a more participatory style of evaluation or research is ideal, but even in situations when this is not possible, providing opportunities for stakeholder groups to participate in designing studies, choosing important questions, or participating in data analysis and interpretation of data are invaluable learning opportunities. Promotion of dialogue about issues important to women and other oppressed groups such as reproductive rights, violence against women, health care, cultural humility, barriers to change, and structural violence can lead to an increased understanding of these issues and possible solutions. In the words of Batliwala and Pittman (2010), we need "to prioritize internal learning as central to organizational and movement strengthening" (p. 4). Feminist evaluators and researchers can become catalysts for change by creating the conditions for robust dialogue and engaged learning during their work. We have much work to do.

REFERENCES

Bamberger, M. (2009, November). *The gender context of program evaluation.* Paper presented at the annual conference of the American Evaluation Association, Orlando, FL.

Bamberger, M., & Podems, D. (2002). Feminist evaluation in international development. In D. Seigart & S. Brisolara (Eds.), *Feminist evaluation: Exploration and experiences* (pp. 83–97). New York: Guilford Press.

Batliwala, S., & Pittman, A. (2010). *Capturing change in women's realities: A critical overview of current monitoring and evaluation frameworks and approaches.* Toronto: Association for Women's Rights in Development. Retrieved from *www.awid.org.*

Bergren, M. (2010, Sept. 19). Reducing preventable child mortality at school. Pediatrics. Retrieved from *pediatrics.aappublications.org/content/126/3/592. abstract/reply.*

Bheda, D. (2011). En "gendering" evaluation: Feminist evaluation but "I am not a feminist." In S. Mathison (Ed.), Really new directions in evaluation: Young evaluators respecting evaluation. *New Directions for Evaluation, 2011*(131), 53–58.

Brisolara, S., & Seigart, D. (2012). Feminist evaluation research. In S. Hesse-Biber (Ed.), *The handbook of feminist research: Theory and praxis*. Los Angeles: Sage.

Chakravarty, D., Cook, J., & Fonow, M. (2012). Teaching, techniques, and technologies of feminist methodology: Online and on the ground. In S. Hesse-Biber (Ed.), *The handbook of feminist research: Theory and praxis* (pp. 693–710). Los Angeles: Sage.

DeVault, M., & Gross, G. (2012). Feminist qualitative interviewing: Experience, talk, and knowledge. In S. Hesse-Biber (Ed.), *The handbook of feminist research: Theory and praxis* (pp. 206–237). Los Angeles: Sage.

Dryfoos, J., & Maguire, S. (2002). *Inside full-service community schools*. Thousand Oaks, California: Corwin Press.

Farmer, P. (2005). *Pathologies of power: Health, human rights, and the new war on the poor*. Berkeley and Los Angeles: University of California Press.

Fauteux, N. (2010, August). Unlocking the potential of school nursing: Keeping children healthy, in school, and ready to learn. In *Charting Nursing's Future*. Washington, DC: Robert Wood Johnson Foundation. Retrieved from *www.rwjf.org/research-publications*.

Fetterman, D. (2000). *Foundations of empowerment evaluation*. Los Angeles: Sage.

Foster, J. (2009). Cultural humility and the importance of long-term relationships in international partnerships. *Journal of Obstetric, Gynecologic, and Neonatal Nursing, 1*, 100–107.

Greene, J. C. (2007). *Mixed methods in social inquiry*. San Francisco: Jossey-Bass.

Greene, J. C. (2011, September). *American Evaluation Association Newsletter.*

Guba, E., & Lincoln, Y. (1989). *Fourth-generation evaluation*. Newbury Park, CA: Sage.

Guo, J., Jang, R., Keller, K., McCracken, A., Pan, W., & Cluxton, J. (2005). Impact of school-based health centers on children with asthma. *Journal of Adolescent Health, 37*, 266–274.

Gustafson, E. (2005). History and overview of school-based health centers in the U.S. *Nursing Clinics in North America, 40*, 595–606.

Hesse-Biber, S. (2012). *The handbook of feminist research: Theory and praxis*. Los Angeles: Sage.

Institute of Medicine. (2011). *The future of nursing: Leading change, advancing health*. Washington, DC: National Academies Press.

Kemmis, S. (2008). *Opening communicative space: Evaluation and the public sphere*. Unpublished paper shared with author in fall 2008.

Kolbe, L. (2005). A framework for school health programs in the 21st century. *Journal of School Health, 75*, 226–228.

Kruger, B., Toker, K., Radjenovic, D., Comeaux, M., & Macha, K. (2009). School nursing for children with special needs: Does number of schools make a difference? *Journal of School Health, 79*, 337–346.

Lamontagne, P. (2009, April 13). Editorial: Make room for nurse practitioners. *Montreal Gazette*, p. A2.

Lear, J. (2007). Health at school: A hidden health care system emerges from the shadows. *Health Affairs, 26*, 409–419.

Lykes, M., & Herschberg, R. (2012). Participatory action research and feminisms: Social inequalities and transformative praxis. In S. Hesse-Biber (Ed.), *The handbook of feminist research: Theory and praxis* (pp. 331–368). Los Angeles: Sage.

MacDougall, C. (2008, March). *Healthy schools: Overview and opportunities.* Paper presented at North Bay Community Conference, North Bay, Ontario, Canada.

Mertens, D. (2008). *Transformative research and evaluation.* New York: Guilford Press.

Moses, K., Keneally, J., Bibby, H., Chiang, F., Robards, F., & Bennett, D. (2008). Beyond bandaids: Understanding the role of school nurses in NSW. *Proceedings of School Nurses Association of NSW Annual Conference.* Retrieved from *www.caah.claw.edu.au/projects/summary-report.pdf.*

Nabors, L., Troillett, A., Nash, T., & Masiulis, B. (2005). School nurse perceptions of barriers and supports for children with diabetes. *Journal of School Health, 75,* 119–124.

Nafisi, A. (2004). *Reading Lolita in Tehran.* New York: Random House.

New South Wales Nurses and Midwives Association. (2006, October). Nurse practitioners advance against the odds. *Union News.* Retrieved February 13, 2013, from *www.nswnma.asn.au/news/6377.html.*

Parker, R. (1993). *Another point of view: A manual on gender analysis training for grassroots workers.* New York: UNIFEM.

Patton, M. Q. (1997). *Utilization-focused evaluation.* Thousand Oaks, CA: Sage.

Patton, M. Q. (2002). *Qualitative research and evaluation methods.* Thousand Oaks, CA: Sage.

Pennington, N., & Delaney, E. (2008). The number of students sent home by school nurses compared to unlicensed personnel. *Journal of School Nursing, 24*(5), 290–297.

Pheterson, M. (2008). School-based health centers help keep students healthy—and in school. *New York Nurses Network,* 15–17.

Poppendieck, J. (1998). Sweet charity?: Emergency food and the end of entitlement. Quoted in P. Farmer (2005). *Pathologies of power: Health, human rights, and the new war on the poor.* Berkeley and Los Angeles: University of California Press.

Resha, C. (2010). Delegation in the school setting: Is it a safe practice? *Online Journal of Issues in Nursing, 15*(2). Available at *www.nursingworld.org.*

Richards, I. (2010). Uneasy bedfellows: Ethics committees and journalism research. *Australia Journalism Review, 31*(2), 35.

Ricketts, S., & Guernsey, B. (2006). School-based health centers and the decline in black teen fertility during the 1990s in Denver, Colorado. *American Journal of Public Health, 96,* 1588–1592.

Robert Wood Johnson Initiative at the Institute of Medicine. (2010). *The future of nursing: Leading change, advancing health.* Retrieved from *www.nap.edu/catalog/12956.html.*

Scudder, L., Papa, P., & Bray, L. (2007). School-based health centers: A model for improving the health of the nation's children. *Journal for Nurse Practitioners, 3,* 713–720.

Seigart, D. (1999). *Participatory evaluation and community learning: Sharing knowledge about school-based health care*. Unpublished dissertation, Cornell University, Ithaca, NY.

Seigart, D., & Brisolara, S. (Eds.). (2002). Feminist evaluation: Explorations and experiences. *New Directions for Evaluation, 2002*(96).

Sidebottom, A., Birnbaum, A., & Nafstad, S. S. (2003). Decreasing barriers for teens: Evaluation of a new teenage pregnancy prevention strategy in school-based clinics. *American Journal of Public Health, 93*, 1890–1892.

Siegel, E., & Bachmann, M. (2009). "Sex clinics" in schools will result from health care reform. *Huffington Post*. Retrieved March 29, 2013, from *www.huffington-post.com/2009/10/01/bachmann-sex-clinics-will_n_306292.html*.

Strauss, A., & Corbin, J. (1990). *Basics of qualitative research: Grounded theory procedures and techniques*. Newbury Park, CA: Sage.

Strozer, J., Juszczak, L., & Ammerman, A. (2010). *2007–2008 National School-Based Health Care Census*. Washington, DC: National Assembly on School-Based Health Care.

Summers, L., Williams, J., Borges, W., Ortiz, M., Schaefer, S., & Liehr, P. (2003). School-based health center viability: Application of the COPC model. *Issues in Comprehensive Pediatric Nursing, 26*, 231–251.

Tervalon, M., & Murray-Garcia, J. (1998). Cultural humility versus cultural competence: A critical distinction in defining physician training outcomes in multicultural education. *Journal of Health Care for the Poor and Underserved, 9*(2), 117–125. Retrieved March 29, 2013, from *http://info.kp.org/community-benefit/assets/pdf/our_work/global/Cultural_Humility_article.pdf*.

Thomas, K. (2012, Sept. 7). *Tiny lifesaver for a growing worry*. New York Times. Retrieved March 29, 2013, from *www.nytimes.com/2012/09/08/business/mylan-invests-in-epipen-as-child-allergies-increase.html?pagewanted=all*.

Veugelers, P., & Fitzgerald, A. (2005). Effectiveness of school programs in preventing childhood obesity: A multilevel comparison. *American Journal of Public Health, 95*, 432–435.

Weber, L., & Castellow, J. (2012). Feminist research and activism to promote health equity. In S. Hesse-Biber (Ed.), *The handbook of feminist research: Theory and praxis* (pp. 434–455). Los Angeles: Sage.

CHAPTER 11

Feminist Research Approaches to Empowerment in Syria

Alessandra Galiè

Introduction

This chapter presents the findings of an assessment of the empowerment of 12 women farmers from three Syrian villages involved in a participatory plant breeding (PPB) program coordinated at the International Centre for Agricultural Research in the Dry Areas (ICARDA). The findings show that PPB has the potential to enhance women's recognition as farmers, facilitate their access to relevant plant varieties and information, increase their access to opportunities, and support their decision making. The assessment also shows the difficulties and pitfalls of some of the strategies adopted by the program. Moreover, this chapter discusses how these findings were used to make the PPB program's activities more gender-equal. It reviews some of the advantages of the application of the chosen methodology and techniques in the sociopolitical culture and technical context of the research and in the framework of feminist evaluation.

The Context

Agriculture is increasingly seen as an engine to enhance growth, reduce poverty and improve livelihoods (World Bank, Food and Agriculture Organization of the United Nations [FAO], International Fund for Agricultural Development [IFAD], 2009). New pathways of Agricultural Research for Development (AR4D) are needed to enhance food security vis-à-vis current and future challenges (e.g., population increase, climate change) and to target poor farmers from marginal areas who have benefited the least from the achievements of AR4D to date (International Assessment of Agricultural Knowledge, Science, and Technology for Development [IAASTD], 2009). Worldwide, rural women have been shown to have a substantial role in agriculture and household food security through their role in food production, processing, and food cultures (Jiggins, 2011; World Bank, FAO, & IFAD, 2009). Yet rural women have generally limited access to and control of resources and information, and access to opportunities and markets (Turrall, 2012). Gender-based inequalities existing at ground level have been shown to constrain the efficacy of efforts to enhance agricultural production and food security (World Bank, FAO, IFAD, 2009). Increasingly, efforts have been made both to include gender concerns in AR4D and to address women's empowerment throughout the project cycle (World Bank, FAO, IFAD, 2009).

PPB for crop improvement is today accepted as a useful approach to meet the current and future challenges of AR4D (World Bank, 2008). PPB aims to enhance rural livelihoods by breeding plant varieties that better reflect farmers' crop and trait needs. Ample evidence shows that farmers' needs are shaped by their local agroecological and socioeconomic circumstances, and are affected by gender (Ceccarelli & Grando, 2007; Paris, Singh, Cueno, & Singh, 2008). Gender considerations are important whenever men and women play a role along the food production-to-consumption chain that might entail specific needs, priorities, and knowledge (Farnworth & Jiggins, 2003). For instance, those in charge of food processing might have preferences related to cooking quality that are different from those in charge of marketing, who might prioritize customers' product requirements. Plant breeding, however, is often considered mainly in terms of its aim to produce "technical outputs" (i.e., improved crop varieties). The way social factors and gender inequality affect technology development and adoption is often overlooked (Ransom & Bain, 2011). At the same time, considering plant breeding as a technical intervention only overlooks its impact on social relations within communities and households.

The lack of gender considerations in PPB raises two issues: the effectiveness of technology development and the equity of development opportunity. Gender-blind plant breeding is likely to overlook the needs of female farmers and not include their crop and trait preferences in the criteria adopted when selecting improved varieties. Lack of access to relevant and good varieties might negatively affect women's ability to perform their key roles in food production, processing, and food cultures. This ultimately affects the effectiveness of AR4D in enhancing rural livelihoods and in supporting the right to food. The exclusion of gender considerations in plant breeding also raises the issue of inequity in development opportunity. Breeding programs often focus on crops and traits with higher market potential in favorable environments and overlook crops and traits that might be essential for the livelihood of women and subsistence farmers. By overlooking the needs of the most marginal farmers and women, while supporting only farmers in favorable conditions, AR4D risks aggravating existing inequalities rather than reducing the gender and poverty gap.

The empowerment of rural women is seen as a key to increasing both the effectiveness of agricultural technology development and to contributing to the equity of development opportunity. "Empowerment" of farm women, it is argued, enhances their capability to collaborate with scientists, and this is believed to increase the effectiveness of agricultural research (Song & Vernooy, 2010). Women's empowerment is also considered to provide women with the means to express their needs and to act in their own interests so that they can benefit from rural and agricultural development (De Schutter, 2009). In spite of its importance, however, empowerment is hardly ever analyzed in rigorous ways. This flaw might be caused by the elusive nature of the concept, the difficulty of capturing it in a definition, and, consequently, the technical challenge of establishing proper indicators to monitor and measure it. Overlooking the impact of projects on the empowerment of its stakeholders can reduce the understanding of how projects affect power relations in any given situation; it can limit the understanding of social change dynamics that affect research aims and processes; and it can miss the opportunity to refine strategies to bring about gender justice.

Background to the Research

In Syria, small-scale farming supports the livelihoods of the majority of the rural poor. Yet agriculture's share of gross domestic product is only just over 20% associated with low added value per agricultural worker and low capital stocks per agricultural worker (IAASTD, 2009). Syrian small-scale farming is characterized by a wide range of agroecological conditions and agronomic systems that are often organized based on a gender division of labor (United Nations Development Programme [UNDP], 2006). Along the food production-to-consumption chain women are mainly involved in manual activities (e.g., weeding, fertilizing, hand planting and harvesting, and food processing) and men mainly in mechanized and marketing activities. In the last decades, women's share of agricultural work has increased because agriculture has increasingly been unable to support rural livelihoods and many men, mostly the young, have moved to urban areas or abroad in search of cash incomes (Abdelali-Martini, Goldey, Jones, & Bailey, 2003). Women, children, and the old have remained in the villages. This has resulted in the feminization of agricultural labor; women have increasingly become involved in farming activities on-farm to avoid hiring labor from outside as well as being hired off-farm to work as daily laborers. The available data indicate that about 44% of the women in farming households work in agriculture as paid laborers, and most of the remainder contribute unpaid labor to the family farm (IAASTD, 2009; Ransom & Bain, 2011; World Bank, FAO, IFAD, 2009).

While women's roles in food production and provision have increased, the control of the farm has generally been assigned to a man in the family who stayed back on the farm (Abdelali-Martini et al., 2003). At the same time, rural women in Syria have limited access to and control of productive resources essential for farming (e.g., land, water, and seed) because property is mostly in men's names and inputs are provided by the centralized public system to title holders only (UNDP, 2006). Moreover, because marketing is predominantly a male activity, women also have limited access to sources of seed varieties and information, and control over the revenues generated through the sale of the agricultural produce (UNDP, 2006). IAASTD (2009) argues that feminization of agriculture can represent a further marginalization of small-scale farms because rural women have mostly limited education and restricted access to resources and opportunities.

The high variability of agroecological and socioeconomic conditions in farming systems in Syria, and the changing composition of household farm labor, would entail breeding programs to adopt strategies that successfully target this diversity and address the needs of all those who are involved in farming. However, the Syrian national system for agriculture is centralized and the research agenda and the breeding priorities are usually determined by breeders in research institutes without the involvement or consultation of farmers to assess their real needs. The agroeconomic environments where crops are grown for improvement do not reflect the circumstances of farmers from the most dry and marginal areas and many of the products of formal research are not appropriate to their farming conditions (Ceccarelli & Grando, 2007). Sociocultural factors that affect farmers' preference and resources are not taken into account. Moreover, despite the different access to resources, roles in the food chain, and decision-making processes, women and men have in Syrian farming, crop improvement lacks a gender component and is targeted to male farmers only, thereby overlooking the needs of women farmers. In the case of wheat and barley (two of the most important crops), for example, variety improvement is usually focused on yield increase only.

Other relevant traits that might be relevant to women's income-generating activities (e.g., stem quality for handicraft) to their manual work (e.g., spike height for manual harvesting), and to house nutrition (e.g., food-processing qualities) might be overlooked, making the variety less relevant for women's needs and activities (Galiè, 2012).

PPB combines the knowledge of farmers and researchers to produce varieties that reflect the range of concerns farmers take into account when choosing their preferred variety and the resources they have access to (Almekinders & Hardon, 2006; Aw-Hassan, Martini, Galiè, & Rischkowsky, 2010). This makes PPB effective in responding to multiple farmers' needs at ground level also in marginal areas characterized by a high variability of agroecological and sociocultural opportunity. It also makes PPB well suited to address gender-based preferences in variety development. Evidence shows that PPB has positive effects on the empowerment of farmers (Ceccarelli & Grando, 2007; Paris et al., 2008). However, the impact of PPB on women farmers and gender relations has been little analyzed (Farnworth & Jiggins, 2003; Paris et al., 2008). The processes by which PPB can enhance women's empowerment have also received limited attention.

A barley PPB program was started at the International Centre for Agricultural Research in the Dry Areas (ICARDA) in 1996 in collaboration with the General Commission for Scientific and Agricultural Research (GCSAR)—the Syrian national research institution for breeding—and with the extension offices located in the larger villages. However, from its inception, the PPB program adopted a gender-neutral approach, that is, it was open, in principle, to the participation of both women and men but it did not address their distinct needs and preferences. After 10 years of PPB activities, it was found that only male farmers were involved in the program. In 2006 a women pro-active approach was started in order to achieve gender-balanced PPB. This meant that the PPB program actively encouraged the participation of women in growing barley trials in their or their family's fields; in selecting and scoring the lines they preferred based on their needs and preferences; and in participating in the meetings of PPB male and female farmers to decide what lines to select for growing in the following year, and how to name the varieties selected after 4 years of trials. The women were also involved in other PPB activities such as international conferences and farmers' exchange visits.

This women pro-active effort provides the basis of the study reported in this chapter that set to assess the process by which participation in the PPB might affect the empowerment of the newly involved women farmers. The study addressed the research question: "How can the PPB in Syria affect the empowerment of the women farmers participating in the program?" (Galiè, 2013). This chapter discusses the further question: "How can an evaluation of women's empowerment as affected by PPB enhance the programs' gender-equitable approach?"

Assessing changes in empowerment as affected by development programs addresses the concerns expressed by feminists that most gender frameworks document gender inequalities without challenging them (Bamberger & Podems, 2002). Numerous programs implicitly accept the gender status quo and address women's practical needs without challenging underlying gender inequalities such as the access to and control of resources (Bamberger & Podems, 2002). In some cases an assumption is made that documenting gender inequalities is sufficient for programs to adapt and address gender concerns. Feminist evaluation, on the contrary, aims to analyze the impact of programs on gender structures and inequities, to provide a voice for women and the most vulnerable groups who are often not heard in the development process, and to integrate these new perspectives in development programs with the aim of increasing the equity of development outcomes (Bamberger & Podems, 2002).

This chapter builds on the assessment of how participation in PPB was felt by the women themselves to impact on their empowerment (Galiè, 2013). It discusses the role of this assessment in providing information that can be helpful to improve strategies that enhance the empowerment of women farmers in PPB. The study is especially important because it shows how feminist evaluation of empowerment can enhance the effectiveness and equity of PPB for small-scale farmers in a region where there is relatively limited research on women in agriculture.

Conceptual Framework

Feminist evaluation focuses on gender inequities and social justice (Sielbeck-Bowen, Brisolara, Seigart, Tischler, & Whitmore, 2002). Social justice captures the aspiration to create a just society or institutions and to remove clearly identifiable injustices (Sen, 2010). *Social justice* is defined as "fairness and equity as right for all in the outcomes of development, through processes of social transformation" (Reeves & Baden, 2000, p. 31). Gender equality is intrinsic to social justice because it argues for the right of both women and men to equally enjoy the outcomes of development based on their diverse needs and aspirations. To achieve equality of development outcomes women and men might need different means and treatment because they might have distinct needs, preferences, and also entitlement to resources and opportunities (Reeves & Baden, 2000). The right of women to access equal development opportunities is stated by the UN Convention on the Elimination of All Forms of Discrimination Against Women (CEDAW) that establishes the right of rural women to participate in the elaboration and implementation of development planning at all levels; to access appropriate technologies, information, and rural services; and to obtain formal and informal training to enhance their technical proficiency (retrieved from *www.un.org/womenwatch/daw/cedaw/text/econvention.htm#article14*).

Feminist evaluation argues that gender inequalities exist at all levels of society, are systemic and structural, and embedded and reinforced by societal norms and institutions. Kabeer (2010) discusses how development interventions reflect the worldviews of those who design them and are therefore often based on the same structures of unequal power distribution that characterize our world. As a result, development interventions do not always promote greater social justice and have rarely promoted gender justice (Kabeer, 2010). On the contrary, gender-blind development has often resulted in the marginalization of women, particularly poor women, and aggravated existing inequalities rather than supplying opportunities to promote social and gender justice (Kabeer, 2010; Srinivasan & Mehta, 2003). To progress toward social justice, feminist evaluation aims to make explicit the existence of gender inequities in development and examine opportunities to reverse them (Sielbeck-Bowen et al., 2002).

Empowerment is crucial for social justice because the realization of life choices relates to the ability to make strategic decisions and to act to implement them. Empowerment through participatory technology is an important step away from "technology transfer" in agriculture (Bartlett, 2005; Gonsalves, Becker, Braun, Campilan, & De, 2005). Empowerment can be defined as "a process to acquire the ability to make strategic life choices" (Kabeer, 1999). In Sen's (1990) words, empowerment is "replacing the domination of circumstances and chance by the domination of individuals over chance and circumstances" (p. 44). Kabeer thinks of empowerment mainly in terms of "challenging power relations" (Kabeer, 2003). Chambers (1993) defines empowerment as "to take more control over their lives and secure a better livelihood with ownership and control of productive assets as key elements." Fernea (2003) locates discourses of empowerment in the Middle East where, she argues, "family feminism" is more appropriate than "Western feminism" because the former values equally women's productive and reproductive roles in the family while the latter underplays the importance of women's reproductive role.

Most scholars see agency as a key factor of empowerment and self-determination. *Agency* is the ability to define goals and act upon them to achieve chosen outcomes (Kabeer, 1999, p. 435; see also Bartlett, 2005). Kabeer (1999) argues that to choose what life to live alternatives need to be both conceivable and materially possible. On the contrary, constraints to the capacity of exercising agency include the lack of alternative choices and the lack of opportunities to materialize these choices. Referring to Bourdieu's (1977) idea of *doxa*—"the aspects of tradition and culture which are so taken for granted that they have become naturalized . . . and exist beyond discourse and argumentation" (Kabeer, 1999, p. 441)—Kabeer states that the availability of choice depends on the availability of "competing ways of being and doing." Therefore, to exercise choice, a critical consciousness is needed that questions the social order and conceives alternatives.

The study this chapter describes adopted the concept of empowerment formulated as "a process by which an individual acquires the capacity for self-determination, that is, of living the life that she or he has reason to value" (adapted from Sen, 1990; Kabeer, 2010). The study operationalized the concept of empowerment by defining indicators with the respondent women farmers in order to reflect women's pragmatic realities and concerns. Thereby the study identified four indicators of empowerment: "recognition," "access to resources," "access to opportunities," and "decision making." These indicators relate to three basic principles of self-determination identified by Santarius and Sachs (2007): "recognition," "distribution of resources," and "access to opportunities." "Recognition" is understood as both the self-awareness and public acknowledgment of the roles and identities individuals chose to take in society. "Distribution of resources" is a material expression of recognition and refers to the right of individuals to access and control resources that are necessary for survival. "Opportunities" are necessary for individuals to make use of the resources they access, to live their chosen identity, and ultimately to actualize their right to self-determination. Decision making was adopted as a fourth cross-cutting indicator because it is considered key in the definition of empowerment and self-determination, as indicated by the respondents (Galiè, 2013).

The Research Area

In Syria food security has been a national priority since the 1980s. Small-scale agriculture is the main engine of the Syrian economy and a major support for rural livelihoods, particularly in marginal dry areas. Half of the rural labor force is employed in agriculture and 70% of land-holders own less than 3 hectares (IFAD, 2009: *www.ifad.org/operations/projects/regions/pn/factsheets/sy.pdf*). The agricultural sector is highly centralized based on a national plan where the government establishes the hectares to be cultivated under each of the so-called strategic crops (wheat, barley, cotton, sugar, beets, tobacco, lentils, and chickpeas), sets the price of seed, and also the quantity of irrigated and rain-fed areas based on national priorities and the availability of natural resources. The

FEMINIST RESEARCH IN PRACTICE

government is involved in both providing the seed for the strategic crops and marketing them. The new National Framework for Regional Planning (2011–2015) places great emphasis on agriculture, in the light of climate change, declining water reserves, and land degradation. Despite progress in achieving national self-sufficiency in some of the strategic crops, the rural sector has been affected by a series of setbacks (e.g., drought, depletion of water resources, salinization, soil erosion, and fast population growth) that, over the last decades, have undermined the livelihoods of rural households. In 2010 between two to three million people were living in extreme poverty, of whom the majority were small farmers (De Schutter, 2010).

Agricultural planners have identified five agroecological zones in Syria based on annual precipitation:

- Zone 1 has an average annual rainfall over 350 mm.
- Zone 2 has an average rainfall between 250 and 350 mm.
- Zone 3 has annual precipitation between 250 and 200 mm.
- Zone 4 has annual rainfall between 200 and 150 mm.
- Zone 5 has annual rainfall below 150 mm.

At the start of this study in 2006, the PPB barley program was operating in 24 villages spread across seven provinces that stretch across zones 2, 3, and 4, that is, including the marginal areas affected by recurrent drought and resulting crop losses. In each village, between eight and 10 male farmers were involved in the PPB work consistently across the 4 years of the selection procedures undertaken by farmers. These villages formed the "population" from which the respondents in this study were recruited.

Methodology

This research is a small-N study (George & Bennett, 2005; Mahoney & Goertz, 2006), as appropriate to situations where few or no previous studies have been conducted and little information exists. Flyvbjerg (2006) argues that the largest amount of information about a given problem is rarely provided by a random sample but more likely obtained through the strategic selection of cases and their in-depth analysis and description. By developing "a lot of information about a few" the groundwork is laid for follow-up studies from which generalizations could be made. As a small-N study, the respondent women were interviewed every week for 4 or up to 6 months a year over 4 years (2006–2010). This intensive interaction over a long period produced richly textured information that may be extrapolated and interpolated, with caution, to other situations understood to be broadly similar.

The research was conducted based on participatory exercises (e.g., resource mapping and activity calendars) (Chambers, 1992), participant observation (Geertz, 1984), and semistructured interviews (Food and Agriculture Organization of the United Nations [FAO], 1990) with single-sex groups in three Syrian rural villages over 4 years (2006–2010). The methodology adopted in this research is in line with the feminist guidelines for conducting evaluation research presented by Bamberger and Podems (2002). The researcher engaged in a long-term, participatory, and emotional relationship with the respondents that were treated as equals; ethical concerns for the implication of the research were a high priority. The research was continuously reflexive and consciousness raising. The information discussed and the knowledge produced were beneficial for the respondent women as stated by them. Perceptions and feelings were an acknowledged integral part of the research. Finally, the evaluation moved beyond gender disaggregation and addressed critical gender issues (see below).

Respondent Selection

The respondent women were drawn from three villages that were purposively selected to represent points along a continuum of participation in the PPB program (Table 11.1). The villages of Ajaz and Souran are located in agroecological zone 2. Here, relatively favorable temperatures and rainfall, irrigation facilities, and good market access favor intensive land use and make agriculture a main source of income, complemented by nonfarm and off-farm activities. Conditions for smallholder barley growing are relatively favorable (two barley seasons every 3 years (FAO & National Agricultural Policy Centre [NAPC], 2006). In the village of Lahetha the harsh ecologic environment and the lack of water for irrigation make agriculture highly susceptible to abiotic stress. Livelihoods mainly rely on nonfarm income and casual employment. Barley cultivation is marginally possible but provides a second source of income only in years of higher rainfall (FAO & NAPC, 2006).

Twelve main women respondents from 10 small-scale farm households were selected based on their interest in the PPB program, their involvement in agriculture, or their interest in the research itself (see Table 11.1 for an overview of respondents). The women in these households participated in an intensive interaction with the researcher throughout the 4 years of the research in both repeat written exercises and oral discussions. Five respondents from four households were drawn from

TABLE 11.1. An Overview of PPB Project Respondents

Ajaz (nonparticipating in PPB)

- **Location:** North-west, Idleb province
- **Agroecological zone:** 2
- **Rainfall:** 320 mm
- **Population:** 550
- **Main religion:** Sunni Islam
- **Main crops:** barley, wheat
- **Female respondents:** five respondents from four households: four women (written exercises and oral discussions); one woman (oral discussion); two to five "additional" women (oral discussions) from same or different households
- **Male respondents:** 12 men (oral discussions) of whom nine were related to the main respondent women

Souran (involved in PPB since 1996)

- **Location:** North-west, Hama province
- **Agroecological zone:** 2
- **Rainfall:** 300 mm
- **Population:** 32,000
- **Main religion:** Sunni Islam
- **Main crops:** barley, wheat, chickpeas
- **Female respondents:** two respondents from one household: one woman (written exercises and oral discussions); one woman (oral discussion); two to five "additional" women (oral discussions) from same of different households
- **Male respondents:** five men (oral discussions) of whom one was related to the main respondent women, four PPB participants

Lahetha (involved in PPB since 2003)

- **Location:** South-west, Sweida province
- **Agroecological zone:** 4
- **Rainfall:** 174 mm
- **Population:** 3,500
- **Main religion:** Druse
- **Main crops:** barley
- **Female respondents:** five respondents from five households: five women (written exercises & oral discussions); two to five "additional" women (oral discussions) from same or different households
- **Male respondents:** seven men (oral discussions) of whom three were related to main respondent women, four PPB participants

the village of Ajaz. Ajaz was chosen as a village nonparticipating in PPB activities, but within the spectrum of PPB activities, because male farmers had expressed an interest in PPB but for logistical reasons collaboration had not started. In the case of Souran, the men from 10 households were long-term participants in PPB. Two women respondents were drawn from one of these households. Five women respondents from five households were drawn from the village of Lahetha. In Lahetha eight men from eight households had been PPB participants over the medium term. Two women belonged to two households that were already participating in PPB. Three women were drawn from households new to the PPB.

The choice of involving women from households from two villages characterized by different agroecological zones, religion, and length of involvement in the PPB activities, as in the case of Souran and Lahetha, was thought to increase the contextualized understanding of the observed changes and their attribution to the PPB program. Similar changes taking place in most different cases increase the attribution of the change to one common cause (George & Bennett, 2005). The similarities between Ajaz and Souran were thought to increase the attribution to the PPB program of changes that took place in Souran only given that Ajaz was not involved in the PPB program.

Complementary Research Activity

A diagnostic study (Galiè, 2007) was conducted in 2006 to assess the reasons for the nonparticipation of women in the PPB program until then and their interest in the program. This study provided useful insights that informed much of the research that followed.

Action research (Almekinders, Beukema, & Tromp, 2009) took place alongside and in addition to the studies reported in this thesis. In fact, the researcher in collaboration with the PPB team and the interested farm women developed ways in which to involve them in PPB activities. Information drawn from the action research activity contributed to shape the research reported in this chapter.

Participant observation during PPB activities (Geertz, 1984) took place over four cropping seasons. These activities included yearly meetings to evaluate and select crops, an exchange between Jordanian and Syrian women farmers organized in 2006, and the International Farmers' Conference organized at ICARDA by the PPB program in 2008 (Galiè et al., 2009). This conference, that brought together 50 farmers (14 women and 36 men) from nine countries in the region and 12 researchers (seven men and five women), focused on the potential value of farmers' knowledge for agricultural research and plant breeding in particular. An evaluation of the conference focused on the change in behavior of the participants and their networks, and was particularly critical to generate additional information on gender issues in agriculture and knowledge (Galiè et al., 2009).

A male MA student carried out seven semistructured interviews with 24 men in the same three villages in 2009 (Table 11.1) to explore men's opinion about the intrahousehold division of agronomic labor and their understanding of women's role as farmers.

Data Collection

The research started in 2006 with a diagnostic study to understand the reasons why women farmers in villages participating in the PPB program had not become involved (Galiè, 2007). The understanding provided by the diagnostic study informed the research question explored between 2007 and 2010. Three stages of fieldwork were organized in these 4 years: 2007–2008, 2009, and 2010. Stage 1 was a baseline study carried out in all three villages. Stages 2 and 3 consisted of repeat interviews to assess changes in selected indicators of empowerment over the 2 years.

Four indicators of changes in empowerment were selected with the respondents on the basis of both their difficulties in joining the PPB program up until 2006, and of the question "What would allow you to make of your life what you wish it to be like?" The women identified the following indicators: (1) recognition of women as farmers; (2) access to productive resources—seed in particular—and information; (3) access to opportunities; and (4) decision making. Changes in these indicators were explored with the respondent women through a number of exercises conducted over 3 years during women-only meetings with the help of a female translator. The "recognition of women as farmers" indicator was studied through family structures and activity (Guijt & Shah, 2006) and semistructured group interviews (FAO, 1990). Changes in the "access to productive resources" indicator were studied through resource maps (Guijt & Shah, 2006) and the sustainable livelihood framework (Mancini, Van Bruggen, & Jiggins, 2007). As part of the sustainable livelihood framework the women were asked to score and discuss their perception of how much of each capital (social, human, natural, physical, and financial) they possessed.

Matrix analysis (Miles & Huberman, 1994) was used to assess the women's perceptions of changes in the intrahousehold decision-making indicator. The women's daily activities were matched with their perception of the power dynamics affecting them. The final indicator, "access to opportunities," was studied by means of rich pictures (Attenborough, 2006) where the women represented their wishes for an "ideal future" and their assessment of a "likely-to-happen future," and discussed their opportunities to reach their desired life path. Semistructured interviews complemented each of these exercises in providing more complete and in-depth information.

Data Analysis

All fieldwork interviews were written up, transcribed in digital format, and verified by one female assistant and by the respondents. Visual material including pictures and video interviews complemented the written material. The findings were analyzed descriptively (Patton, 1980) and quantitatively. The software package Atlas.ti (Development GmbH 1993–2009) was also used to organize, code, aggregate, and disaggregate both the written and visual material, and to triangulate findings elicited through the various methods.

Main Findings

Recognition of Women as Farmers

The findings show that the self- and public recognition of the respondent women as farmers entailed a complex interplay of fluid identities, defined in relation to other family members and affected by societal norms of what women's roles are supposed to be (Galiè, 2013). They also show that PPB affected both the self- and public recognition of women as farmers involved in the program. In 2007–2008 the study found that in the three villages, despite their substantial role in farming, the respondent women and particularly the younger ones considered themselves and were considered by women and men alike as "helpers," while the men were called "farmers." Married women were generally considered "housewives," while only women beyond 60 years and female heads of households who worked on farming full time declared they were "farmers."

The PPB affected these perceptions in Souran and Lahetha. Between 2007 and 2010 the number of women defining themselves as "farmers" in Lahetha and Souran increased. However, in written exercises also the number of men defined as "farmers" increased—even when the men were not involved in farming. The women from Lahetha argued that their participation in the PPB program and its public activities (such as the International Farmers' Conference) had increased their visibility as farmers in the village. The different views on women's role in farming became the topic of a lively discussion that took place during a PPB meeting among male farmers, extension agents, and ICARDA facilitators in 2009. The evaluation of the International Farmers' Conference revealed that some female and male family members were positively impressed by the number of women invited to the event that, they asserted, had increased their awareness of the key role of women in Syrian farming.

In Ajaz, the perceptions of women as farmers did not change across the 4 years. Two women mentioned that the lack of recognition of their agricultural work by their menfolk implied a heavy workload—because they were expected to perform all household duties regardless of their farm work. One young unmarried woman who managed the family farm faced the hostility of the village (i.e., mocking and exclusion from marriage arrangements) because she performed activities usually assigned to men, that is, driving the tractor and dealing with a retailer. Two other women mentioned that in some households in the village the work of women in the family fields was acknowledged by their menfolk who, in return for this work, assigned to the women a piece of land they could manage and profit from.

The women agreed that the identity "farmer" was appropriate for men only, as not in line with the roles of mothers and housewives women are expected to take. This affected, they maintained, their ability to declare "publicly" their role in agriculture (Galiè, Jiggins, & Struik, 2012).

Access to Resources

The baseline study in 2007 revealed that none of the respondent women, nor their womenfolk neighbors, owned any property, and that all property was in the men's name. This situation had not changed in 2010. The sustainable livelihood framework (SLF) revealed that in all three villages across the 4 years agriculture was considered by the women as the most important source of livelihoods for their households. Unmarried women considered off-farm agriculture as the only source of cash income they had access to and control over.

Natural capital for the respondent women in PPB villages included environmental factors (e.g., soil, water) and PPB seed. The women from Lahetha maintained that the PPB program had provided them with varieties that better fit their environment and needs. However, during semi-structured interviews in 2009 and 2010 the women complained about having received from the extension office quantities of PPB seed smaller than those received by the male farmers. They also complained about their fields being repeatedly discarded as PPB trial hosts for no apparent valid reason. In Souran the scoring of natural capital was high in 2008 because of the PPB seed that was considered "not just OK, but very good."

The PPB was shown to affect the social capital positively in the Souran household, by providing good seed that helped the household build a reputation as a reliable seed provider. In 2009 a problem in the distribution of PPB seed among the village PPB farmers affected negatively their ability to sell the seed, with negative consequences, they maintained, on their reputation as seed providers and consequently on their social capital. PPB affected negatively the social capital of the young unmarried women from Souran after her unsupervised participation to a conference in Aleppo was criticized by the village. In Lahetha, participation in this conference by five older women—as in other PPB activities—was thought to influence their social capital positively, mainly by providing opportunities for collaboration with other farmers from the region and the village. In Ajaz changes in social capital took place only as a consequence of major public events, that is, a national increase in fuel prices and a drought that affected the exchange of goods with nomadic groups.

PPB was believed by the respondent women from Souran and Lahetha to affect their human capital positively by increasing their self-confidence in speaking in public and by providing access to valuable agricultural information and exposure to new and international surroundings (e.g., travel to Aleppo, ICARDA, Amman; meeting Jordanian farmers). However, in 2009 the scoring for human capital in Lahetha decreased as the women participated in two international events and were exposed to new people with different skills. Human capital stayed constant in Ajaz across the 3 years.

The influence of PPB and also of this research on human capital was also evident in a list of potential training needs mentioned by the women from Souran and Lahetha. This became increasingly longer and articulated in 2009 and 2010 and included, among others, "access to information," "knowledge of technological devices," "English courses," and "computer courses" (Galiè, 2013). The women from Ajaz only mentioned generic skills and "English language" probably as a result of intensive collaboration with the researcher. PPB was not mentioned to influence women's financial capital even though the sale of PPB seed was considered an essential revenue for the household in Souran. Physical capital varied in all villages for reasons external to the PPB program and related to the status of the infrastructure in the area.

Access to Opportunities

The rich pictures used to contrast women's aspiration for a "dream future" and expectations of a more achievable "realistic future" revealed the ideal image of a woman the respondents were trying to conform to, and also their feelings of having limited opportunities, particularly for education and for self-determination. Sometimes the respondents critically mentioned social norms adopted by the village and their family as constraints to alternative future options, while at other times they asserted that these social norms characterized the identity of their society and culture and were not to be subverted. PPB did not seem to affect women's expectations for the future.

Generally, the married women from Ajaz and Souran had wishes mainly for their children to get educated, get married, and have children. The younger women from Ajaz and Souran wished in both dream and realistic futures across the 4 years to marry a good man and become good mothers and wives. They thought their future depended on what their husbands would decide for them in terms of jobs, number of children, and the ability to travel. The women felt ashamed of formulating wishes for the dream future different from their expected future because, some argued, that might reveal ambitious attitudes on their part that are not appropriate to modest women. The young woman from Souran maintained that she preferred to refrain from dreaming of an ideal future to avoid disappointment at the actual life she was likely to live. She added that in the village they knew what life path they could expect and that if they had been exposed to new cultures and places they might have had different wishes.

The five women from Lahetha wished in both their dream and realistic futures to have a farm with irrigation water, to see their children conclude their studies, and to marry. The realistic rich picture in 2010 included more women as managers of commercial activities.

Decision Making

All the women respondents from the three villages over the 3 years declared that they had less decision making than their male counterparts about family management and farming. The married women from Ajaz mostly agreed that they had some decision-making power but that the last decision stayed with their menfolk. One young woman who was de facto managing the family farm thought in 2009 that she had the same decision-making power as her younger brother until he lived abroad; at his return she continued doing the same farm work but he was the main decision maker. She added, though, that her brother would not take decisions she would not agree about. The young woman from Souran felt that she had the least decision-making power in household management, which rested mostly with her mother and partly with her brothers. As a consequence of her exposure to ICARDA PPB varieties and information, however, in 2008 she decided what varieties to plant in the family field.

The married women from Lahetha declared they shared most decisions with their husbands. The widows felt they had almost all decision making. The widows felt that the information obtained through the PPB had made them able to make decisions about farm management more independently. The married women felt that the PPB had increased their ability to share decision making about agriculture with their husbands, who also valued their opinion more.

Analysis and Discussion

This chapter set out to address the question: "How can an evaluation of women's empowerment as affected by the PPB enhance the program's gender-equitable approach?" The findings of the evaluation showed that in Syria, like elsewhere, women's role as farmers was generally understated by women and men when talking publicly about the organization of their household. The findings also showed some of the practical implications of the nonrecognition at the household level as identified by the women of Ajaz. On these bases, the PPB started to assess pragmatically who was involved in agronomic management—rather than addressing the "farmers"—in order to decide whom to involve in the program. The findings illustrated that participation in the PPB program could increase the recognition of women's role as farmers both in terms of self-awareness and of public recognition particularly through public international events. They also revealed that the importance of the PPB in supporting the recognition of women as farmers might be mostly valuable when followed by a public questioning of traditional gender roles by asking questions such as: "Who can collaborate with the PPB program?," "Who works in agriculture?," and "Who has knowledge?"—as in the discussion that took place in Lahetha. According to Kabeer (1999), questioning the *doxa* is a first step to stimulate critical consciousness to conceive alternatives toward discursive and finally material alternatives in a path to self-determination.

The study revealed the difficulties of implementing gender-equal norms within the program. The sustainable livelihood framework demonstrated that the PPB can provide varieties that respond to women's needs; it can enhance women's access to resources, that is, seed and information, thereby supporting the second principle of self-determination identified by Santarius and Sachs (2007). However, the study also revealed some of the difficulties women faced in obtaining an equal share of the PPB benefits (as in the case of the gender-discriminating distribution of PPB seed in Lahetha, of the selection of field hosts, or the wrong seed delivered in Souran). This highlighted the need for the PPB to create explicit gender-equal distribution mechanisms and to monitor their actual implementation to avoid the customary gender-discriminating rules that were reproduced in the sharing of the benefits of the PPB program.

In terms of life opportunities the PPB did not affect expectations for the future. The respondent women saw their future roles mostly as mothers and wives and in some cases only as farmers and entrepreneurs. These findings raise the question whether family feminism is appropriate to the Middle East, as argued by Fernea (2003), because its "image of women" is more aligned with traditional gender roles. Can accessing new spaces and exploring new meanings of women and farmers entail new understandings of empowerment that question traditional models, as mentioned by the young woman in Souran? In this framework, and given the limited set of life opportunities mentioned by the respondents as available to them, the PPB could open up opportunities to experience new contexts and conceive different life paths. Also, the very exploration of desires and opportunities to realize them was found to stimulate alternative thinking and increase informed decisions (Annas, 2003), as indicated by changes in women's perceptions of their training needs.

Decision making about farm and household management was shown by the findings to be mostly in the hands of men. However, the findings revealed a diversity of situations shaped continuously by variables such as household composition, age, gender, status, experience, and gender-based perceptions of how decision making ought to be organized. The findings indicated that the PPB needed to include both women and men involved in farming along the food production-to-consumption chain; to participate in variety development to ensure that all decision makers were involved in variety selection; and that all had access to relevant varieties and related information. The involvement of all farm decision makers in setting breeding priorities has been argued for as a strategy to increase the likelihood that improved varieties reflect everybody's needs and are therefore more likely to be adopted by households (Ashby & Lilja, 2004).

Together with addressing these practical needs (i.e., enhancing access to good seed) the PPB was found to be able to address more strategic needs as advocated by feminist evaluation (Bamberger & Podems, 2002). By including all the "doers" in farming, the PPB was found to open up decision-making opportunities commensurate with women's roles in food provision, production, and food cultures even in cases when women had little decision making and wished to have more. This was considered important to provide all women and men with equal opportunities to benefit from crop improvement. Involving all doers in the farm was found particularly important to support women's empowerment rather than reinforcing already existing gender-based power structures by providing more opportunities to the men who already had an advantaged access in comparison to women. The case of the women in Souran shows that their sale of PPB barley seed had become an important source of revenues despite the fact the barley is usually considered a male crop. It also showed how the involvement of a young woman in PPB activities increased her decision making at the household level. However, the dependence of both the sale of seed and the young woman's social capital on the support of the village farmers warned the PPB program about the need to ensure that its women's pro-active strategies found support at both the village and household level.

The PPB was found to affect women's access to opportunities to participate in decision making about crop development and also in international and regional events. International and public events in particular were found to constitute opportunities that could affect strongly the empowerment of farm women by affecting their recognition as farmers, their human and social capital, and their decision making. These events became important in the agenda of the PPB program as additions to field and breeding activities. The sustainable livelihood framework, however, showed how the PPB activities could be experienced as empowering by some women and "disempowering" by others (as in the case of the changes in social capital perceptions after the Aleppo Conference). This suggested that to successfully support the empowerment of participating women, the PPB needed to target its activities to the diversity of women's experiences and needs and pay particular attention to supporting the participation of young women. Ex-ante and ex-post assessments undertaken with the women farmers on the occasion of major public events were suggested as important means for the PPB to preempt disempowering circumstances and better target future activities.

The Methodology

The choice of this study to adopt a definition of empowerment based on the principle of self-determination was shown appropriate to transcend specific models of life that might be context- or culturally specific: empowerment as a means for self-determination rests on and reifies individuals' choices. Furthermore, in the experience of this study, conceiving empowerment as self-determination allowed the concept of empowerment to become more easily graspable and life-relevant for women farmers in comparison to complex theoretical definitions that are exclusive to social theorists. Discussing with the respondent women "What would allow you to make of your life what you wish it to be like" allowed a shared exploration and understanding of women's life aims and a discussion on hindrances to achieve these aims. It also allowed the women farmers to identify the indicators of empowerment that best reflected their own worldviews.

This study chose to adopt impact indicators identified by the respondents for three main reasons. Because of the complex nature of the concept of empowerment and the specificity in time and space of gender issues, women's empowerment is best analyzed through a grounded approach that places women in their individual context (Cornwall & Anyidoho, 2010). Also, the critical change approach applied to evaluation (Patton, 2002) argues that evaluators are "change agents." They work to "critique social inequities, raise consciousness, and strive to change the balance of power in favour of those less powerful, if nothing else through increasing their capacity to represent their own interests effectively through evaluation" (Patton, 2002, p. 103). Therefore, local identified indicators of empowerment were thought by the researcher to increase the relevance of this evaluation for the women respondents. Moreover, feminist evaluation argues that "knowledge and values are culturally, socially and temporarily contingent" (Sielbeck-Bowen et al., 2002, p. 6) and that placing program stakeholders as the knowers at the center of the evaluation activity helps provide multiple explanations of reality (Sielbeck-Bowen et al., 2002). This is particularly relevant in an evaluation of changes in empowerment where the latter is defined mostly as changes in inner perceptions.

Assessing changes in women's perceptions distinguishes this research from quantitative approaches to crop improvement that are most common. Feminist evaluation argues that emotions, intuition, and relationships are legitimate sources of knowledge (Sielbeck-Bowen et al., 2002). Zueger (2005) argues that the "subjective reality" of people is their "functional reality" since what people perceive is what makes up their life. Bamberger and Podems (2002) argue that feminist concerns about understanding the life experiences and perspectives of individuals and groups, and about questions such as "whose voice is heard" and "who designed, conducted, interpreted and disseminated the study" could contribute to international development. Integrating these voices, life experiences, and perceptions in monitoring and evaluating the impact of agricultural research for development can contribute to progress in the path toward enhancing the empowerment of the women involved.

At this point in time when Syria, like other countries in the Middle East, is experiencing popular demand for changes in its governance systems, the importance of integrating gender considerations in agricultural research for development and plant-breeding activities in particular might receive new attention. Kandiyoti (1991) maintains that in case of "growing popular discontent . . . governments may make the tactical choice of relinquishing the control of women to their immediate communities and families, thereby depriving their female citizens of full legal protection" (p. 276). New spaces for institutional reform and new opportunities might open up for approaches such as the ICARDA gender-sensitive participatory breeding program to be adopted by national breeding institutes. This would constitute a step toward the enhancement of food security and toward socially and gender-equitable development.

Conclusions

This chapter demonstrates how the findings of an evaluation of empowerment of women contributed to enhancing the equitable approach of the PPB program in Syria. The findings showed that decision-making processes and control over resources in the households of the respondent women overall advantaged their menfolk. However, they also showed that the reality of women's disadvantage on the ground is multifaceted and results from complex interactions between household and community members and from individual circumstances and the ability to negotiate. Nonetheless, the public display of women's and men's roles in the household was simplified in accordance with stereotypical gender roles. The findings suggested that, by working on the basis of "public displays," the PPB run the risk of "institutionalizing" traditional gender roles and further obscuring alternative understandings and performances of "women" and "farmers" that might exist at ground level. Conversely, the study showed the space that the PPB could open for new understandings to be conceived.

By showing how the PPB could empower women, the study reported in this chapter demonstrated that the impact of interventions such as the PPB are far from being just "the provision of technical outputs," that is, improved seed. The PPB can affect the recognition of farmers, their access to seed, information, and opportunities, and decision making, thereby affecting the power dynamics within households and among individuals and their life circumstances. Therefore, gender-blind PPB in Syria was considered to entail not only reduced effectiveness of the breeding activity by excluding the needs and priorities of women farmers from seed development; it was argued to affect also their right to self-determination by supporting only the capabilities and life circumstances of men, thereby aggravating existing inequalities. A women pro-active approach was adopted by the PPB to enhance a gender-balanced involvement of Syrian farmers and support a more equal access to development opportunities offered by the PPB program.

By highlighting the potentialities of the PPB in empowering women, this study opens the ground for more holistic evaluations of breeding programs that include both technology effectiveness and equity of development concerns. At the same time, the research shows the different positionalities that the respondent women have within their households and communities that entail individual paths of empowerment. In so doing, the study warns against simplifications and blue print approaches to the "empowerment of women." The study also shows some of the pitfalls of approaches that do not take into account the complexities of women's life contexts. Thereby, it makes a case for feminist evaluation to show the impact of gender-blind agricultural technology programs on social change dynamics, and to suggest possible strategies to target its address-ees, thereby increasing the equity of development outcomes and contrib-uting to social and gender justice. Finally, the study also provides one methodology for such a feminist evaluation of empowerment. It argues that the utilization of self-selected indicators for the evaluation of empow-erment respects the specificity of time and space of gender issues and avoids imposing external values across cultural contexts, as advocated by feminist evaluators.

The current civil war in Syria and popular demand for more equi-table forms of governance—that can arguably be partly related to the lack of rural and agricultural development opportunity—reinforce the points made above. They show the appropriateness of both equitable development opportunity and technology-effectiveness considerations in programs of AR4D. In this context feminist evaluation is needed to raise awareness about the potential social inequity effects of development interventions, particularly those that in the name of the "neutrality of technology" do not question their social impact. This research showed also the reasons why—in a context where some social groups are overall disadvantaged, such as rural women in Syria—it might be appropriate for a development intervention such as the PPB to question its interaction with, rather than reinforce, the status quo. At the same time, feminist evalu-ation is needed to enhance local understandings of empowerment that can support individuals' right to self-determination. In fact, the effects of this very evaluation of empowerment on the perceptions by the respon-dent women of their needs and future desires indicate the potential role of feminist evaluation in increasing the capability of the respondents to make informed decisions and voice their needs.

REFERENCES

Abdelali-Martini, M., Goldey, P., Jones, G., & Bailey, E. (2003). Towards a femi-nization of agricultural labour in northwest Syria. *Journal of Peasant Studies, 30*(2), 71–94.

Almekinders, C. J. M., Beukema, L., & Tromp, C. (2009). *Research in action: Theo-ries and practices for innovation and social change* (Mansholt Publication Series, 6). Wageningen, The Netherlands: Wageningen Academic Publishers.

Almekinders, C. J. M., & Hardon, J. (Eds.). (2006). *Bringing farmers back into breed-ing: Experiences with participatory plant breeding and challenges for institution-alisation* (Agromisa Special, 5). Wageningen, The Netherlands: Agromisa Foundation.

Annas, J. (2003). Women and the quality of life: Two norms in one. In M. Nuss-baum & A. Sen (Eds.), *The quality of life* (pp. 279–296). Delhi: Oxford India.

Ashby, J. A., & Lilja, N. (2004). Participatory research: Does it work?: Evidence from participatory plant breeding. In *Proceedings of the 4th International Crop Science Congress*. Retrieved from *www.cropscience.org.au/icsc2004/pdf/1589_ashbyj.pdf*.

Attenborough, K. (2006). Soft systems in a hardening world: Evaluating urban regeneration. In W. Bob & I. Imam (Eds.), *Systems concepts in evaluation: An expert anthology* (pp. 75–88). Inverness, CA: EdgePress.

Aw-Hassan, A., Martini, M., Galiè, A., & Rischkowsky, B. (2010). *Perspectives on gender-responsive action research.* Paper presented at the workshop "Repositioning gender-responsive participatory research in times of change," Program on Participatory Research and Gender Analysis, CIAT, Colombia.

Bamberger, M., & Podems, D. R. (2002). Feminist evaluation in the international development context. In D. Seigart & S. Brisolara (Eds.), Feminist evaluation: Explorations and experiences. *New Directions for Evaluation, 2002*(96), 83–96.

Bartlett, A. (2005). *No more adoption rates!* Paper presented at the PRGA Impact Assessment Workshop, October 19–21, 2005, CIMMYT Headquarters, Mexico.

Bourdieu, P. (1977). *Outline of a theory of practice.* Cambridge, UK: Cambridge University Press.

Ceccarelli, S., & Grando, S. (2007). Decentralized-participatory plant breeding: An example of demand driven research. *Euphytica, 155*(3), 349–360.

Chambers, R. (1992). Rural appraisal: Rapid, relaxed and participatory. *IDS Discussion Paper, 311*(311), 1–68. Institute of Development Studies, Brighton. Retrieved from *http://community.eldis.org/txFileDownload/f.59b4ab37/n.Dp311.pdf*.

Chambers, R. (1993). Challenging the professions: Frontiers for rural development. Intermediate Technology Development Group. Retrieved from *www.amazon.com/exec/obidos/ASIN/1853392081/webservices-20?dev-t=DRJ66LDC6TEVA& camp=2025&link_code=xm2*.

Cornwall, A., & Anyidoho, N. A. (2010). Women's empowerment: Contentions and contestations. *Development, 53*(2), 144–149.

De Schutter, O. (2009). *Seed policies and the right to food: Enhancing agrobiodiversity and encouraging innovation. Assembly* (Vol. 42473).

De Schutter, O. (2010). *Mission to Syria from 29 August to 7 September 2010.*

Farnworth, C. R., & Jiggins, J. (2003). *Participatory plant breeding and gender analysis* (PPB Monograph, p. 116). Cali, Colombia: CGIAR Systemwide Program on Participatory Research and Gender Analysis (PRGA).

Fernea, E. W. (2003). Family feminism or individual feminism?: Different histories, different paths to gender equity. *Hawwa, 1*(2), 131–151.

Flyvbjerg, B. (2006). Five misunderstandings about case-study research. *Qualitative Inquiry, 12*(2), 219–245.

Food and Agriculture Organization of the United Nations (FAO). (1990). *The community's toolbox: The idea, methods and tools for participatory assessment, monitoring and evaluation in community forestry.* Bangkok, Thailand: Author.

Food and Agriculture Organization of the United Nations (FAO). (2011). *The state of food and agriculture: Women in agriculture: Closing the gender gap for development. Lancet* (Vol. 2). Rome: Author. Retrieved from *www.ncbi.nlm.nih.gov/pubmed/22408551.*

Food and Agriculture Organization of the United Nations (FAO) and National Agricultural Policy Centre (NAPC). (2006). Women's role in agriculture and gender related issues in Syria. Damascus, Syria. Retrieved from *www.napcsyr.org/dwnld-files/working_papers/en/18_womenrole_ss_en.pdf.*

Galiè, A. (2007). *Diagnostic study.* Unpublished.

Galiè, A. (2012). Equal access for women to seeds and food security in Syria. In S. Turrall (Ed.), Innovative approaches to gender and food security. *Insights, 2012*(82).

Galiè, A. (2013). Empowering women farmers: The case of participatory plant breeding in ten Syrian households. *Frontiers: A Journal of Women's Studies, 36*(1), 58–92.

Galiè, A., Hack, B., Manning-Thomas, N., Pape-Christiansen, A., Grando, S., & Ceccarelli, S. (2009). Evaluating knowledge sharing in research: The International Farmers' Conference organized at ICARDA. *Knowledge Management for Development Journal, 5*(2), 108–126.

Galiè, A., Jiggins, J., & Struik, P. (2012). Women's identity as farmers: A case study from ten households in Syria. *Journal of Life Sciences, 64–65*, 25–33.

Geertz, C. (1984). From the native's point of view: On the nature of anthropological understanding. In R. A. Shweder & R. LeVine (Eds.), *Culture theory: Essays on mind, self, and emotion* (pp. 123–136). New York: Cambridge University Press.

George, A., & Bennett, A. (2005). *Case studies and theory development in the social sciences.* London: MIT Press.

Gonsalves, J., Becker, T., Braun, A., Campilan, D., de Chavez, H., Fajber, E., et al. (2005). *Participatory research and development for sustainable agriculture and natural resource management: A sourcebook.* International Development Research Centre, International Potato Center (CIP)-Users Perspectives with Agricultural Research and Development (UPWARD), Laguna, Philippines, and International Development Research Centre, Ottawa, Canada.

Guijt, I., & Shah, M. K. (Eds.). (2006). The myth of community: Gender issues in participatory development. Warwickshire, UK: Intermediate Technology Publications.

International Assessment of Agricultural Knowledge, Science, and Technology for Development. (2009). *Agriculture at a crossroads.* Washington, DC: Island Press. Retrieved from *www.agassessment.org.*

Jiggins, J. (2011). *Science review SR: 48, Gender in the food system* (Foresight Project). London: Government Office for Science.

Kabeer, N. (1999). Resources, agency, achievements: Reflections on the measurement of women's empowerment. *Development and Change, 30*, 435–464.

Kabeer, N. (2003). *Gender mainstreaming in poverty eradication and the MDGs.* Retrieved from *www.idrc.ca/en/ev-28774-201-1-DO_TOPIC.html.*

Kabeer, N. (2010). Women's empowerment, development interventions and the management of information flows. *IDS Bulletin, 41*(6), 105–113.

Kandiyoti, D. (Ed.). (1991). Women, Islam and the state. Basingstoke, UK: Macmillan.

Mahoney, J., & Goertz, G. (2006). A tale of two cultures: Contrasting quantitative and qualitative research. *Political Analysis*, *14*(3), 227–249.

Mancini, F., Van Bruggen, A. H. C., & Jiggins, J. L. S. (2007). Evaluating cotton integrated pest management (IPM) farmer field school outcomes using the sustainable livelihoods approach in India. *Experimental Agriculture*, *43*(01), 97.

Miles, M. B., & Huberman, A. M. (1994). *Logical analysis/matrix analysis: Qualitative data analysis* (2nd ed.). Newbury Park, CA: Sage.

Mosedale, S. (2005). Assessing women's empowerment: Towards a conceptual framework. *Journal of International Development*, *17*(2), 243–257.

Paris, T. R., Singh, A., Cueno, A. D., & Singh, V. N. (2008). Assessing the impact of participatory research in rice breeding on women farmers: A case study in eastern Uttar Pradesh, India. *Experimental Agriculture*, *44*(1), 97–112. Retrieved from *http://journals.cambridge.org/action/displayAbstract?fromPage=online&aid=1589868&fulltextType=RA&fileId=S0014479707005923.*

Patton, M. Q. (1980). *Qualitative evaluation methods*. London, UK: Sage.

Patton, M. Q. (2002). Feminist, yes, but is it evaluation? In D. Seigart & S. Brisolara (Eds.), Feminist evaluation: Explorations and experiences. *New Directions for Evaluation*, *2002*(96), 97–108.

Ransom, E., & Bain, C. (2011). Gendering agricultural aid: An analysis of whether international development assistance targets women and gender. *Gender and Society*, *25*, 48–74.

Reeves, H., & Baden, S. (2000). *Gender and development: Concepts and definitions*. Bridge Report, Brighton, UK: Institute of Development Studies.

Sachs, W., & Santarius, T. (Eds.). (2007). *Fair futures, limited resources and global justice*. London, UK: Zed Books.

Sen, A. (1990). Development as capability expansion. In K. Griffin & J. Knight (Eds.), *Human development and the international development strategy for the 1990s* (pp. 41–58). London, UK: Macmillan.

Sen, A. (2010). *The idea of justice*. London, UK: Penguin Books.

Sielbeck-Bowen, K. A., Brisolara, S., Seigart, D., Tischler, C., & Whitmore, E. (2002). Exploring feminist evaluation: The ground from which we rise. *New Directions for Evaluation*, *2002*(96), 3–8.

Song, Y., & Vernooy, R. (2010). Seeds of empowerment: Action research in the context of the feminization of agriculture in southwest China. *Gender Technology and Development*, *14*(1), 25–44.

Srinivasan, B., & Mehta, L. (2003). Assessing gender impacts. In H. A. Becker & F. Vanclay (Eds.), *The international handbook of social impact assessment: Conceptual and methodological advances* (pp. 161–178). Cheltenham, UK: Elgar.

Turrall, S. (Ed.). (2012). *Insights 82: Innovative approaches to gender and food security*. Institute of Development Studies, University of Sussex, Brighton, UK.

United Nations Development Programme (UNDP). (2006). *The importance of gender mainstreaming in Syria TOOLKIT*. Retrieved from *www.pogar.org/publications/other/undp/gender/syria-gender-toolkit-06e.pdf.*

World Bank (2008). *World development report: Agriculture for development.* Retrieved from   *http://siteresources.worldbank.org/INTWDR2008/Resources/WDR_00_ book.pdf.*

World Bank, Food and Agriculture Organization of the United Nations (FAO), & International Fund for Agricultural Development (IFAD). (2009). *Gender in agriculture sourcebook.* Washington, DC: World Bank Publications.

Zueger, R. C. (2005). *Participatory development projects in the Andes: Looking for empowerment with Q-methodology.* Paper presented at the PRGA Impact Assessment Workshop, October 19–21, 2005, International Maize and Wheat Improvement Center (CIMMYT) Headquarters, Mexico.

CHAPTER 12

Feminist Research Approaches to Studying Sub-Saharan Traditional Midwives

Elaine Dietsch

Introduction

There are many feminisms and contending models of feminist research (Olesen, 2008), but the primary goal of all feminisms has always been and will likely always be to correct the invisibility and distortion of female experience in ways that seek to transform women's unequal social status (Dietsch, 2003; Harding, 1987). The purpose of this chapter is to describe how one research project, "The Experience of Being a Traditional Midwife," reflects feminist research values and guidelines. The value of the traditional midwives' (TMs') ways of learning, knowing, and teaching was evident in the data they provided but could only be made visible if a feminist/critical approach rather than a descriptive approach was taken to the research process (Dietsch & Mulimbalimba-Masururu, 2011a).

A synopsis of the study is provided prior to discussion on how it was informed, influenced, and underpinned by feminist research ideology. Feminist values guiding the conceptualization, design, implementation, data collection, analysis, and dissemination of findings from the study are made explicit. The contribution feminist research values and guidelines made to the study are explored. The study is undeniably feminist in spirit, intent, and practical outworking, but was not labeled as such in its proposal, implementation, or dissemination; the reasons for this will be reflexively considered. To conclude, lessons learned from working within a feminist research framework are shared with the reader.

Study Synopsis

In late 2009 a research project to explore the experience of being a TM in Kenya was conducted. The aim of the project was to learn not only *about* but also *from* the TMs' experiences. The term "traditional midwife" was adopted for the study, rather than "traditional birth attendant," which is the nomenclature used in World Health Organization (WHO) reports and most global literature. The word "midwife" means to be "with woman" (Fraser & Cooper, 2009); in the 5 years prior to the research project, I had worked alongside TMs and had often observed their exemplary midwifery skills. The term "traditional midwife" was chosen to validate the participants as midwives and, importantly, to reflect the term used by women and participants themselves, *mkunga* (a Kiswahili word meaning "midwife").

The experience of being a TM is culturally complex but embedded in a system where only midwifery knowledge gained through an authoritative, formal, institutionalized setting is considered legitimate by those empowered to decree who is or is not allowed to define themselves as a midwife by accord of the International Confederation of Midwives (2011).

The project was labeled a service-based, qualitative study, and it soon became evident that it needed to be a study based on a critical framework. The principles of research founded on critical inquiry will be explained in greater depth in the section relating to data analysis. Service-based research, like feminist research, focuses on ethically sound, culturally safe research methods that place an emphasis on identifying and reducing power differentials between researchers and participants (Dietsch, 2006). Service-based research focuses on exploring issues that are important to the participants themselves and are likely to bring about positive and more equitable outcomes for them. In this instance, anticipated beneficiaries include not only the participating TMs but also the women and their newborns who access their services in the area in inland Kenya where the project was located.

The research setting is in rural Kenya, close to the Ugandan border; the people living here depend mainly on small, subsistence agricultural projects for their survival. Primarily Bukusu, communities speak their Bukusu mother tongue as a first language and Kiswahili as a second but universal language; English, when it is spoken, is the district's third language. Women are less likely than men to be conversant in English, as literacy and education levels are significantly lower for females than for males. There is no electricity or running water in most of the villages where the TMs reside and practice. Already considered one of the most socioeconomically disadvantaged areas of Kenya, the postelection violence of early 2008 further threatened the area when arson, looting, rape, and murder became widespread among the local population and the internal refugees en-route as they tried to flee to the relative safety of Uganda. In late 2008 the district's struggling economy was further decimated by serious drought, which still continues. Famine, fuel shortages, and political unrest in 2008 and 2009 were exacerbating the disadvantage experienced by TMs and the women they serve in the region (Dr. Luc Mulimbalimba-Masururu, personal communication, February 7, 2009; Wadhams, 2008).

The literature review conducted prior to the study concluded that current global policies favoring only skilled (professional) birth attendance evolved without rigorous evidence that maternal and newborn mortality rates would decrease if TMs were discouraged from supporting birthing women (Bullough et al., 2005; Costello, Azhand, & Barnett, 2006; Kruske & Barclay, 2004). Until 1987, the World Health Organization (WHO) and allied agencies still supported the training and resourcing of TMs (usually referred to as "traditional birth attendants" [TBAs] in the literature, but for the purposes of consistency, they will be referred to as TMs in this chapter) as a strategy to reduce the maternal mortality rate (Kruske & Barclay, 2004). However, in 1987 there was a shift in WHO, the United Nations Population Fund (UNFPA), the United Nations Children's Fund (UNICEF), the World Bank, the International Planned Parenthood Federation, and the Population Council policies. By 1997, the Safe Motherhood Technical Consultation decreed that TMs were not considered skilled because they lacked the capacity to manage obstetric complications (Safe Motherhood Interagency Group, 2002). Only professionally trained and licensed/registered doctors, nurses, and midwives could consider themselves as skilled birth attendants (SBAs) and should support a woman during labor and birth (WHO/UNFPA/UNICEF/World Bank, 1999). There were counterarguments from a number of researchers (e.g., Bullough et al., 2005; Darmstadt et al., 2009; Kruske & Barclay, 2004) that these new WHO/UNFPA/UNICEF/World Bank (1999) policies that impacted sub-Saharan African women more than any other groups of women, were based on lower-grade evidence that is historical, observational, and experiential rather than systematic. In effect, TMs were erroneously blamed for the Maternal and Newborn Mortality Rate (MNMR) (Kruske & Barclay, 2004) as contrary to expectations, policy changes have not resulted in the anticipated improvement in MNMR which is increasing in a number of sub-Saharan African nations and the impact of the HIV/AIDS epidemic is only partly responsible for this increase (Hogan et al., 2010; United Nations, 2009). While the focus remains on birthing women being supported only by SBAs in enabling, institutional environments, social factors such as poverty, gender inequity, war/regional conflict, unsafe and unavailable emergency care, inadequate transportation, malnutrition, and low levels of literacy are deemed unimportant (Dietsch, 2010; Harrison, 1997). Counter to emerging evidence, policies persist that effectively discourage governments from training and resourcing TMs (Kruske & Barclay, 2004) who are the preferred caregiver for the majority of birthing women in this area of inland Kenya (Dietsch & Mulimbalimba-Masururu, 2011b). The knowledge, expertise, and role of the TMs is being increasingly devalued by governments and global agencies at the same time as their services are being increasingly sought by women (Dietsch & Mulimbalimba-Masururu, 2010; Tritten, 2009). However, ignoring social factors impacting on maternal and newborn mortality rates and the power exerted over TMs need not remain unchallenged. This feminist research project continues to expose an invisible power differential and otherwise inaudible oppression.

Changes to global health policy ignored healthy women's preferences to birth in their own community with a trusted TM. These changes portray birthing with a SBA in an institution equipped to manage major obstetric complications as the single most important factor to prevent maternal deaths (WHO/UNFPA/UNICEF/World Bank, 1999). By definition, this diminishes the importance of the role that TMs play in supporting the majority of women in this region. Furthermore, even if it were possible for all women to access such a staffed and equipped facility (highly unlikely, given current resources and spending priorities), there is no guarantee of safety, and women continue to lose their lives at rates not comprehendible to Western readers (Dugger, 2011).

Concurrent with the implementation of Global Health Policy change (WHO/UNFPA/UNICEF/World Bank, 1999), maternal mortality increased between 2000 and 2008 in a number of southern sub-Saharan African countries including Mozambique, Namibia, South Africa, and Swaziland. The maternal mortality in 16 countries including the Central African Republic, the Democratic Republic of Congo, Gabon, Malawi, Mozambique, Zambia, Botswana, Lesotho, Namibia, South Africa, Swaziland, Zimbabwe, Chad, Côte d'Ivoire, Liberia, and Nigeria have increased from the 1980 rates (Hogan et al., 2010). Costello et al. (2006) and Hogan et al. (2010) argue that the HIV/AIDS epidemic is not entirely responsible for this increase in mortality.

In the interests of women and their newborns in resource-poor nations, it is imperative that the context in which women birth and social determinants that impact on their mortality and morbidity be urgently considered and addressed. These social determinants include but are not limited to poverty; gender inequity, including limited access to education and high labor expectations for females; violence against women; malnutrition and shortage of safe drinking water; and inadequate infrastructure including transport and communication deficits (Chandy, Steinholt, & Husum, 2007; Cox, 2009). Mathole, Lindmark, and Ahlberg (2005) argue that significant and sustainable reductions in maternal and mortality rates will only occur when these deficits are righted and TMs are not perceived as universally unskilled and dangerous but treated as colleagues and potential lifesavers, a viable option for healthy, childbearing women who choose to use their services.

Research Methods

Data for the project were collected from 84 participants (83 female and one male), self-identifying as TMs (*mkunga*) during interviews and from field notes taken during and immediately after interviews. Eighteen individual and 10 group interviews took place in homes, halls, and fields. In this context, interviewing participants together in a group was not a focus group with predefined aims but rather a pragmatic necessity as many more participants than expected walked for many miles to be interviewed. It would have been unethical to deny potential participants their right to be interviewed and heard. However, if the interviews had been conducted individually, they would have gone on until after dark and exposed participants, the researcher, and the interpreter to unnecessary dangers. Group interviews were also a very culturally acceptable way of interviewing.

Interviews were semistructured; these were audio-taped and their English components transcribed verbatim. As a researcher, my Bukusu language skills are nonexistent and my Kiswahili language competence is so rudimentary it can not be used for interviewing purposes. Participants were therefore interviewed with the assistance of one or more interpreters. Interpreters were at least trilingual, speaking Bukusu, Kiswahili, and English. All participants were at least bilingual in Bukusu and Kiswahili, the latter two languages being used interchangeably by interpreters and participants alike. The role of the interpreter as a key component of this project required careful consideration, including who would interpret and how the interpretations would occur. Interpreters inevitably assign meaning to words in both languages that may or may not be congruent with the researcher's intent (Pitchforth & van Teijlingen, 2005; Wong & Poon, 2010). It is possible for the feminist researcher to base all her or his work on a sound, philosophical platform only to realize that the interpreter did not share the same ideology. Following each interview, the interpreter(s) and I would review the interview and transcript to ensure inflections and attitudes that supported and affirmed participants were evident and the interview process was not being used to exert power over and intimidate participants. I noticed that the more time I spent with the interpreters, the more competent we all became in conversing and esteeming the participant's choice of language. For example, early in the research process I realized that the main interpreter was not always translating literally the participant responses, but was rather using the terminology that she had learnt from previous interviews (a simple example, "the mama was bleeding, bleeding, bleeding" was translated as "the woman hemorrhaged"), which the interpreter had erroneously deemed to be more professional or acceptable to me. Time spent forming a relationship between the interpreters and me, our sharing of values, philosophies, and ideologies prior to and while working together in data collection was time very well spent.

Data collection utilized semistructured interviews and only two predetermined questions:

1. "Please tell me about your role as a traditional midwife."
2. "How have birth kits impacted your practice?"

As part of the consent process, potential participants were advised that it was their story, their experience that was to be highly valued. Although prompts were available for the interviewer to use to encourage participants to share their experience of being a TM during interviews, in reality these prompts were never required. As cited above, interview questions only related to participant's experience of being a TM and participants were never asked to share their own birthing experiences. However, it became evident that the participants had a strong desire to share their own experiences of being a birthing woman as well as a TM. A very small number of participants shared that they had birthed alone, a few had birthed in an institution, but most had birthed with the assistance of a TM. Participants were not denied the opportunity to share their own birthing stories and their relationship to the person who had been their TM. Their experiences, whether as a TM or as a birthing woman, provided rich data about TM experiences, roles, and practices. Only one participating TM was male and so had not experienced childbirth himself. This man had assisted his wife (also a TM) to safely birth 10 healthy children. After the birth of his eighth child, he had been invited by his neighbors to be a TM for them. Although highly unusual to have a male TM, this man appeared to be well accepted by both the men and the women of his village. The other participants (probably reflecting the attitudes of the male TM's neighbors) equated his role with the SBAs at the nearby hospital, who were reportedly also more receptive to him than to the female TMs when on occasions he transferred a woman to the hospital in an emergency. Importantly, it would seem that the male gender of this TM afforded him with a prestige equivalent to the SBAs in the region, and greater than with his TM colleagues.

The scene will be set, so readers are better able to visualize the environment where the TMs support women to birth. Try to imagine . . . a woman in established labor walking, sometimes many kilometers, sometimes at night, sometimes during the day along rough tracks, to the TM's home. She is usually but not always accompanied by a female companion, often her mother, mother-in-law, or sister, but sometimes she walks alone. The walk may be in the wet season or it may be in the dry season. Relocating to the TM is considered a cultural necessity for the woman. A common belief is that if a man is aware his partner is in labor, it will make for a more prolonged and painful labor. However, there is an additional consideration: many men do not like their partner to birth inside "his" home and so, if the woman does not go to the TM's home, she may be forced to labor outside and alone. Less often the woman will go to a government or private hospital to birth, but the journey, the walk, will usually be even further in these instances. One participant explained:

> "At times the husbands, when they see their wives doing such a job, they don't like, so it becomes a problem . . . sometimes when the woman goes in to labor, the husband does not like her to stay in the home." (Participant, group interview 1)

The TM's home is like most others in the villages, a simple dwelling with only one or two rooms in total. Most, but not all TMs, have husbands and children who live with them. If it is a two-room dwelling, the family members will vacate into the second room in deference to the laboring woman who is seeking the support of the TM. Only babies and toddlers will remain with their mother, the TM. If it is a one-room home, then any family members will stay outside as long as the woman is laboring, often sleeping under trees, bushes, or a makeshift tarpaulin (if they are fortunate enough to have one). Sleeping outside is particularly problematic during the rainy season in this region where mosquito-borne malaria is endemic. Male partners and children of TMs were not interviewed for this research project, but from observation they appear to accept that the first priority for occupation of their home is afforded to the laboring woman and her TM. This may in part be due to the fact that the minimal income received by the TM is usually the family's only or main source of income. The TM's home is usually made of mud, with a thatched roof and compacted cow dung floors and almost always kept meticulously clean. Many TMs do not have a bed for themselves to sleep on or the woman to labor on and so the woman labors and births on the floor, sometimes lying, sometimes semisitting, but increasingly in more upright positions.

> "The black sheet, kneeling on that . . . that is how a woman would give birth, kneeling." (Participant, group interview 9)

Fees paid to the TM for her combined antenatal, intrapartum, and post-natal care vary enormously from 200 shillings ($4) to 500 shillings ($10). But all participants spoke of how common it was for women to pay them nothing, or offer payment in kind, such as a chicken.

It is difficult for the Western reader to imagine the extent of this materially impoverished environment. Likewise, it may be difficult for many to appreciate the kindness and patience these TMs (and by implication, the TM's family) show to laboring women, the connection they have with them, and the evidence-based midwifery care they often provide. Acts of kindness include but are not limited to providing nourishment and hydration for the laboring woman and washing her. The woman is washed not only after the birth but also on arrival at the TM's home after her long walk to get there.

> "So you wash her and you give her tea and you give her porridge, but that does not happen in the hospital." (Participant, group interview 9)

Regardless of the cultural context, maternal mobility in labor has multiple physiological advantages and improves maternal and newborn health outcomes (Baker, 2010; Lawrence, Lewis, Hofmeyer, Dowswell, & Styles, 2009). Kitzinger (2005) describes the benefits for women and their newborns when laboring women are enabled to follow what she describes as their own "birth dance." The TMs spoke of being a "mamma" to the laboring woman, encouraging her mobility through dancing with her.

> "[I am] a mamma to her . . . cannot force the mother to give birth . . . [we are] dancing." (Participant, group interview 2)

Data were thematically analyzed and exemplars in the participants' own translated words were identified for both analysis and presentation purposes. Data analysis was attended through a critical lens. In practical terms this meant:

- Identifying that the role and experience of the TMs are mediated by power relations in the society where they live. There are a number of mediating powers in this context including but not limited to global health authorities such as the WHO; professional bodies such as the International Confederation of Midwives (ICM); and SBAs, all of whom operate within a largely (but not absolutely) patriarchal, male-preferring, and male-dominant environment.

- Recognizing the role that privileged groups play in oppressing the subordinate TM.
- Disentangling the project's research findings from the ideology that perpetuates the "accepted wisdom" that birth with a SBA in an institution is necessarily and always safer for women and their newborns than birth with a TM.
- And very importantly, an ever-present awareness that I, as a well-educated, affluent, professional, Western researcher could unconsciously reproduce the class and racial oppression experienced by the TMs.

The impetus of this study was to provide participants with a vehicle to describe their experience of being a TM, that is, to make their role visible to others outside their realm of practice and to make their voice audible. The primary theme identified during data analysis was that being a TM meant being in relationship with women (Dietsch & Mulimbalimba-Masururu, 2011b). Related subthemes included that being a TM is about caring: being patient, kind, humble, and calm. Being a TM is about practicing intuitively: for example, following the woman's progress and not intervening in accord with prescribed time limits placed on a woman's labor and cervical dilation. Other themes included TMs' relationships with SBAs and working in an impoverished environment.

Founding the Study on Feminist Research Ideology

While not labeled as a feminist project, the research was informed and influenced by feminist research methodology and ideology. The project was conceptualized in response to my own personal experience and observations while working with TMs in Kenya and the Democratic Republic of Congo on a short-term, annual basis since 2004. What I saw and previously reported on (Dietsch, 2005; Dietsch & Mulimbalimba-Masururu, 2006) were TMs who provided safe, woman-centered care in an impoverished environment. In contrast, what was being promoted in much of the health literature and by conventional wisdom was the antithesis of this, where TMs (referred to as TBAs) were often portrayed as unskilled and incompetent (Armour, 2009; Fronczak, Arifeen, Moran, Caulfield, & Baqui, 2007; Goodburn & Campbell, 2001; Izugbara, Ezeh, & Fotso, 2009). By inference, TMs are erroneously seen as the cause of and the scapegoat for much of the unacceptably high maternal and newborn mortality rates in most third-world, resource-poor nations (Kruske & Barclay, 2004). This distortion required redress and I had confidence in the TMs themselves that their stories and their experience would be the vehicle best suited to correcting the distortion. A secondary consideration was to explore how resources were being used by the TMs and how those resources (birth kits funded through the Australian Government Aid Agency) might be improved. The research project entitled *The Experience of Being a Traditional Midwife in an Area of Inland Kenya and the Impact of AusAID Provided Resources (Birth Kits) on Their Practice* was proposed.

The project received CSU Institutional Ethics Committee (IEC) Approval. The feminist nature of the study was implicit but not explicit in both the CSU Competitive Grant and the IEC application documents that described the philosophical framework for this study actively seeking to acknowledge and respect TMs' local knowledge and experience. It is only in retrospect and in preparation of this chapter that I realize it did not occur to me to explicitly refer to the project as a feminist study from the outset. Both the grant and the IEC applications referred to a service-based research philosophy and discussed the importance of employing culturally appropriate research methods that place an emphasis on identifying and reducing power differentials between researchers and participants.

The service-based research ethics (Dietsch, 2006) employed were akin to feminist ethics espoused by Preissle (2007) in that they placed value on the experiences of participants, sought to replace ignorance with knowledge, and purposed to relieve participant oppression. The primary difference is that while feminist research ethics has a gender focus and seeks to reconfigure androcentric knowledge (Preissle, 2007), service-based research may seek to relieve participant oppression which may or may not have a gender focus. Both service-based research and feminist research ethics critique the politics of the research project itself as well as the oppression and marginalization of the participants within the health care arena and public health discourse. The challenge was to conduct this study in a way that did not exacerbate, reproduce, or create new power imbalances over the TMs participating.

Two interrelated ethical concepts governed the project from proposal, through data collection, analysis, and the dissemination of findings; these were the needs to engage in a continual process of reflection founded on the principles of cultural humility and to employ service-based research ethics including those based on a feminist ethos. *Cultural humility* is defined as a continual process of self-reflection and self-critique in order to redress power imbalances and to develop mutually beneficial and equitable partnerships with communities and individuals (Foster, 2009; Tervalon & Murray-Garcia, 1998). Service-based research values mirrored feminist research values and were employed for the purposes of ensuring a nonhierarchical relationship between participants and researcher (Liamputtong, 2007)—an attitude of cultural humility was seen as a strategy to help achieve this goal. The participants were acknowledged as being the experts in their own practice environment and culture and were identified as being far from the unskilled TM (referred to as a traditional birth attendant) stereotyped in the literature (see Bisika, 2008, as an example). Cultural humility was the conscious process adopted in this study to overcome any tendency toward researcher ethnocentrism or any notion of superiority that could have led to cultural incompetence and/or insensitivity. In practice, this meant taking time to self-reflect and critique my words and actions following each interview and at each stage of the data collection, analysis, and reporting process.

Data was collected in keeping with principles common to both service-based and feminist research. Feminist research values the trust and reciprocity kindled by long-term relationships, and I had developed close relationships with a significant number of participants during my annual faculty practice since 2004. However, the empathy built between many of the participants and me had the potential to be misappropriated by me for the sake of optimizing data collection. The positive nature of my relationship with participants was not unethical and our relationship could not and should not be denied. However, in the interests of both the project's and the participants' integrity and rights, the nature of the relationship needed to be made transparent. Significantly, before, during, and after each interview it was important to reflect on my motivation and whether our relationship was being used in a manipulative way to gather data that may not otherwise have been forthcoming.

It was during data analysis and reporting that the importance of looking at the data through a critical lens became most apparent; assumptions made in privileged, Western literature and discourse that were contrary to the findings of this project needed to be exposed. In practice, this meant choosing to expose gender inequities where they occurred; for example, none of the female participants owned or could even access a watch or a mobile phone to enhance communication in an emergency, but it was very common for their male partners to own both watches and mobile phones. Most of the participants in this study were illiterate and had never studied a textbook but their illiteracy did not negate their knowledge base. They had studied women and birth. Experience had taught them not only physiology, but the power of patience, kindness, and humility as a means of bringing about positive outcomes for birthing women and their newborns. The participants were confident in themselves and birthing women. Their confidence was not founded on knowledge from a medical perspective or an authoritative source but was rather an embodied knowledge in that it had emerged from practice, experience, and reflection. In both Western and Kenyan hospital settings, a woman's own subjective knowledge, and a midwife's knowledge of physiological birth gained through experience, are considered of less value than the use of birth technology and medical knowledge that are acknowledged as privileged and authoritative (Dietsch & Mulimbalimba-Masururu, 2011a; Gould, 2000; Jordan & Aikins Murphy, 2009). Participating TMs esteemed the uniform, certificate, name badge, birth technology, and the privileges of the SBA working in the hospital maternity unit, but not at the expense of their own self-worth nor of providing compassionate woman-centered midwifery care. The TMs considered it a privilege to wash the laboring woman who had often walked long distances to seek out her service, to provide the woman with porridge and tea, to dance with her, and to encourage her to adopt physiological birthing positions (Dietsch & Mulimbalimba-Masururu, 2011b).

The participants in this study valued both their own and the woman's knowledge and experience, which they perceived as being devalued by professional caregivers. The dominant ethos, power, and prestige afforded by technology legitimizing authoritative knowledge, certification, and uniform were not challenged. The fact that participating TMs maintained their confidence in women, birth, and themselves reflects their resilience as women in an androcentric culture, the support they provide each other, and the esteem they receive from women in their villages (Dietsch & Mulimbalimba-Masururu, 2011b).

This study was designed, implemented, and its findings continue to be disseminated with the aim of articulating for and with women explanations they have provided about phenomena affecting their lives. Findings are disseminated in global health forums, peer-reviewed professional literature, midwifery conferences, and to those involved in resource (birth kit) distribution. This research project has benefited both myself and the participants. As a midwifery research academic it has enabled me to write numerous articles in peer-reviewed journals, present findings at conferences, participate on global health forums, and write this chapter, all of which enhance my professional standing. Outcomes from the research that benefit the participants and the women they serve include but are not limited to the funding of village women and TMs to make up the birth kits and disseminate them in their own communities, the building of strategically placed birth huts, and provision of midwifery education seminars.

The Contribution of Feminist Research Values and Guidelines to the Study

Feminist research considers the woman's view as particular and privileged (Olesen, 2008) and the woman is seen as more than a source of data: she is first and foremost exquisitely a person (Dietsch, 2003; Rose, 1990). However, the fact that all but one of the participants in this study were female and that their voices were valued does not make this a feminist study. This study is feminist because it illuminates aspects of the TMs' experience that have previously been suppressed or ignored within the powerful, biomedical discourse that dominates the global health policy agenda; it exposes gender inequity and esteems the participants and their role in providing a highly valued and much-demanded health service by women in rural Kenyan villages.

It is too simplistic to say that the TMs are oppressed by a male system because they are female. Their most obvious oppressors are other females. Most SBAs are female, licensed nurses and midwives working within institutions and, on occasions, are reported to abuse and assault women and TMs when they seek emergency care (Bowser & Hill, 2010). Furthermore, reports of emotional and physical violence were frequently described by many of the participants,

> "The nurses in the hospital . . . they beating of you . . . the beat the women, beat!" (Participant, group interview 20, p. 2)

Although common in this area, abuse of women in hospitals is not unique to Kenya. Abuse of women by health professionals, the majority of whom are female, has been reported in countries as diverse as Australia (Dietsch, Shackleton, Davies, Alston, & McLeod, 2010a) and the Democratic Republic of Congo (Vanderlaan, 2009). As Bowser and Hill's (2010) report indicates, the behavior of some nurses and midwives can be misogynist and although this may be due, in part, to their oppression as a group (as described by Freire, 1972), misogynist acts need to be revealed so that strategies can be developed to reduce them (Bowser & Hill, 2010).

In this study, the TMs shared instances where the female hospital staff identified not with the women or the TMs but with the institution that bestowed power on them. There is a hegemonic hierarchical ordering of power that is in the interests of SBAs and institutional systems to maintain over the TMs. The professional midwives are labeled SBAs by global health agencies and have prestige due to their licensure, income, superior formal education, uniform, and recognition by the authorities, including the International Confederation of Midwives (2011) that is denied to the TMs.

For three decades innumerable feminist writings have argued that the biomedical sciences that underpin global health agency policy is value-laden, a-contextual, patriarchal, and androcentric (Broom, 1995; Raymond, 1982; Smith, 2008). The biomedical sciences, in contrast to the social sciences, continue to grow more powerful as a privileged discourse in global health agency policy (Kruske & Barclay, 2004). Global health agency policy agendas and the influences of the biomedical sciences remain invisible and largely unquestioned because they are considered ideological, functional, and pastoral as they purport to being beneficent and serving the needs of others and because there is no conscious or individual malicious intent. Though never the intent, the privileging of a biomedical over a social discourse and action is maleficent in outcome and may be costing women and newborns their lives (Arps, 2009; Chalo, Salihu, Nabukera, & Zirabamuzaale, 2005; Chandy et al., 2007; Cox, 2009; Dugger, 2011; Shen & Williamson, 1999; Stewart, 2006; Tuguminize, 2005; Weiser et al., 2007; Win, 2007). However, ignoring the social factors impacting on maternal and newborn well-being and the power exerted over TMs need not be a static phenomena. This research project, guided by feminist research values, continues to expose the domination and oppression for what it is.

Feminist Research: A Victim of Academic Fashion?

As stated, this project was undeniably feminist in purpose, content, and intent but was never labeled "feminist" but rather as a "critical study," informed by service-based research principles. The question as to why I did not label it a feminist study has caused me to be reflexive about my own place in the feminist research agenda and factors that influenced my decision.

I had previously not consciously considered that the trend for feminist research to be subsumed under research relating to gender and/or from a critical theoretical framework had impacted my own research practice. For the purposes of writing this chapter, I needed to determine if there was evidence to support my belief that fewer overtly feminist studies were being published or if this perceived trend was anecdotal and a priori. A simple search was undertaken on the Cumulative Index to Nursing and Allied Health Literature (CINAHL) database to compare articles with critical + research; gender + research; feminist + research as "MW? in subject heading." The trends in Table 12.1 indicate that there has been a steady and significant decrease in the proportion of feminist research articles published compared with gender research and critical research articles.

My perceptions were verified, but as a woman and academic self-identifying as a feminist these perceptions should not have influenced my research or my writing. In the context of this study and on reflection, the feminist label was never intentionally abandoned; it was, however, not consciously considered even though I was fully aware that the project would adhere to feminist ethics at all times.

I had given no thought as to what research label was likely to be more palatable to funding agencies. At the risk of sounding superficial, it would

TABLE 12.1. Trends in Critical, Gender, and Feminist Research Articles Published 1995–2010

Year	CINAHL critical research articles	CINAHL gender research articles	CINAHL feminist research articles	% of feminist research articles	% of gender research articles	% of critical research articles
1995	146	11	14	8.2%	6.4%	85.4%
2000	197	14	17	7.5%	6.1%	86.4%
2005	245	26	20	6.9%	8.9%	84.2%
2006	277	54	30	8.3%	15%	76.7%
2007	266	43	22	6.6%	13%	80.4%
2008	351	79	21	4.7%	17.5%	77.8%
2009	301	53	10	2.7%	14.6%	82.7%
2010	164	30	5	2.5%	15%	82.4%

seem that feminist research has fallen out of academic fashion and I had become an unquestioning victim of that fashion. It is not known and it is beyond the scope of this chapter to determine if research labeled as "feminist" receives equal funding and publication consideration as gender research or critical research theory. However, it would seem that feminist research, which always aims to expose the invisible, has become invisible itself under the umbrella of "gender" and critical research theory.

Lessons Shared

No simple formulaic advice can or should be offered to anyone considering conducting feminist, cross-cultural research in resource-constrained nations. This chapter has offered the reader some thoughts to consider before embarking on similar research. It was the depth of the relationship between myself as researcher and the participants, and the reciprocal respect we had for one another, that breathed life into the data collection, analysis, and dissemination processes. I believe that any critical research (including projects grounded on a feminist ethos), if conducted without relationship in the cross-cultural context, are at risk of becoming at best merely voyeuristic, and at worse exploitative. Feminist researchers enter the field and engage with participants for many reasons and these must be carefully self-critiqued prior to proposing any research where both the power and the resource differential between the researcher and the participant are so great. Altruistic intent is no safeguard against exacerbating power differentials and leaving participants feeling (rightly or wrongly) that they were used only to further the researcher's academic status or provide her or him with an exotic experience.

A practical consideration is financial. While not idealizing, deifying, or objectifying sub-African women, it is a fact that I have found that the generosity and hospitality of women in the sub-Saharan nations is beyond anything found in western communities. The African women have so little but desire to share whatever they have with visitors to their community. Culturally, generous sharing of time, hospitality, and possessions with visitors is esteemed. It is essential that any feminist research undertaken provides benefits to, but does not cost, participants and/or their community. While there are always costs to the participant in terms of time burden and the potential for emotional distress when some experiences are relived or retold, financial costs should not be a part of any research especially where there is existing participant economic deficits and distress. Lack of researcher preparation may leave women and communities having to use their own resources to support the research project or the researcher, which is inexcusable.

Lessons Learned

By way of conclusion, there are a number of lessons I have personally learned from working cross-culturally within a feminist research framework. First is the ease with which I identified culturally foreign practices as oppressive compared with no less oppressive practices embedded within my own culture. For example, I am very quick to critique the actions of the man who refuses to allow his partner to labor and birth in "his" home. His actions are abhorrent and obviously abusive as the woman believes she has no alternative but to walk in labor, often many kilometers, to a safe place to birth. However, it is much easier to justify, on the grounds of economic rationalism and risk assessment, my own government's policy of closing maternity units in rural areas and giving women no choice but to travel away from their homes and communities to birth (Dietsch et al., 2008). Women are evacuated from their family and support networks (Dietsch et al., 2011) and forced to drive many kilometers, often on very unsafe roads, to access maternity services (Dietsch, Shackleton, Davies, Alston, & McLeod, 2010b). I am led to question whether the African man's practice or the Australian government's policy is any more or less oppressive than the other!

Feminist research at its core seeks to expose oppression and power exerted over women. Power belongs to those who have the capacity to provide or withhold resources from another, thereby maintaining the power status quo (Dacher, Gruenfeld, & Anderson, 2003). In the context of global midwifery, the title "midwife" is a highly valued resource but it is formally withheld from anyone who has not satisfactorily completed a midwifery educational program (International Confederation of Midwives, 2011). In the research setting of Kenya, the health professionals in institutions refer to themselves as *daktari* (doctor) or *mwuguzi* (nurse), but never *mkunga* (midwife). The term *mkunga* is the domain of the TM in this area of Kenya (Dietsch & Mulimbalimba-Masururu, 2011a) but the *mkunga* is not accepted as a legitimate midwife by those with the power to define who or who may not be considered a midwife. In the health literature, health professionals supporting women during labor and birth no matter how or less experienced, competent or incompetent, are termed SBAs and the only legitimate birth attendants (Harvey et al., 2004; Kruske & Barclay, 2004). In contrast, no matter how skilled or knowledgeable, the person without the required admittance "to a midwifery educational program, duly recognised in the country in which it is located, has successfully completed the prescribed course of studies in midwifery and has acquired the requisite qualifications to be registered and/or legally licensed to practice midwifery" has no right to the title midwife (International Confederation of Midwives, 2011). The International Confederation of Midwives is the peak midwifery body to which I proudly belong. Its membership is overwhelmingly female and would adhere to feminist principles and philosophy but such is the occult nature of power to the powerful that the potential for oppression of women was not considered when the definition of midwifery was first adopted in 2005 and then amended very slightly in 2011 (International Confederation of Midwives, 2011). The 2005 congress was attended before this study was conducted but after I had had the privilege of working with TMs in 2004. I was aware of many of the TMs' skills and yet did not consider the need to advocate on their behalf. As part of the meetings responsible for defining midwifery at the 2005 congress, this has been a painful lesson for me to learn and one that I hope not to replicate.

A further lesson learned from this feminist research project has been that the hegemonic hierarchical ordering of ownership of legitimate and perceived superior knowledge and title not only supports the domination of biomedical over social discourse but it serves to devalue and deskill the TMs who are the source of birthing support for two-thirds of the women in sub-Saharan Africa (Dietsch & Mulimbalimba-Masururu, 2011a; Krueger, 2009). A more positive lesson has been the knowledge that power, domination, and oppression are not static phenomena but dependent on human agency for their perpetuation (Foucault, 1980). The participating TMs in this study are eager to learn practices that can assist them to ensure positive outcomes for women and their newborns from health professionals. They, in turn, have much to teach health professionals about best midwifery practice. The current status quo does not always support a reciprocal learning and teaching model but instead a very unbalanced paradigm where it is the health professional who is perceived to have all the knowledge, practices, and resources of value. The oppression experienced by the participating TMs in this study need not be fixed. The historical and social conditions that contribute to the oppression, having been recognized and named now, have the potential to be overcome.

ACKNOWLEDGMENTS

Dr. Luc Mulimbalimba-Masururu, Medical Director, Mission in Health Care and Development, Kenya and the Democratic Republic of Congo, played an invaluable role in the research process, including the recruitment and attainment of informed consent of the participants, data analysis, and providing advice on cultural security for participants at every phase of the research pathway. I acknowledge and appreciate the time, generosity, and courage of each of the traditional midwives who participated in the project. This research project was funded through a Charles Sturt University Competitive Grant and Centre for Inland Health, Research Fellowship.

REFERENCES

Armour, K. (2009). Maternal mortality here and abroad. *Nursing for Women's Health, 13*(3), 187–190.

Arps, S. (2009). Threats to safe motherhood in Honduran Miskito communities: Local perceptions of factors that contribute to maternal mortality. *Social Science and Medicine, 69*, 579–586.

Baker, K. (2010). Midwives should support women to mobilize during labour. *British Journal of Midwifery, 18*(8), 492ff.

Bisika, T. (2008). The effectiveness of the TBA programme in reducing maternal mortality and morbidity in Malawi. *East African Journal of Public Health, 5*, 103–110.

Bowser, D., & Hill, K. (2010). *Exploring the evidence for disrespect and abuse in facility-based childbirth: Report of a landscape analysis.* (USAID Translating Research into Action). Boston: Harvard School of Public Health.

Broom, D. (1995). Masculine medicine, feminine illness: Gender and health. In D. Lupton & M. Najman (Eds.), *Sociology of health and illness: Australian readings* (2nd ed., pp. 99–112). Melbourne: MacMillan.

Bullough, C., Meda, N., Makowiecka, K., Ronsmans, C., Achadi, E., & Hussein, J. (2005). Current strategies for the reduction of maternal mortality. *BJOG: An International Journal of Obstetrics and Gynaecology, 112*(9), 1180–1188.

Chalo, R., Salihu, H., Nabukera, S., & Zirabamuzaale, C. (2005). Referral of high-risk pregnant mothers by trained traditional birth attendants in Buikwe

County, Mukono District, Uganda. *Journal of Obstetrics and Gynaecology, 25,* 554–557.

Chandy, H., Steinholt, M., & Husum, H. (2007). Delivery life support: A preliminary report on the chain of survival for complicated deliveries in rural Cambodia. *Nursing Health Science, 9,* 263–269.

Costello, A., Azhand, K., & Barnett, S. (2006). An alternative strategy to reduce maternal mortality. *Lancet, 368*(9551), 1477–1479.

Costello, A., Osrin, D., & Manandhar, D. (2004). Reducing maternal and neonatal mortality in the poorest communities. *British Medical Journal, 329,* 1166–1168.

Cox, K. (2009). Midwifery and health disparities: Theories and intersections. *Journal of Midwifery and Women's Health, 54*(1), 57–64.

Dacher, K., Gruenfeld, D., & Anderson, C. (2003). Power, approach and inhibition. *Psychological Reviews, 110,* 265–284.

Darmstadt, G., Lee, A., Cousens, S., Sibley, L., Bhutta, Z., Donnay, F., et al. (2009). 60 million non-facility births: Who can deliver in community settings to reduce intrapartum related deaths? *International Journal of Gynecology and Obstetrics, 107*(Suppl. 1), S89–S112.

Dietsch, E. (2003). *The "lived experience" of women with a cervical screening detected abnormality: A phenomenological study.* Unpublished PhD diss., Bathurst, Australia: Charles Sturt University.

Dietsch, E. (2005). Excellence in adversity: A story of a Kenyan birth attendant. *MIDIRS Midwifery Digest, 15*(4), 478–482.

Dietsch, E. (2006). Service-based research: Is it feasible? Is it ethical? Is it really research? In G. Whiteford (Ed.), *Voice, identity and reflexivity* (pp. 127–133). Albury, Australia: Charles Sturt University.

Dietsch, E. (2010). The experience of being a traditional midwife: relationships with skilled birth attendants. *Rural and Remote Health, 10*(online), 1481.

Dietsch, E., Davies, C., Shackleton, P., Alston, M., & McLeod, M. (2008). *Luckily we had a torch: Contemporary birthing experiences of women living in rural and remote NSW.* Wagga Wagga, Australia: Charles Sturt University.

Dietsch, E., Martin, T., Shackleton, P., Davies, C., Alston, M., & McLeod, M. (2011). Australian Aboriginal kinship: A means to enhance maternal well-being. *Women and Birth, 24*(2), 58–64.

Dietsch, E., & Mulimbalimba-Masururu, L. (2006). We ask that the world please hear us. . . . Women from the Democratic Republic of Congo (DRC) share their stories of survival. *MIDIRS Midwifery Digest, 16*(4), 467–469.

Dietsch, E., & Mulimbalimba-Masururu, L. (2010). Reconsidering the value of traditional birth attendants: A literature review. *African Journal of Midwifery and Women's Health, 4*(3), 133–138.

Dietsch, E., & Mulimbalimba-Masururu, L. (2011a). Learning lessons from a traditional midwifery workforce in Western Kenya. *Midwifery, 27,* 324–330.

Dietsch, E., & Mulimbalimba-Masururu, L. (2011b). The experience of being a traditional midwife: Living and working in relationship with women. *Journal of Midwifery and Women's Health, 56*(2), 161–166.

Dietsch, E., Shackleton, P., Davies, C., Alston, M., & McLeod, M. (2010a). "You can drop dead": Midwives bullying women. *Women and Birth, 23*(2), 53–59.

Dietsch, E., Shackleton, P., Davies, C., Alston, M., & McLeod, M. (2010b). "Mind you, there's no anaesthetist on the road": Women's experiences of labouring en route. *Rural and Remote Health, 10*(online), 1371. Available at *www.rrh.org-au/publishedarticles/article_print_1371.pdf.*

Dugger, C. (2011). *Maternal deaths focus harsh light on Uganda. New York Times.* Retrieved on August 3, 2011, from *www.nytimes.com/2011/07/30/world/africa/30uganda.html?_r=1&hpw.*

Foster, J. (2009). Cultural humility and the importance of long-term relationships in international partnerships. *Journal of Gynecologic, Obstetric and Neonatal Nursing, 38,* 100–107.

Foucault, M. (1980). *Power/knowledge: Selected interviews and other writings 1972–1977.* (C. Gordon, Ed., C. Gordon, L. Marshall, J. Mepham, & K. Soper, Trans.). Brighton, UK: Harvester Press.

Fraser, D., & Cooper, M. (2009). The midwife. In Diane Fraser & Margaret Cooper (Eds.), *Myles textbook for midwives* (15th ed., pp. 3–10). Edinburgh: Elsevier.

Freire, P. (1972). *Pedagogy of the oppressed.* Harmondsworth, UK: Penguin Books.

Fronczak, N., Arifeen, S., Moran, A., Caulfield, L., & Baqui, A. (2007). Delivery practices of traditional birth attendants in Dhaka slums, Bangladesh. *Journal of Health, Population and Nutrition, 25*(4), 479–487.

Goodburn, E., & Campbell, O. (2001). Reducing maternal mortality in the developing world: Sector-wide approaches may be the key. *British Medical Journal, 322,* 917–920.

Gould, D. (2000). Normal birth: A concept analysis. *Journal of Advanced Nursing, 31,* 418–427.

Harding, S. (1987). Introduction: Is there a feminist method? In S. Harding (Ed.), *Feminism and methodology* (pp. 1–14). Bloomington: Indiana University Press.

Harrison, K. (1997). Maternal mortality in Nigeria: The real issues. *African Journal of Reproductive Health, 1*(1), 7–13.

Harvey, S., Ayabaca, P., Bucagu, M., Djibrina, S., Edson, W., Gbangbade, S., et al. (2004). Skilled birth attendant competence: An initial assessment in four countries, and implications for the Safe Motherhood movement. *International Journal of Gynecology and Obstetrics, 87*(2), 203–210.

Hogan, M., Foreman, K., Naghavi, M., Ahn, S., Wang, M., Makela, S., et al. (2010). Maternal mortality for 181 countries, 1980–2008: A systematic analysis of progress towards Millennium Development Goal 5. *Lancet, 375,* 1609–1623.

International Confederation of Midwives. (2011). *International definition of the midwife.* International Confederation of Midwives Council Meeting, July, 2011, Durban, South Africa. Retrieved April 4, 2012, from *www.internationalmidwives.org/Portals/5/2011/Definition%20of%20the%20Midwife%20-%20 2011.pdf.*

Izugbara, C., Ezeh, A., & Fotso, J. (2009). The persistence and challenges of homebirths: Perspectives of traditional birth attendants in urban Kenya. *Health Policy and Planning, 24,* 36–45.

Jordan, R., & Aikins Murphy, P. (2009). Risk assessment and risk distortion: Finding the balance. *Journal of Midwifery and Women's Health, 54,* 191–200.

Kitzinger, S. (2005). *The politics of birth.* Edinburgh: Elsevier.

Krueger, G. (2009). *A critical appraisal looking at traditional birth attendants: Their potential impact on the health of mothers and newborns in developing countries and the policy on traditional birth attendants.* Unpublished masters in international health thesis, Switzerland, University of Basel, Basel.

Kruske, S., & Barclay, L. (2004). Effect of shifting policies on traditional birth attendant training. *Journal of Midwifery and Women's Health, 49*(4), 306–311.

Lawrence, A., Lewis, I., Hofmeyer, G., Dowswell, T., & Styles, C. (2009). Maternal positions and mobility during first stage labour. *Cochrane Database of Systematic Reviews*, issue 2.

Liamputtong, P. (2007). *Researching the vulnerable: A guide to sensitive research methods.* London: Sage.

Mathole, T., Lindmark, G., & Ahlberg, B. (2005). Competing knowledge claims in the provision of antenatal care: A qualitative study of traditional birth attendants in rural Zimbabwe. *Health Care for Women International, 26*(10), 937–956.

Olesen, V. (2008). Early millennial feminist qualitative research: Challenges and contours. In N. Denzin & Y. Lincoln (Eds.), *The landscape of qualitative research* (pp. 311–370). Los Angeles: Sage.

Pitchforth, E., & van Teijlingen, E. (2005). International public health research involving interpreters: A case study from Bangladesh. *BMC Public Health, 5*, 71.

Preissle, J. (2007). Feminist research ethics. In S. Hesse-Biber & S. Nagy (Eds.), *Handbook of feminist research: Theory and practice* (pp. 515–532). London: Sage.

Raymond, J. (1982). Medicine as patriarchal religion. *Journal of Medicine and Philosophy, 7*(2), 197–216.

Rose, J. (1990). Psychologic health of women: A phenomenologic study of women's inner strength. *Advances in Nursing Science, 12*(2), 56–70.

Safe Motherhood Interagency Group. (2002). *Skilled core during childbirth: Information booklet.* New York: Family Core International.

Shen, C., & Williamson, J. (1999). Maternal mortality, women's status, and economic dependency in less-developed countries: A cross-national analysis. *Social Science and Medicine, 49*, 197–214.

Smith, L. (2008). On tricky ground: Researching the native in the age of uncertainty. In N. Denzin & Y. Lincoln (Eds.), *The landscape of qualitative research* (pp. 113–143). Los Angeles: Sage.

Stewart, K. (2006). Can a human rights framework improve biomedical and social scientific HIV/AIDS research for African women? *Human Rights Review, 7*(2), 130–136.

Tervalon, M., & Murray-Garcia, J. (1998). Cultural humility versus cultural competence: A critical distinction in defining physician training outcomes in multi-cultural education. *Journal of Health Care for the Poor and Underserved, 9*(2), 117–125.

Tritten, J. (2009). Traditional midwifery. *Midwifery Today, 20*, 5.

Tuguminize, L. (2005). The role of TBAs in midwifery care: The Ugandan experience. *British Journal of Midwifery, 14*, 276–278.

United Nations. (2009). *Millennium Development Goals indicators: The official United Nations site for MDG indicators.* New York: United Nations. Retrieved

November 30, 2009, from *www.millenniumindicators.un.org/unsd/mdg/Series-Detail*.

Vanderlaan, J. (2009). Trip to the Congo. *Midwifery Today, 20*, 46–47, 69.

Wadhams, N. (2008). A massacre in a Kenyan church. *Time World*. Retrieved July 30, 2011, from *www.time.com/time/world/article/0,8599,1699181,00.html*.

Weiser, S., Leiter, K., Bangsberg, D., Butler, L., Percy-de Korte, F., Zakhe, H., et al. (2007). Food insufficiency is associated with high-risk sexual behaviour among women in Botswana and Swaziland. *PLoS Medicine, 4*(10), 260–598.

WHO/UNFPA/UNICEF/World Bank. (1999). *Reduction of maternal mortality: A joint statement*. Geneva: World Health Organization.

Win, E. (2007). Not very poor, powerless or pregnant: The African women forgotten by development. In A. Cornwall, E. Harrison, & A. Whitehead (Eds.), *Feminisms in development: Contradictions, contestations and challenges* (pp. 79–85). Brighton, UK: University of Sussex: Zed Books.

Wong, J., & Poon, M. (2010). Bringing translation out of the shadows: Translation as an issue of methodological significance in cross-cultural qualitative research. *Journal of Transcultural Nursing, 21*(2), 151–158.

FINAL REFLECTION

Feminist Social Inquiry: Relevance, Relationships, and Responsibility

Jennifer C. Greene

Introduction

What does a reaffirmation of core feminist principles and commitments signal for contemporary social research and evaluation? What does feminist inquiry signify today, and why is it important for our societies? This brief commentary will engage these questions toward a synthesis of both aspiration and practice as voiced by the contributors to this volume. I write this commentary as a scholar of social science methodology and of evaluation theory and practice. I also write as a feminist, but not a feminist scholar. So, my comments engage the substance of these chapters from the standpoints of contemporary challenges in methodology and evaluation, and contemporary issues in our societies. I endeavor to make connections between the arguments and passion of the authors in this volume and a social inquiry practice of relevance and consequence in today's troubled world.

I came of age in the 1960s in the United States—a time of considerable political turmoil and social protest. Interlaced with the movements for civil rights for racial and ethnic minorities, for an end to the Vietnam War, and for an end to the "military industrial complex" was the "women's liberation movement," a political and cultural activism for equal rights and opportunities for women. This was heady stuff, even (or perhaps especially) for students at a small liberal arts college for women. The featured speaker at my college graduation in 1971 was Kate Millet, a renowned feminist of that era. For me, the personal was totally political at that time, as I was coming of age amid a tumultuous political and cultural transformation of the American landscape.

Fast forward to March 2013. The U.S. Supreme Court this week is deliberating the constitutionality of same-sex marriage, a civil rights happening almost unimaginable just a few months ago, a happening widely celebrated by long-time advocates of equal rights for LGBT (lesbian, gay, bisexual, and transgender) colleagues and friends. Regarding equal rights for women, Title IX of the U.S. Education Amendments of 1972, which stated that "no person in the United States shall, on the basis of sex, be excluded from participation in, be denied the benefits of, or be subjected to discrimination under any education program or activity receiving Federal financial assistance" and which has substantially transformed athletic and other domains of opportunity for women, is ancient history for most of today's young women and girls. In many fields of endeavor and responsibility, women, especially in Western countries, have been afforded substantial opportunities and have attained significant accomplishments.

Yet, also in today's world, a Pakistani girl, Malala Yousufzai, was shot in the head by the Taliban for openly advocating for education for all girls (*http://thelede. blogs.nytimes.com/2012/10/09/pakistani-activist-14-shot-by-taliban*). Gang rape is a culturally unpunished activity on public buses and streets in India (*www.bbc.co. uk/news/world-asia-india-20753075*; *www.cnn.com/2013/01/13/world/asia/ india-new-gang-rape*). And millions of women and girls in countries worldwide— east, west, north, and south—remain locked into impoverished and harsh lives with little agency, efficacy, or hopes of self-actualization (*http://womensrightsworld-wide.org*; *www.fordham.edu/Campus_Resources/eNewsroom/topstories_2331. asp*; *www.fwhc.org/stats.htm*).

So, yes, absolutely! A volume on feminist approaches to social research and evaluation remains timely and important, even urgent, in the face of continuing radical gender inequities and unconscionably limited life chances. The particular character of 21st-century feminist inquiry offered in this volume will be engaged next.

An Activist, Caring Vision of Social Inquiry with Women's Well-Being as a Point of Departure

We are fortunate to be social researchers and evaluators in a time of incredible pluralism in our fields. Long past the time when social inquiry was constituted by the "proper methods properly applied" (Smith & Heshuius, 1986), we have experienced in recent decades an explosion of philosophical, methodological, and sociopolitical developments in our fields. We have become lifelong learners in the process, delving into the philosophical traditions of postpositivism, constructivism, and critical social science (Guba, 1990); activist frameworks like feminism, critical race theory, and participatory action research; the ever-challenging poststructuralism and postmodernism; and more recently materialism and postqualitative research (St. Pierre & Lather, 2013). As we have probed the contours, concepts, and language of these philosophical and assumptive frameworks for social inquiry, we have also learned about the methodologies and methods, as well as the values, commitments, and stances, that accompanied each one. And we have tried them on for size and fit, assessing their look, functionality, and purpose.

So today we have a significant, sometimes dizzying plurality, of ways of thinking about the nature of our social world, what constitutes warranted knowledge, and how best to attain that knowledge (Lincoln & Guba, 2000). And most social inquirers today do not swear allegiance to one particular framework, but rather construct their own blend of aspects of multiple assumptive and methodological frameworks. The eminent Donald Campbell, after all, was an ontological realist (believing that the social world exists independently of our knowing it) and an epistemological relativist (believing that we can only know the social world from our own standpoint within in), and he embraced both quantitative and qualitative methodologies (Campbell, 1974/1988, 1975/1988). I believe we construct our own framework based on the particular character of our field of inquiry, our personal commitments and values, and our aspirations for the place of our work in the world. Among the requirements I have for my inquiry framework are *relevance* to my work as an educator and educational evaluator, an intentional emphasis on the *relational fabric* of inquiry practice, and a commitment to (and *responsibility* for) an inquiry practice of constructive consequence in the world, an inquiry practice that directly, even if modestly, strives to make the world a better place.

Because these personal inquiry framework requirements resonate with my readings of the chapters in this volume, I will use them to structure the comments that follow. My connection of a particular author to a particular point does not mean that other authors did not also make this point; rather the connections are illustrative.

Relevance

The authors in this volume argue persuasively that feminist social inquiry is a powerful way of engaging meaningfully with contemporary social issues of persistent and urgent importance. It is powerful in part because feminist research and evaluation can take on multiple countenances, informed by multiple theories and philosophical assumptions. Sharon Brisolara (Chapter 1) reports on three sets of theories guiding contemporary feminist inquiry: standpoint theories that attend to silenced and heretofore invisible voices; poststructural theories that offer a structural perspective on the inequitable ways in which the social realities of different classes of people are constructed and maintained; and postcolonial theories that reject definitions and constructs from outside "colonial" thought and, in doing so, reclaim resistance for themselves.

That is, there have been several waves of feminist thought over the years and there remain several genres of feminist assumptions and perspectives on how women's issues can best be conceptualized and empirically studied. This diversity within feminist thinking makes it applicable to multiple domains of human endeavor—from persistent inequities in educational opportunities and achievement for women in developed countries to persistent threats to the life chances and very survival of especially rural women around the globe. Across this diversity are two core shared commitments. First, feminist inquiry "begins with an acknowledgment and examination of the structural nature of inequities beginning with gender as a point of departure" (Brisolara, Chapter 1, pp. 22–23). Feminist inquiry, that is, is anchored in commitments to gender equity and to the well-being of women and girls. And citing Elson (2011, p. 3), Katherine Hay (Chapter 8, p. 202) observes "that a feminist lens can challenge the idea of 'rational economic man' and can help us to 'rethink the criteria we can use to evaluate economic and social policies and to construct better ones that are more likely to realize the dreams of social justice and women's rights.' "

Second, feminists today well recognize and embrace the intersectionality of privilege and especially discrimination and oppression. Women and girls not only suffer significant disadvantage compared to men and boys, but women and girls who are racial or ethnic minorities in their own countries, who are poor, who are disabled, who live in underserved communities, who observe minority faiths, and so forth suffer multiplicative disadvantage due to the intersections of these minority statuses. In this volume, Brisolara (Chapter 1, p. 20) observes that "intersectionality . . . helps to elucidate how race, class, and gender are integrated and 'mutually constitutive' (Davis, 2008)." And Donna Mertens (Chapter 4), under the broad justification of inquiry conducted in service of social justice, argues that

> Evaluators who work in communities with a goal of furthering human rights for women and the people who share their life spaces need to be aware of and able to implement approaches to evaluation that are responsive to the bases of differential experiences, including geographic regions; economic levels; religion; race/ethnicity; disability; deafness; refugee, immigrant, or indigenous status; tribal affiliations; or sexual identity. (pp. 95–96)

It is these core commitments that make feminist social inquiry directly engaged with today's most pressing social issues and thus highly relevant to today's troubled world. These commitments are especially relevant to and can directly inform my own inquiry work as an educational evaluator. I remain fully convinced that education is the surest pathway to meaningful social change, including fair and equitable life opportunities for all peoples, even if education is perhaps the slowest such pathway. I further believe that my own educational evaluation practice should emphasize the ways in which the program being evaluated is serving the full diversity of learners in that context, in particular those who are least well served. Feminist inquiry commitments and thereby feminist inquiry methodologies strategies can well support these ambitions.

Relationships

Although still a quiet conversation, talk about the social and relational dimensions of social inquiry is heard in multiple locations today. That this talk is heard in feminist inquiry circles is no surprise. Relationships are central to most women's lives, and many female social science inquirers incorporate the social, the relational, and the interactive into their inquiry scholarship and practice.

In the field of evaluation, Tineke Abma has been a leading scholar on this issue. In an evaluation handbook chapter, Abma (2006) argued that

> The social relations between the evaluator and various stakeholders are most importantly the kinds of relationships the evaluator establishes in the field and the "roles" and "identities" he or she takes on (Ryan & Schwandt, 2002). These are important in evaluation because they (1) are partly constitutive of the character and contours of the evaluative knowledge that is generated, and (2) communicate particular values and norms. (pp. 186–187)

The relational dimensions of evaluation thus refer to how the evaluator *is* in the context being evaluated—the character of the evaluator's presence, the relationships established, the conversations held, and so forth. Abma continues her discussion by outlining four different positions in evaluation theory and practice related to these social relationships. Two of the four are consonant with this volume's presentation of feminist inquiry: (1) an interpretivist or dialogic evaluation approach in which social relationships are cultivated as part of the hermeneutic or educative ambitions of the evaluation, and (2) a critical social science or participatory evaluation approach in which structural changes in the relational, and thus also the power dimensions, of the context are the evaluation's aspirations.

Some time ago, Bessa Whitmore wrote a newsletter article entitled, "It's the Process That Counts" (Whitmore, 1991). Consonant with her participatory and feminist evaluation commitments, Whitmore argued in this article that such commitments are enacted in the evaluation's processes—the social relations, communications, and interactions that take place in an evaluation—rather than in the evaluation's methods or results. Whitmore's chapter in the present volume (Chapter 3) details, and illustrates with highly instructive examples, multiple aspects of a feminist evaluator's *role*, which directly bears on the evaluation process and thus the social–relational dimensions of evaluation practice. As one example, Whitmore argues that one dimension of the feminist evaluator's role is as a collaborator.

> The evaluator as collaborator assumes an equal relationship with stakeholders, . . . strives to make space for all voices, shares power and control, . . . shares her or his own experience and perspectives and welcomes those of stakeholders. . . . One option is to build a collaborative evaluation team, consisting of stakeholders committed to the process. This will involve attending to the relationships among team members and consciously working to build trust and confidence with one another. This role reflects the valuing of cooperation rather than competition, and democratic participation. (p. 70)

Tristi Nichols (Chapter 7) also attends to the relational dimensions of feminist inquiry in this text by presenting a feminist–ecological model for evaluation. Nichols cites Grasswick (2008, p. 141) in observing that "the feminist ecological model considers power and power dynamics in their many forms individually and systematically, in individual, relational–social, and social–structural contexts." And further, also from Grasswick (2008, p. 151), Nichols states that the connections among gender "as intertwined with other axes of oppression and social stratification are only one aspect of the deeply relational nature of ecological thinking that Code [author of a related article] recommends."

Further, in her research study on traditional midwives (TMs) in sub-Saharan Africa, Elaine Dietsch (Chapter 12) engages with the continuing critical importance of inquirer reflexivity in feminist inquiry. Specifically:

> The challenge was to conduct this study in a way that did not exacerbate, reproduce, or create new power imbalances over the TMs participating. . . . [So,] two interrelated ethical concepts governed the project from proposal, through data collection, analysis, and the dissemination of findings; these are the needs to engage in a continual process of reflection founded on the principles of cultural humility and to employ service-based research ethics including those based on a feminist ethos. (p. 320)

Dietsch further emphasizes the centrality of the relational character of her research study.

> It was the depth of relationship between myself as researcher and the participants, the reciprocal respect we had for one another that breathed life into the

data collection, analysis, and dissemination processes. I believe that any critical research (including projects grounded on a feminist ethos), if conducted without relationship in the cross-cultural context, are at risk of becoming at best, merely voyeuristic and at worse, exploitative. (p. 325)

A good share of my own research on evaluation this past decade has featured a values-engaged, educative approach to evaluation. Central to this approach are the relational and communicative aspects of the evaluator's presence and work, as it is through these aspects that particular values are communicated. Connecting with these contemporary feminist ideas about the sociorelational dimensions of evaluation can well inform our continuing work on values engagement in evaluation. Reflections on some of our field work that tested our developing ideas about defensibly engaging with values in evaluation included the following:

> In the end, our experience, both conceptually and practically, highlights the need for attention to the relational and communicative aspects of evaluation, specifically, evaluation's interpersonal interactions, including the language, attitudes, and procedures drawn upon to develop and sustain trusting relationships, convey commitments, state objectives, share ideas, express interpretations, make decisions, and the like for particular evaluative purposes. These aspects influence the character of values engagement. . . . Focusing on these aspects has reinforced our belief that evaluators must assume *responsibility* for explicating and justifying the values being advanced in their work. (Hall, Ahn, & Greene, 2011, p. 206; emphasis added)

It is to this third and last characteristic of contemporary feminist inquiry—that of responsibility—that I now turn.

Responsibility

Beyond the integrity of the study—both substantively and methodologically— inquirer responsibility for me encompasses two important aspects of our work. First, inquirers are responsible for clearly stating and conveying the assumptions, stances, and values being advanced in a given research or evaluation study. Because these are active choices among a wide array of inquiry framework and methodology possibilities, inquirers need to openly present and justify the choices made. Second, inquirers are responsible for the purpose, direction, and intended uses of the research or evaluation being conducted. Nearly all inquirers wish to contribute to societal well-being, yet this goal takes many different forms— generating knowledge and informing theory, improving an activity's or program's design or implementation, providing information for or democratizing decision making, educating the general citizenry, critiquing discriminatory or oppressive structures and practices, and catalyzing action and social change. Especially in evaluation, these different purposes shape very different evaluation studies. And perhaps more consistently in evaluation than in research, these different purposes invoke different roles for evaluation in society.

I aspire for my own evaluation practice to be of consequence in the contexts in which I work. The consequences I most value are enabling practitioners to think critically and reflectively about their own practice and advancing the interests of those who are least well served in that context. As with my discussions above about relevance and relationships, many of the presentations in this volume resonate with these personal commitments about consequence.

Multiple authors in this volume present feminist inquiry as an activist practice. Brisolara (Chapter 1) offers as one of eight principles for feminist inquiry the following: "Action and advocacy are considered to be morally and ethically appropriate responses of an engaged feminist evaluator" (p. 30). This principle was further elaborated as follows: "Advocacy with or for people central to the evaluation, such as facilitating action on evaluation findings, is one of the most important intended outcomes of the evaluation. In order for advocacy to be ethical, the evaluator must discuss possible actions with participants most likely to be affected by advocacy and respect their experiences and concerns" (p. 32). Empowering action is a major agenda for Mertens's (Chapter 4) transformative paradigm and of Whitmore's (Chapter 3) participatory inquiry framework. Reflecting on their evaluation experiences in South America, Silvia Salinas-Mulder and Fabiola Amariles (Chapter 9) argue that feminist evaluators should concentrate on attending to the power relationships evident in the context, the program being evaluated, and the evaluation process (much like Abma). This is even though—or perhaps because—gender-responsive evaluation is not widely accepted in South America. Salinas-Mulder and Amariles further argue that "the evaluation task, where the evaluator is a subjective, interpretative, and powerful actor (not an objective spectator), is thus simultaneously technical, strategic, and ultimately political" (p. 225).

Feminist action and advocacy agendas come alive in the case studies reported in this volume. Donna Podems (Chapter 5) recounted how a feminist evaluation of a mental health institution in South Africa persisted in documenting the value of the work of a nonprofit agency (NPO) in this context, despite a lack of access to the institution's patients. The documentation obtained constituted strong evidence that the NPO's staff were providing critically vital services to patients and thereby served to maintain and strengthen the viability of the NPO's work in the institution's eyes. This activist agenda was supported by Podems's feminist evaluation approach. Denise Seigart's (Chapter 10) multinational study of school-based health care invoked an educative action agenda. "Since feminist evaluators value an action orientation, it was the intent during this study to foster dialogue and community learning about various models for providing care for children, particularly with regard to the care provided for girls and young women" (p. 267). The depth and relevance of this learning is evident in the examples provided by Seigart. Alessandra Galiè (Chapter 11) presents her work with Syrian women farmers involved in a Participatory Plant Breeding (PPB) program. "The findings show that PPB has the potential to enhance women's recognition as farmers, facilitate their access to relevant varieties and information, increase their access to opportunities, and support their decision making" (p. 284), though not without some limitations. Action in this study involved both educative and structural dimensions.

In these multiple but politically and conceptually coherent ways, the authors in this volume advocate for and powerfully illustrate the consequential potential of feminist research and evaluation.

Reprise

Feminist and gender-responsive social inquiry remain important resources for equity-oriented researchers and evaluators, as the battle for equal rights and opportunities for women is still joined. This volume offers conceptual, practical, and political concepts and strategies for enacting a feminist study. The concepts and strategies fulfill my aspirations for an evaluation practice that is relevant, relationally oriented, and consequentially responsible. I have confidence that other social researchers and evaluators can take inspiration from the substance and passion of the chapters in this volume for their own vision of feminist, gender-responsive, activist, and consequential social inquiry.

REFERENCES

Abma, T. A. (2006). The social relations of evaluation. In I. F. Shaw, J. C. Greene, & M. M. Mark (Eds.), *The Sage handbook of evaluation* (pp. 184–199). London: Sage.

Campbell, D. T. (1974/1988). Evolutionary epistemology. In E. S. Overman (Ed.), *Methodology and epistemology for social science, selected papers, Donald T. Campbell*. Chicago: University of Chicago Press.

Campbell, D. T. (1975/1988). "Degrees of freedom" and the case study. In E. S. Overman (Ed.), *Methodology and epistemology for social science, selected papers, Donald T. Campbell* (pp. 393–434). Chicago: University of Chicago Press.

Guba, E. G. (Ed.). (1990). *The paradigm dialog.* Thousand Oaks, CA: Sage.

Hall, J. N., Ahn, J., & Greene, J. C. (2011). Values-engagement in evaluation: Ideas, illustrations, and implications. *American Journal of Evaluation, 33*(2) 195–207.

Lincoln, Y. S., & Guba, E. G. (2000). Paradigmatic controversies, contradictions, and emerging confluences. In N. K. Denzin & Y. S. Lincoln (Eds.), *Handbook of qualitative research* (2nd ed., pp. 163–188). Thousand Oaks, CA: Sage.

Smith, J. K., & Heshuius, L. (1986). Closing down the conversation: The end of the quantitative–qualitative debate among educational inquirers. *Educational Researcher, 15*(1), 4–12.

St. Pierre, E., & Lather, P. (2013). Post-qualitative research. Special issue. *Qualitative Studies in Education, 26*(6).

Whitmore, E. (1991). Evaluation and empowerment: It's the process that counts. *Harvard Family Research Center Networking Bulletin on Empowerment and Family Support.* Cambridge, MA: The Harvard Family Research Center.

Glossary

AEA or **American Evaluation Association:** The leading professional organization for evaluators (*www.eval.org*).

American Evaluation Association's Guiding Principles for Evaluators: A set of statements intended to guide the work of professional evaluators for evaluators themselves and to inform stakeholders about the principles they should be expected to uphold.

Androcentric/androcentricism: The practice, conscious or otherwise, of placing male human beings at the center.

AR4D: Agricultural research for development.

Axiology: The branch of philosophy associated with the nature of ethics.

Beneficiaries: In the context of development aid, the term "beneficiaries" refers to the persons and communities that are the target of the project outputs. As a preassumed "condition," it does not usually imply an evaluation of whether people really benefited.

CEDAW: The United Nations Convention on the Elimination of All Forms of Discrimination against Women.

Civil Society: The hallmark of a democratic society is the freedom of individuals to associate with like-minded individuals, express their views publicly, openly debate public policy, and petition their government. "Civil society" is the term that best describes the nongovernmental, not-for-profit, independent nature of the organizations that allow for this type of broad citizen participation. It is through the advocacy efforts of civil society organizations (CSOs) that people are given a voice in the process of formulating public policy. Organizations including human rights groups, professional associations, religious institutions, pro-democracy groups, environmental activist organizations, business associations, labor unions, media organizations, and think tanks play a vital role in educating the public and the government on important local and national issues.

Conversatorio (Conversatorie): Flexible and informal round table discussions with key actors and informants (as opposed to the more structured and strict technique of focus groups), to gather people with diverse backgrounds and perspectives to discuss a particular issue of the evaluation.

Cultural Competence: Disposition and ability to learn about cultures and to act in accord with their norms and practices.

Electoral Assistance: Includes free and fair elections, which are indispensable to democracy. Although other elements of democracy can develop before competitive elections are held, a country can not be truly democratic until its citizens have the opportunity to choose their own representatives.

Empowerment: A process by which an individual acquires the capacity for self-determination, that is, of living the life that she or he has reason to value.

Epistemology: The branch of philosophy associated with the nature of knowledge.

Epistemological: The study of the nature and scope of knowledge and theories of knowledge.

Evaluand: The subject of an evaluation, typically a program or system rather than a person.

Gender: Socially constructed to describe a range of characteristics related to and differentiating, typically, masculinity and femininity.

Gender Analysis: A systematic approach to examining factors related to gender by identifying and understanding the different roles, relationships, situations, resources, benefits, constraints, needs, and interests of men and women.

Governance: A broad concept in that many citizens of developing countries recognize the intrinsic value of democracy (e.g., elections, human rights, and representation). However, they are also concerned with a government's ability to function. In general, governance issues pertain to the ability of government to develop an efficient and effective public management process. Because citizens lose confidence in a government that is unable to deliver basic services, the degree to which a government is able to carry out its functions at any level is often a key determinant of a country's ability to sustain democratic reform.

Herstory: A term used to describe history or historical accounts written from a *feminist* perspective; typically herstory emphasizes the roles and/or experiences of women and is told from a woman's point of view.

Incidencia Política (**Advocacy**): A Spanish expression widely used in Latin America to mean the rights-based efforts of communities and interest groups to persuade decision makers to change norms, plans, and policies or to formulate and implement new ones.

International Development: Refers to multiple strategies for contributing to human development and improving the quality of life for people. Typically refers to foreign aid, poverty reduction strategies, public health, and education policies and programs offered to or implemented within countries in the southern hemisphere or nations previously colonized by Western nations.

Methodology: The study and analysis of the methods applied to/within a particular field.

Millennium Development Goals: International development goals established by the United Nations in 2000; member nations agreed to meeting these goals by 2015.

NGO: Nongovernmental organization; sometimes synonymous with nonprofit organizations, often used in reference to such organizations in international development contexts.

NPO: Nonprofit organization.

Ontology: Related to the nature of being, reality, or existence.

Participatory Plant Breeding (PPB): Participatory plant breeding (PPB) for crop improvement is a science-based procedure in which professional plant breeders and researchers from various disciplines collaborate with farmers in the design—and not merely in the final testing—of locally adapted varieties that meet farmers' needs, priorities, and local market opportunities.

Paternalistic: A pattern of treating or governing people in a fatherly manner, especially by providing for their needs without giving them rights or responsibilities.

Postmodern: Refers to philosophic, literary, cultural, social, and scientific thought critical of the assumptions and universalizing tendency of Western thought.

Recognition: Acknowledgment of the identities and associated roles individuals freely chose to take in society. Recognition refers both to self-awareness of inward ontological transformations and perceptions of one's self and of one's public self.

Reference Group: A group organized with diverse internal and external actors to support external evaluation teams by providing ideas and feedback from different perspectives in key moments of the evaluation process.

Reflexivity: The ability to recognize the influence of socialization on personal views and biases.

Rule of Law: Respect for the rule of law and a well-developed justice system are underpinnings of a democratic society and a modern economy. Effective rule of law resolves conflicts and fosters social interaction in accord with legal norms and widely accepted societal values. It also enhances predictability, equitable treatment, and a respect for basic human rights; provides services in accord with societal demand and expectations; and helps curb the arbitrary exercise and abuse of power by other branches of government, elites, and other privileged groups. In all these regards, justice-sector institutions must perform their functions effectively. At the same time their operations must be transparent, accountable, and in compliance with the law.

Sex: An analytic category referring to biological, anatomical distinctions in men, women, and intersexed persons.

Terms of Reference (ToR): The document that sets out a road map for the achievement of the evaluation goals and describes the task assigned to the evaluation team.

Theory of Change: An approach toward social change based on identifying and making explicit assumptions about underlying cause–effect relations that enable transformation.

TIG or **Topical Interest Group:** The primary organizing groups within the American Evaluation Association, the leading professional organization for evaluators.

Transformative Paradigm: Philosophical framework that prioritizes human rights and social justice.

UN or **United Nations:** The United Nations is "an international organization founded in 1945 after the Second World War by 51 countries committed to maintaining international peace and security, developing friendly relations among nations and promoting social progress, better living standards and human rights" (retrieved from *www.un.org*).

UNEG or **United Nations Evaluation Group:** A professional network that connects units within the United Nations system responsible for evaluation.

UNIFEM: The United Nations Development Fund for Women, an entity with a mission to foster women's empowerment and gender equality.

WAD: Women and development.

WID: Women in development.

Women in Development: Projects focused on women in the southern hemisphere.

Author Index

Subject Index

About the Editors

Sharon Brisolara, PhD, is owner of Evaluation Solutions, an evaluation organization located in Northern California. Her work has focused on collaborative health promotion, youth development, poverty reduction, and international development efforts. Dr. Brisolara's areas of expertise (and passions) include feminist evaluation, qualitative research, participatory processes, mixed method approaches, and evaluation capacity building. She also regularly teaches sociology and program evaluation at local universities and community colleges.

Denise Seigart, PhD, is Chair of the Undergraduate and Graduate Nursing Programs at Boise State University in Boise, Idaho. She has been a nurse, teacher, administrator, and advocate of feminist evaluation for many years. Dr. Seigart's research interests include feminist and participatory approaches to evaluation of health care services for women and children, for the purpose of fostering community learning.

Saumitra SenGupta, PhD, has worked in mental health services research in California and nationally for over 15 years and currently works for the California Mental Health External Quality Review Organization. He has served in a number of capacities, including as a faculty member of the University of Arizona Medical School and a research psychologist for San Francisco County Mental Health Services. Dr. SenGupta is an expert in quantitative and qualitative research methods and utilizing mental health information systems for such research. He has held several leadership positions at the American Evaluation Association and is a member of the *American Journal of Evaluation* editorial board.

Contributors

Fabiola Amariles, MS, Learning for Impact, Weston, Florida

Sharon Brisolara, PhD, Evaluation Solutions, Shasta, California

Elaine Dietsch, PhD, School of Nursing, Midwifery and Indigenous Health, Charles Sturt University, Wagga Wagga, New South Wales, Australia

Alessandra Galiè, PhD, International Livestock Research Institute, Nairobi, Kenya

Jennifer C. Greene, PhD, Department of Educational Psychology, University of Illinois at Urbana–Champaign, Champaign, Illinois

Katherine Hay, PhD, Bill and Melinda Gates Foundation, New Delhi, India

Sandra Mathison, PhD, Faculty of Education, University of British Columbia, Vancouver, British Columbia, Canada

Donna M. Mertens, PhD, Department of Education, Gallaudet University, Washington, DC

Tristi Nichols, PhD, Manitou Incorporated, Peekskill, New York

Donna Podems, PhD, Centre for Research on Evaluation, Science and Technology (CREST), Stellenbosch University, Stellenbosch, South Africa

Silvia Salinas Mulder, MA, Independent Consultant, La Paz, Bolivia

Denise Seigart, PhD, undergraduate and graduate nursing programs, Boise State University, Boise, Idaho

Rebecca Selove, PhD, Center for Prevention Research, Tennessee State University, Nashville, Tennessee

Saumitra SenGupta, PhD, California Mental Health External Quality Review Organization, Sacramento, California

Kathryn Sielbeck-Mathes, PhD, Centerstone Research Institute, Nashville, Tennessee

Elizabeth Whitmore, PhD, School of Social Work, Carleton University, Ottawa, Ontario, Canada